T0200352

Electromagnetic Fields and Radiation

Electromagnetic Fields and Radiation

Human Bioeffects and Safety

Riadh W. Y. Habash

University of Ottawa
Ottawa, Ontario, Canada

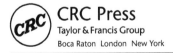

CRC Press
Taylor & Francis Group
Boca Raton London New York

CRC Press is an imprint of the
Taylor & Francis Group, an **informa** business

CRC Press
Taylor & Francis Group
6000 Broken Sound Parkway NW, Suite 300
Boca Raton, FL 33487-2742

First issued in paperback 2019

© 2002 by Taylor & Francis Group, LLC
CRC Press is an imprint of Taylor & Francis Group, an Informa business

No claim to original U.S. Government works

ISBN-13: 978-0-8247-0677-7 (hbk)
ISBN-13: 978-0-367-39654-1 (pbk)

This book contains information obtained from authentic and highly regarded sources. Reasonable efforts have been made to publish reliable data and information, but the author and publisher cannot assume responsibility for the validity of all materials or the consequences of their use. The authors and publishers have attempted to trace the copyright holders of all material reproduced in this publication and apologize to copyright holders if permission to publish in this form has not been obtained. If any copyright material has not been acknowledged please write and let us know so we may rectify in any future reprint.

Except as permitted under U.S. Copyright Law, no part of this book may be reprinted, reproduced, transmitted, or utilized in any form by any electronic, mechanical, or other means, now known or hereafter invented, including photocopying, microfilming, and recording, or in any information storage or retrieval system, without written permission from the publishers.

For permission to photocopy or use material electronically from this work, please access www.copyright.com (http://www.copyright.com/) or contact the Copyright Clearance Center, Inc. (CCC), 222 Rosewood Drive, Danvers, MA 01923, 978-750-8400. CCC is a not-for-profit organization that provides licenses and registration for a variety of users. For organizations that have been granted a photocopy license by the CCC, a separate system of payment has been arranged.

Trademark Notice: Product or corporate names may be trademarks or registered trademarks, and are used only for identification and explanation without intent to infringe.

**Visit the Taylor & Francis Web site at
http://www.taylorandfrancis.com**

**and the CRC Press Web site at
http://www.crcpress.com**

Family is life's gift.

I dedicate this book to Najat and to our favorites Gandhi, Mara, Marina, and Mikeli.

Preface

OBJECTIVES

Since the start of life on Earth until the beginning of the twentieth century, weak, natural low-frequency electric and magnetic fields (in addition to the earth's static geomagnetic field) determined the earth's electromagnetic (EM) environment. These natural fields come from two main sources: the sun and thunderstorms. However, since the beginning of the twentieth century, our environment has contained a variety of fields and waves, of natural origin and technically produced.

Electromagnetism is a basic force of nature, just like nuclear energy and gravity. It is found almost everywhere. Currently, this energy is utilized in various ways, though we still lack the full understanding of its fundamental properties. Many inventions of the late twentieth century, ranging from everyday home and office appliances to cellular phones, are so important and so advantageous; we wonder how we ever lived without them. These inventions have become an integral part of our modern life. We just need to know that they are safe.

In recent years, there has been a developing awareness that EM fields produced by everything, ranging from power lines to cellular phones are implicated in a variety of illnesses, including cancer. This has become a very controversial issue. Authorities are sending conflicting messages due to insufficient knowledge. That is probably, a situation of crises, when authorities claim this is not an important matter and the public does not have to worry about using a cellular phone or living next to a cellular base station or power line. A closer look shows that it may not be wise to ignore the potential health hazards of electromagnetic fields. Effects are produced by very low magnitude forces, which are not easy to explain. The effects may be divided into various categories, according to their nature and functions.

Over the years, a lot of cutting-edge research regarding these effects has been carried out. Researchers are now trying to identify the various types of effects that may lead to health risks to humans. Nonionizing electromagnetic fields are one of the newer environmental hazards that may lead to adverse effects on human health. Such effects must be carefully considered and are of prime importance in protecting the public.

This book is divided into two self-contained parts and one introductory chapter. Part I deals with extremely low frequency (ELF) fields, while Part II deals with radio frequency radiation (RFR). These two parts are composed of twelve chapters, each consisting of several sections dealing with distinct aspects of electromagnetic fields and radiation.

Chapter 1: Introductory Topics

This chapter is an introduction to electromagnetic fields and radiation. It includes basic scientific information—the familiar reader may skip most of it. It is included in order to enable this book to stand on its own. Further details of the basics may be found in any electromagnetic textbook. This chapter focuses on the fundamental scientific information that is associated with the use of electromagnetic energy. In so doing, a general overview is provided of the related scientific terms that are being used. Brief sections on the historical development of the subject and my perception of the controversy over possible electromagnetic health effects are discussed. Literature resources, which may be useful for the reader, are also included.

Part I: Extremely Low-Frequency Fields

Part I is composed of Chapters 2, 3, 4, and 5. The purpose of this part is, first to describe the characteristics of extremely low-frequency (ELF) fields. Second, to discuss the current research strategies and their implications for three central ideas: sources of ELF field exposure; human health issues including laboratory investigations and epidemiological studies; and safety standards and approaches for managing the exposure. If your interest lies only with radio frequency radiation (RFR), Part I may be safely skipped. Of course, you are encouraged to read this part for more information.

Chapter 2: Sources of Electric and Magnetic Fields

In this chapter, we will only look at a small part of the EM spectrum, the ELF portion. This is the part of the spectrum where much research has been carried out, although substantial work has also been done in relation to the RFR portion. We should note that in the ELF range, electric and magnetic fields are not coupled or interconnected in the same way they are at higher frequencies, therefore, it is more correct to refer to them as electric and magnetic fields rather than electromagnetic fields. The reader is provided with details of ELF exposure sources such as transmission and distribution lines, substations, transformers, video display terminals (VDTs), and other related appliances. This chapter also focuses on the major problems that are associated with the coupling of fields generated by the above sources and other objects.

Chapter 3: Bioeffects of ELF Fields

In this chapter, I follow a classification of biological levels while describing the ELF bioeffects. This involves studies on free radicals, cells, tissues, organs, whole organisms, and the population. Also, I emphasize research studies to identify possible biological effects and health implications on the human body due to exposure to electric and magnetic fields. Significant attention has been given to study the relationship between exposure to ELF fields and cancer. A distinction is made between experimental studies of cells, taken either from living organisms, from cell cultures, or of grown cells for the purpose of shedding light on possible interaction mechanisms, and studies of animals, to clarify possible interaction mechanisms. Assessment of risk could be applied to humans.

Chapter 4: Epidemiological Assessment Studies

Chapter 4 provides a comprehensive scenario for the development of epidemiological studies. Some of these studies have suggested that a link may exist between exposure to ELF fields and certain types of cancer, primarily leukemia, brain cancer, and breast cancer. Other studies have found no such link. In addition, many noncancer epidemiological studies have also been considered.

Chapter 5: Regulatory Activities and Safety Trends

This chapter delves into the details of major engineering issues related to the safety and ELF exposure. These issues are regulatory activities and health safety standards, electric and magnetic field measurement methods, field measurement surveys, and field management techniques. This chapter reviews a majority of the older as well as the emerging, protection guidelines for electric and magnetic field exposure. Information about the possible mitigation measures that might be considered is also described.

Part II: Radio Frequency Radiation

Part II places a strong emphasis on radio frequency radiation (RFR). The discussion covers physical properties, sources, bioeffects and health hazards, human exposure guidelines and safety standards, RF site survey, RF modeling techniques, instrumentation and measurement, and dosimetry. This part is independent of Part I and may be read without reading Part I.

Chapter 6: Sources of Radio Frequency Radiation

Chapter 6 explains basic technical information about the nature and characteristics of RFR. It deals with the development and exposure aspects of various RF sources, such as high-powered broadcast radio and television stations, radar, mobile radio equipment, paging systems, cellular, PCS, and satellite transmitters, and consumer, medical, and industrial equipment.

Chapter 7: Introduction to Bioelectromagnetics

In Chapter 7, the reader learns in detail the interaction mechanisms of RFR with biological systems. This chapter deals with the key electrical and magnetic parameters that decide the amount of energy absorption at the biological material. Key propagation mechanisms are explained mathematically rather than intuitively.

Chapter 8: Bioeffects of Radio Frequency Radiation

Chapter 8 investigates the biological effects and possible health implications of RFR. Comprehensive physical effects, cellular, animal, and human studies are provided, as these have a critical importance in the overall risk evaluation process. This chapter considers a fair number of studies with conflicting results in order to avoid any inclination toward any particular side in the debate.

Chapter 9: Human and Epidemiological Studies

This chapter reviews three categories of study. First, many human laboratory studies of RF exposures are considered. These studies are classified according to the biological effect rather than exposure environment. Second, a review of the available epidemiological studies appears prudent, particularly with the publication of few studies relevant to cellular communication environments. Third, RF exposure of individuals is also considered at the end of the chapter.

Chapter 10: RF Regulations and Protection Guidelines

This chapter outlines the history and development of RF regulatory activities worldwide. A wide range of the current safety standards and the basis for setting-up these standards are presented. Special emphasis is placed on the development of standards in North America, Europe, and Asia Pacific.

Chapter 11: Incident Field Dosimetry

Chapter 11 considers the first part of dosimetry, including evaluation of RFR through either modeling and/or measurement, and highlights those aspects relevant for cellular communications. This includes the evaluation of incident fields from RFR sources in the near- and far-field regions.

Chapter 12: RF Site Surveys

This chapter presents RF measurement surveys of various sites including mobile systems, cellular base stations, broadcast antennas, traffic radar devices, and heating equipment. Also, this chapter introduces issues related to RF interference, especially those associated with medical equipment.

Chapter 13: Internal Field Dosimetry

This chapter examines various dosimetry techniques for the determination of internal EM fields. In so doing, a case is made for the need to implement various methods to overcome deficiencies of certain techniques. The main quantity to be considered is SAR. The importance of the SAR as the main physical quantity is derived from the fact that SAR provides a measure of internal fields, which could affect a living system by means of thermal, athermal, or nonthermal effects. Many life scientists, however, are not convinced of this consideration. This chapter can also be considered as a tutorial on how to understand the impact of RFR from cellular phones on human head.

INTENDED AUDIENCE

This book is intended for a wide range of audiences interested in understanding the details of EM bioeffects. It is especially useful for:

- Scientists, physicians, and engineers
- Hygienists and environmental specialists
- Electrical equipment designers and operators
- Medical electronics professionals
- Manufacturers and users of portable phones
- Everyone who needs a better hazard-free working environment

This book integrates various aspects of electromagnetic fields such as the biological, medical, biochemical, epidemiological, environmental, risk assessment, and health policy. It is quite a venture into the battling studies to access the research on health effects of electromagnetic fields. Only a few scientists can fully grasp all of these subjects. The author assumes that to understand this book the reader must have a reasonable background in the foundation of various scientific disciplines.

It is not the purpose of this book to provide an in-depth review of the bioeffects of EM fields in relation to human health. Several such reviews have been published over the past few decades. So, what is the purpose of reviewing the research in this book? The answer is simple: to identify and summarize the relevant studies that have been carried out and published; to identify and provide information about on-going studies; and to recommend further areas of research for an assessment of the risk to human health that might arise due to EM exposure.

The information presented in this book is aimed at a broad range of readers. It is believed to be accurate at the time it was written and is, of course, subject to change with the continued advancements in the field. The mention of specific findings, standards, and institutions is for illustration purposes only and does not imply an endorsement of any kind by the publisher or myself.

Importantly, I am not in a position to reveal the truth, but strive to present the evidence. I do not intend to come to any conclusions or alienate myself from a certain idea or group. I have carefully tried to avoid any definite yes/no judgment about health concerns. I present some arguments from both sides of the dividing line in this controversial matter. The reader will have to draw his/her own conclusion as to whether or not he/she is convinced by the investigations.

Finally, I do not claim that this book is a perfect piece of work and errorless. Comments, suggestions, and corrections are greatly appreciated.

ACKNOWLEDGMENTS

I am grateful to several authors whose works I have drawn from. They are the rich resource on whose knowledge I relied while working on this book.

My thanks; also, to many participants in the lectures and seminars I have led in various parts of the world for their polite input and constructive feedback.

I am deeply indebted to the efforts of the elegant staff at Marcel Dekker who gave me valuable suggestions through the publication process. Special thanks are due to my production editor, Ann Pulido. I also would like to thank Theresa Stockton for copyediting the manuscript.

Contents

8   Bioeffects of Radio Frequency Radiation   223

Electromagnetic Fields and Radiation

1
Introductory Topics

1.1 GENERAL

Just as coal enabled the industrial revolution, *electricity* is the unseen fuel of modern life. The dramatic increase in the use of electricity for domestic and industrial purposes proves that electrical energy plays an important part in our society. It is impossible to imagine what our lives would be like without access to this source of energy. Technologies associated with electricity have made our lives easier. Modern society is indeed unworkable without the existence of electrical appliances. Likewise, emerging telecommunication services have greatly enhanced the ability of individuals and groups to communicate with each other and have facilitated the speed of information to persons and machines in both urban and rural environments.

Electricity use is taken for granted. It does not, however, come without risks. People would ideally like this technology to be risk free, but that is impractical in today's society. In particular, there is the potential for shock from contact with electrical conductors. Also, the use of electricity results in the production of electric and magnetic fields or *electromagnetic* (EM) fields. These fields are invisible forces of nature, generated by electricity, which are present whenever electricity exists.

Although EM fields have become an essential part of our life through their numerous applications, there are mounting concerns about the bioeffects that might exist due to exposure to such fields. Since the beginning of the twentieth century, we have been surrounded with a huge sea of man-made EM fields due to the rapid growth of power grids, radio and television (TV) stations, radars, cellular communications, and various appliances at homes and workplaces.

1.2 HISTORICAL PERSPECTIVE

Electromagnetic force, which exists between all charged particles, was not born in a day. It had to go through the long process of being defined. The existing outlook of the role of electromagnetic force in life is not that of the visionary force of earlier days.

The influence of electricity on biology was observed as early as the eighteenth century. While investigating, Luigi Galvani (1737-1798), the known physician and professor of anatomy in Bologna, Italy, announced his discovery that two metals brought into contact with a frog muscle could cause the muscle to incur.

The nineteenth century saw rapid developments in medical applications and physiological effects of electricity and magnetism. Such developments were motivated by the theoretical evolution in EM theory by Faraday, Ampere, Gauss, and Maxwell as well as by the development of alternating current (AC) applications by Jacques Arsenne d'Arsonval (1851-1940), a physician-physiologist with a strong professional interest in electrical engineering and one of the world's early bioengineers, and Nikola Tesla (1856-1943), a Serbian-American inventor and researcher who discovered the rotating magnetic field, the basis of most AC machinery.

Speculations regarding possible bioeffects due to exposure to EM fields began in those times, but rigid investigations started after World War II. By the mid-1970s, much of the concern was directed toward possible health hazards of radio frequency radiation (RFR). In the following years, with the help of the media, public concern diverted from RFR to extremely low-frequency (ELF) fields. Also, attention shifted from the strong electric fields near high-voltage power lines to those relatively weak magnetic fields produced by distribution lines that bring electricity to our homes. During the last few years, concerns regarding RF exposure from cellular phones have grown considerably. These concerns are generated because of the wide use of such equipment worldwide. Moreover, the concerns are largely inflamed by the fact that the cellular phone is placed very close to the user's head.

Observation of the influence of electricity and, accordingly, EM fields on biological systems will continue to be complex and split up over various areas of research such as physics, engineering, biology, medicine, health, environment, and risk assessment and management.

1.3 QUANTITIES AND UNITS

Throughout this book, a quantity of importance is the *field*, which is a region with a corresponding value of some physical quantity at each point of the region. Under certain circumstances, fields produce *waves* that radiate from the source.

1.3.1 Scalar and Vector Quantities

A quantity that has only magnitude and an algebraic sign is called a *scalar* quantity, such as mass, time, and work. While a quantity that has magnitude as well as direction is called *vector* quantity, such as force, velocity, and acceleration. In order to distinguish vectors from scalars, it is advised to use bold letters for vectors. For example, **A** represents a vector quantity while A represents the scalar quantity.

EM problems involve three space variables; therefore, the solution tends to be quite complex. More complexity may arise due to dealing with vector quantities in three dimensions. Vector analysis provides the mathematical means needed for manipulating vector quantities in an effective and suitable way. Using vector analysis saves time and gives wide understanding of the associated physical laws.

In electromagnetics we work with scalar and vector quantities. A field is considered a scalar or vector quantity. For example, electric potential is a scalar quantity, while electric field intensity is a vector quantity.

1.3.2 Units

A measurement of any physical quantity must be expressed as a number followed by a *unit*. A unit is a standard by which a dimension can be expressed numerically. The units for the fundamental dimensions are called the *fundamental* or *base units*. While carrying out EM calculations, there are several systems of base units that are available. However, they may be broken into two main groups. First, the International System of Units (SI) introduced by Griorgi in 1901, including the *meter-kilogram-second-ampere* (MKSA) subsystem representing the four fundamental dimensions *length*, *mass*, *time*, and *electric current*, respectively. Second is the centimeter-gram-second (CGS) system. The units for other dimensions are called *secondary*, or *derived* units and are based on the above fundamental units.

Currently, most the engineers use the practical MKSA system. What is known as the Gaussian system is an unrationalized CGS system, which is mixed in the sense that electric quantities are measured in electrostatic units, while magnetic quantities are measured in EM units. The CGS system is used mainly in the area of physics, where certain simplification in formulas results.

The SI is the standard system used in today's scientific literature. A few CGS system units are also used when appropriate. The complete SI system involves units but also other recommendations, one of which is that multiple and submultiples of the MKSA units be set in steps of 10^3 or 10^{-3}. The fundamental SI units and abbreviations are listed in Table 1-1 [1-4].

Table 1-1 Fundamental SI Units

Quantity	Unit	Abbreviation
Length	meter	m
Mass	kilogram	kg
Time	second	s
Electric Current	ampere	A

In EM theory, there are three main constants, which are related to the properties of the free space (vacuum). They are the *velocity*, *permittivity*, and *permeability* of free space. Velocity of EM waves (including light) in free space is $c = 3 \times 10^8$ meters/second (m/s). Permittivity of free space is $\varepsilon_0 = 8.854 \times 10^{-12}$ farads/meter (F/m). While permeability of free space is $\mu_0 = 4\pi \times 10^{-7}$ henries/meter (H/m).

1.4 FIELD QUANTITIES

The word "field" refers to any quantity whose value depends on its position in space. It also may be defined as an area around a source of electric or magnetic energy within which a force exists and can be measured. Here, we are interested in both electric and magnetic fields. These are vector quantities, meaning they have both magnitude and direction. The simplest situation for introducing the concept of electric or magnetic field is through the *static* field, which is one in which none of the field quantities are varying with time. Any voltage that exists between any two points is constant, while the flowing current is steady.

Wherever electricity is generated, transmitted, distributed, or used, electric and magnetic fields are created, often at significant intensities, due to the presence and motion of electric charges. These artificial fields are generally seen around electric utilities, telecommunication facilities, consumer appliances, industrial and medical equipment, and other common sources. Fields also occur in nature, as in lightning, and in other phenomena such as the northern lights caused by the interaction of solar wind and the earth's magnetic field. Usually, electric and magnetic fields cannot be seen or felt, but they can be measured. Surrounding any wire or conductor that carries electricity, there exists both electric and magnetic fields. These fields often extend for substantial distances around the wire. Today, many man-made sources generate electric and magnetic energy as collective energy in the form of EM waves. These waves consist of oscillating electric and magnetic fields, which may interact differently with matters including biological materials.

Understanding of few simple physical concepts is important for the discussion of any interaction between fields and biological materials. Although early investigations looked basically at the effects of high-level fields, today's studies consider all possibilities of exposure even from low-level fields. In spite of few similarities, electric and magnetic fields have rather different properties and probably different ways of influencing our bodies.

1.4.1 Electric Fields

Electric charges, whether negative (electrons) or positive (protons), are measured in units called coulombs (C). These charges exist both in free space (thunderstorms) and on conductors. When electrons move from one place to another rather than flowing in a line of current, it creates static electricity. In a static field, the positive and negative charges are separated over some distance. People may feel the static electric field while moving across a carpet, when their hair stands up as they near a grounded conductive object. A shock may occur as the current flows through, returning the separated electric charges back to a neutral state.

E, also called electric field intensity, denotes electric field. Electric field exists whenever electric charges are present, which means, whenever electricity is in operation, or when positive and negative charges are separated. The potential difference due to this separation is called *voltage*. The voltage means work measured in joules per coulomb (J/C) needed to move a unit of electric charge between two points. It may be defined by the electric potential difference between two points. The voltage increases as more charges are separated; however, greater energy is released when the charges come together again. **E** fields are intensified by increasing the potential difference or by moving the opposing charges closer together.

The basic unit for **E** field is newtons per coulomb (N/C), which is dimensionally equivalent to volts per meter (V/m). Electric fields could be represented graphically in two ways. First, by assuming **E** produced by a single-point charge Q as shown in Figure 1-1 (a). The arrows show the direction of the **E** field, while its magnitude is higher near the charge and decreases while going away from the charge. Figure 1-1 (b) represents the second way, which shows the **E** field produced by two uniform sheets of charge (a parallel-plate capacitor). Several **E**-field lines originate from positive charges and terminate on negative charges. The **E** field is uniform near the center of the conducting sheets and it bends (fringes) around the edges.

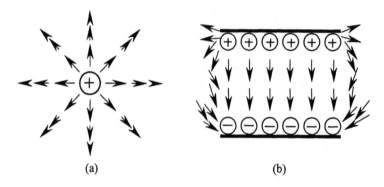

(a)   (b)

Figure 1-1 (a) Electric field lines due to a single point charge. (b) Electric field produced by two uniform sheets of charge.

The movement of electric charges produces *electric current*, which is defined as the rate of change of charge. The current is measured in amperes (A), named after the French mathematics professor Andre-Marie Ampere who, in 1820, found that parallel wires attracted or repelled each other if they carry electric current flowing in the same or opposite direction, respectively. One ampere is equal to one coulomb per second passing a certain reference point. **E** fields are created by still or moving electric charges. It is possible to hear the corona produced by **E** fields of air molecules near extra-high-voltage transmission lines (for example, 230-760 kV). **E** fields are strongest close the device and diminish with distance. They can be shielded or weakened by conductors, buildings, plants, and even the human body.

Electric flux density or *electric displacement*, denoted as **D,** is a measure of the **E** field in terms of equivalent charge per unit area. The unit of **D** is coulombs per square meters (C/m^2). **D** in a dielectric medium (e.g., biological tissues) is directly proportional to **E** as represented by the following equation

$$\mathbf{D} = \varepsilon\,\mathbf{E} \qquad\qquad (1.1)$$

where ε is the permittivity of the dielectric medium in farads per meter (F/m). The term permittivity refers to a fundamental property of the dielectric medium. It may be defined as the electric flux density per unit of electric field intensity within the medium. Basically, dielectric material is an insulating material. The significance of permittivity will be further discussed in Chapter 7 of this book.

Generally, three different quantities describe the permittivity of the medium: ε, ε_0, and a dimensionless quantity known as the *relative permittivity* ε_r or the *dielectric constant*, which is defined as the permittivity relative to that of free space. The three quantities are related by the following equation:

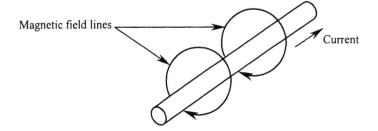

Figure 1-2 Magnetic field lines around a current-carrying conductor.

$$\varepsilon = \varepsilon_0 \, \varepsilon_r \tag{1.2}$$

The dielectric constant of free space is $\varepsilon_r = 1$. This value is assumed for air in most applications. Values of dielectric constant for most biological materials range from 1 (as for vacuum) to about 80 or so.

D and **E** are vectors with the same direction. This is real for all isotropic media, i.e., media whose properties do not depend on direction. The quantities **E** and **D** establish one of two key pairs of EM fields. The other pair consists of magnetic fields.

1.4.2 Magnetic Fields

The **E** field was explained by means of force between charges that act on a line between the charges. With the movement of charges, another kind of force on one another is exerted along the line between the charges. This force stands for the *magnetic field intensity*, denoted as **H**, which is a vector quantity created due to moving charges in free space or within conductors. Magnetic fields run perpendicular to the electric current. This means, while electric current runs in a straight line, magnetic fields surround the line in a circular fashion as shown in Figure 1-2. They control the motion of moving charges. The unit of magnetic field is amperes per meter (A/m). If we have direct current (DC), the magnetic field will be steady, like that of a permanent magnet. If we have AC, the magnetic field will fluctuate at the same frequency as the **E** field; it becomes an EM field, because it contains both **E** and **H** fields.

Significant magnetic fields emanate from sources such as transmission and distribution lines, substations, transformers, network protectors, feeders, switch gears, distribution busways, electric panels, wiring systems, motors, and various electric appliances. Magnetic fields may easily penetrate materials, including people, buildings, and most metals. They are not shielded by most common materials and pass easily through them. In general, magnetic fields are strongest close to the source and diminish with distance. People are not able to sense the presence of magnetic fields. However, high-level magnetic fields may cause a temporary visual flickering sensation called *magnetophosphenes*, which disappear when the source of the magnetic field is removed.

When magnetic field penetrates a cross-sectional area of a medium, it is converted to *magnetic flux density* **B**. It is related to **H** via the vector relation

$$\mathbf{B} = \mu \mathbf{H} \tag{1.3}$$

where μ is the *permeability* of the medium. The term permeability refers to the magnetic property of any material. It is a measure of the flux density produced by a magnetizing current. The full significance of permeability will be discussed in Part I of this book. The basic unit of permeability is henries/meter (H/m). Three different quantities describe the permeability of the medium: μ, μ_o, and a dimensionless quantity known as the *relative permeability* μ_r, which is defined as the permeability relative to that of free space. The three quantities are related by

$$\mu = \mu_o \mu_r \tag{1.4}$$

The relative permeability of free space is $\mu_r = 1$. A material is usually classified as *diamagnetic, paramagnetic,* or *ferromagnetic* on the basis of the value of μ_r. The majority of common materials have μ_r values equal to that of free space or air ($\mu_r \cong 1$ for diamagnetic and paramagnetic substances), unlike their permittivity values. Only ferromagnetic materials such as iron, nickel, and cobalt are exceptional. They have higher values of μ_r.

The traditional unit of magnetic flux density **B** is webers per square meter (Wb/m^2) (weber is the same as a volt-second). It is usually measured in tesla (T), named after Nikola Tesla, or in gauss (G), named after Karl Friedrich Gauss, the nineteenth-century German pioneer in magnetism. In the United States, magnetic field is generally measured in CGS units: oersted (Oe), and gauss (G). In most of the rest of the world, it is measured in tesla (T). Since most ELF environmental exposures involve magnetic field intensities that are only a fraction of teslas or gauss, the commonly units used for measurements are either microteslas (μT) or milligauss (mG). The following conversions may assist while dealing with units:

$$1\ G = 10^{-4}\ T$$
$$1\ A/m = 4\pi \times 10^{-3}\ Oe$$
$$1\ T = 1\ Wb/m^2$$
$$0.1\ \mu T = 1\ mG$$
$$1\mu T = 10\ mG = 0.8\ A/m$$

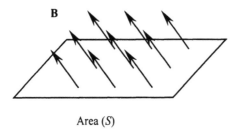

Area (S)

Figure 1-3 Magnetic flux density emerging from an area.

The *magnetic flux* ϕ in webers (Wb) linking the surface S is defined as the total magnetic flux density passing through S. Figure 1-3 shows that **B** is perpendicular to the area S and is constant over that area. Integration is needed to determine **B** if it varies over the surface area. This is defined as

$$\phi = \mathbf{B}\,S = \mu\,\mathbf{H}\,S \qquad\qquad (1.5)$$

1.5 ELECTROMAGNETIC INDUCTION

In 1831, Michael Faraday in London found that a magnetic field could produce current in a closed circuit when the magnetic flux linking the circuit is changing. This phenomenon is known as *electromagnetic induction*. Faraday concluded from his experiment that the induced current was proportional, not to the magnetic flux itself, but to its rate of change.

Consider the closed wire loop shown in Figure 1-4. A magnetic field with magnetic flux density **B** is normal to the plane of the loop. If the direction of **B** is upward and decreasing in value, a current I will be generated in the upward direction. If **B** is directed upward but its value is increasing in magnitude, the direction of the current will be opposite. When **B** is decreasing, the current induced in the loop is in such a direction as to produce a field, which tends to increase **B** [Figure 1-4 (a)]. However, when **B** is increasing, the current induced in the loop is in such a direction as to produce a field opposing **B** [Figure 1-4 (b)]. Therefore, the induced current in the loop is always in such a direction as to produce flux opposing the change in **B**. This phenomenon is called *Lenz's law*. As the magnetic field changes, it produces an **E** field. Integrating **E** field around a loop yields an *electromotive force*, or V_{emf}, measured in volts as follows [1]

$$V_{emf} = \int \mathbf{E} \cdot d\mathbf{I} \qquad\qquad (1.6)$$

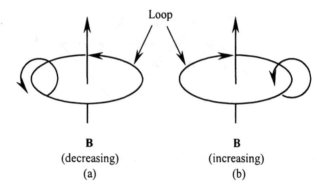

Figure 1-4 Induced currents due to magnetic flux density **B**.

V_{emf} appears between the two terminals, if the loop is open circuit. This is the basic for the operation of an electric generator.

A quantitative relation between the EM force induced in a closed loop and the magnetic field producing V_{emf} can be developed. This is represented by

$$V_{emf} = - \frac{d\phi}{dt} \qquad (1.7)$$

where $\phi = \iint \mathbf{B} . d s$ is the total flux in webers (Wb).

Equation (1.7) may be written as

$$V_{emf} = - \frac{d}{dt} \iint \mathbf{B}. ds \qquad (1.8)$$

where ds is surface element measured in square meter (m^2) and t is time measured in seconds (s).

Although Joseph Henry in Albany, New York also discovered the result shown in Equation (1.8), the credit is still attributed to Faraday. Both Faraday and Henry discovered the above finding independently at about the same time, however, it is known as *Faraday's law* of induction. Faraday's law is well known through its importance in motors, generators, transformers, induction heaters, and other similar devices. Also, Faraday's law provides the foundation for the electromagnetic theory.

The total time derivative in Equation (1.8) operates on **B**, as well as the differential surface area ds. Therefore, V_{emf} can be generated under three conditions: a time-varying magnetic field linking a stationary loop; a moving loop with a time-varying area; and a moving loop in a time-varying magnetic field.

1.6 TIME-VARYING FIELDS

In the preceding section, our primary concern was static fields that are independent of time. In this section, we will deal with dynamic fields, the more general branch of electromagnetics, which involves time-varying fields induced by time-varying sources, which are currents and charge densities.

Let us assume that electric and magnetic fields are varying with time in a certain pattern. An electric field may arise first due to the presence of a charge in the region and second due to the presence of a time-varying magnetic field. Accordingly, the time-varying magnetic field creates an electric field, which is also time varying. This is in fact generated from Faraday's law. When both fields are varying with time, a magnetic field will also arise as a result of the presence of current flowing in a conductor and the presence of a time-varying electric field. The first phenomenon is a result of *Ampere's law*, which states that the line integral of **H** around a closed path is equal to the current traversing the surface bounded by that path.

The English scientist James Clerk Maxwell (1831-1879) presented the second phenomenon. With the existence of this phenomenon, EM wave propagation could be made possible. In addition, Maxwell brought together various laws of electrostatic and magnetic fields. While correlating them, he found that the result derived from Ampere's law was inconsistent in the time-varying field as it was based on stationary closed currents. In order to overcome this problem, Maxwell introduced a certain quantity called *displacement* current, which is proportional to the time derivative of **D**.

In 1873, on the basis of mathematical analysis, Maxwell concluded that light was a propagating wave composed of electricity and magnetism. He arranged his finding into four equations known as *Maxwell's equations*. The original set of Maxwell's equations was written in terms of *potentials* with Cartesian coordinates and, therefore, was difficult to understand. Heaviside and Hertz wrote Maxwell's equations in terms of field quantities, while Lorentz added vector notation. This led to Maxwell's equations in differential form:

$$\nabla \times \mathbf{E} = -\mu \frac{\partial \mathbf{H}}{\partial t} \quad \text{(Faraday's law)} \tag{1.9}$$

$$\nabla \times \mathbf{H} = \sigma \mathbf{E} + \varepsilon \frac{\partial \mathbf{E}}{\partial t} \quad \text{(Ampere's law)} \tag{1.10}$$

$$\nabla \cdot \mathbf{D} = \rho \text{ (Gauss's law for electric fields)} \qquad (1.11)$$

$$\nabla \cdot \mathbf{B} = 0 \text{ (Gauss's law for magnetic fields)} \qquad (1.12)$$

The quantity ∇ (pronounced "del") is a vector operation; σ is the conductivity of the medium; its units are siemens per meter (S/m); and ρ is the volume charge density in coulombs per cubic meter (C/m^3). When ∇ is combined with $\times$, the result ($\nabla\times$) is referred to as the *curl* of the vector quantity that follows. When ∇ is combined with dot, the result ($\nabla.$) is referred to as the *divergence* of the vector that follows.

This section is intended to provide the reader with technologies or applications of Maxwell's equations through qualitative discussion rather than their theoretical implications. Maxwell's equations may be thought of in various ways. Mathematically, they represent a set of partial differential equations. Physically, they are a set of equations that summarize the relationships between electric and magnetic fields. Historically, they may represent one of the major achievements in the area of physics.

Equation (1.9) presents a microscopic form of Faraday's law. It states that a time-varying magnetic field induces an $\mathbf{E}$ field. The magnitude and the direction of the $\mathbf{E}$ field are determined from the curl operation.

Equation (1.10) represents a vector form of Ampere's law. It states that an $\mathbf{H}$ field can be created either by current flowing in a conductor or by a time-varying $\mathbf{E}$ field.

Equation (1.11) constitutes a microscopic form of Gauss's law for electric fields. It shows that an $\mathbf{E}$ field may begin or end on electric charge. It represents Gauss's law for electric fields.

Equation (1.12) represents a microscopic form of Gauss's law for magnetic fields. It indicates that magnetic fields have no point sources on which the field lines could begin or end, meaning that magnetic fields are continuous.

The most important outcome of Maxwell's equations was the prediction of the existence of EM waves. Maxwell proved that EM disturbances originated by one charged body would travel as a wave. Accordingly, Maxwell's equations can be combined to yield the *wave equation* that anticipates the existence of EM waves propagating with the velocity of light.

1.7 ELECTROMAGNETIC ENERGY

This section deals with the flow of *power* carried by electromagnetic waves. Power is the rate at which energy is consumed or produced. It is the product of voltage and current. Power is measured in watts (W). One watt is equal to one joule per second (J/s). However, *power density*, also called the power flux density, is a distribution of power over certain area. Power density is expressed in units of power per area, such as watts per square meter (W/m^2).

Energy is the ability to do work, and it exists in various forms. Energy can be stored as electrical energy. The unit of electrical energy is the same as unit of mechanical energy. It is the joule (J), which is defined as the energy stored by a force of one newton (N) acting over a distance of one meter (m).

The fact that EM energy can travel easily through space without a conducting medium has made it one of the significant tools of modern society. Numerous terms are used for concentrations of EM energy. For any wave with **E** and **H** fields, the term *Poynting vector* **P** is defined

$$\mathbf{P} = \mathbf{E} \times \mathbf{H} \qquad (1.13)$$

The unit of **P** is $(V/m) \times (A/m) = (W/m^2)$, and its direction is along the direction of the wave. **P** represents the instantaneous power density vector associated with EM fields at a given point. **P** is a function of time because both **E** and **H** are functions of time. Equation (1.13) indicates that the rate of energy flow per unit area in a wave is directed normal to the plane containing **E** and **H**. The integration of **P** over any closed surface gives the net power flowing out of the surface. This is referred to as the *Poynting theorem*. The field exposure depends on shape of the source and on reciprocal of the resulting volume factor.

Since EM energy is made up of **E** and **H** fields, it has an effect on the electrically charged particles of atoms, particularly on electrons because of their small masses. In addition, all charged particles in motion have electric and magnetic fields associated with them. When an electron absorbs energy from EM energy, the electron's electric and magnetic fields are altered and its kinetic energy, or energy of motion, increases. The **E** field may transfer energy to electrons through exerted forces, while **H** field does not transmit energy because its exerted forces are always in a direction perpendicular to the velocities of the electrons.

The absorption of energy in a medium is defined as *specific absorption rate* (SAR), which is the rate of energy transferred divided by the mass of the medium. The unit of the SAR is watts per kilogram (W/kg). For a sinusoidal steady-state EM field, SAR is given by

$$\text{SAR} = (\sigma + \omega\varepsilon_o\varepsilon'') \frac{\mathbf{E}^2}{v} \qquad (1.14)$$

where v is the mass density in kg/m^3. The SAR in Equation (1.14) is related to a specific point in the medium. Calculating the SAR at each point in the body and averaging over the whole body obtain SAR for a whole body.

There are cases for which there will be no power flow through the EM field. For example, **P** will be zero when either **E** or **H** is zero or when the two vectors are mutually parallel. Therefore, there will be no power flow in the neighborhood of a device of static charges that has an electric but not a magnetic field.

1.8   ELECTROMAGNETIC FIELDS AND RADIATION

For time-varying fields **E** and **H** are coupled, but in the limit of unchanging fields, they become independent. Practically, from 20-30 kHz and above **E** and **H** cannot be seen separately; they merge to form EM waves. Heinrich Hertz first investigated the existence of EM waves, predicted by Maxwell's equations. Such waves are no longer bound to a conductor, but can propagate freely in space and with losses through biological materials.

EM waves at low frequencies are referred to as EM fields and at very high frequencies are called EM radiation. The term EM field is generally used rather than EM radiation whenever wavelengths greatly exceed distances from exposure sources.

As stated earlier, there are two fields in an EM wave, **E** and **H**, which are both perpendicular to the direction of travel as shown in Figure 1-5. They travel together at very close to 300 million meters per second in air or a vacuum (slower in other materials such as biological tissues). The strengths of **E** and **H** change periodically.

Assume now that **E** and **H** are functions of position and varying with time. This means the field is alternating from plus to minus (going from an extreme value in one direction to an extreme value in the opposite direction) at a rate measured in Hz or cycle per second called *frequency f*. The field may also be characterized by its *wavelength*. The wavelength is the length of one cycle of a signal in meters. It is designated by the symbol λ. The wavelength in air is given by

$$\lambda = \frac{c}{f} \tag{1.15}$$

As the frequency goes up, the wavelength becomes shorter, and more energy is transferred to objects similar in size to the wavelength. Large divisions are commonly used to describe EM radiation as follows:

Kilohertz (kHz)	1,000 cycles per second
Megahertz (MHz)	1,000,000 cycles per second
Gigahertz (GHz)	1,000,000,000 cycles per second

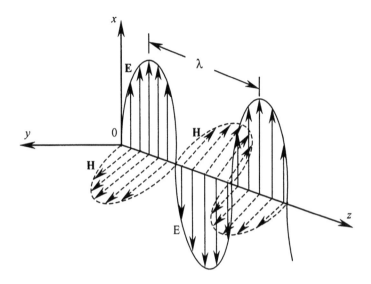

Figure 1-5 An electromagnetic wave propagating in the z-direction.

Amplitude modulation (AM) broadcasting, for example, has a frequency of 1 MHz and a wavelength of about 300 meters. Meanwhile, microwave ovens use a frequency of 2.45 GHz and a wavelength of only 12 centimeters.

An EM wave consists of very small packets of energy called *photons*. The energy in each photon is proportional to the frequency of the wave. The higher the frequency, the larger the amount of energy in each photon. This is defined as

$$eV = hf \qquad (1.16)$$

where h is Planck's constant ($h = 4.135667 \times 10^{-15}$ eV s). Electron volt (eV) is the change of potential energy experienced by an electron moving from a place where the potential has a value of V to a place where it has a value of V+1 volt. The amount of energy a photon has makes it occasionally behave more like a wave and occasionally more like a particle. This is known as the *wave-particle duality* of light. Low-energy photons (such as RFR) behave more like waves, while higher energy photons (such as X-rays) behave more like particles.

In the *near-field region* (distance less than one wavelength from the source), magnetic fields are decoupled. When a transmission line is energized without a load, it creates an **E** field and when the current flows, an **H** field comes into existence. At the *far-field region* (distance greater than one wavelength from the source), primarily at high frequencies, both **E** and **H** are related with the assumption that the characteristic impedance of the plane wave is 377 ohm.

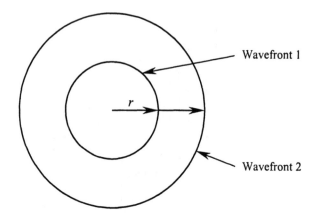

Figure 1-6 Wavefronts at given instants of time.

The term *EM radiation* applies to the dispersal of EM energy. Once generated, EM fields radiate in all directions, depending on how they have been converged. As the field opens, the power spreads, and the energy could be reflected, transmitted, or absorbed as it comes into contact with different types of material. The term radiation should not be alarming, as it does not imply radioactivity, which is the radiation of atomic particles due to the spontaneous decay of an unstable substance.

If EM waves were radiated equally in all directions from a point source in free space, a spherical *wavefront* should result. A wavefront may be defined as a plane joining all points of equal phase. The wave travels at the speed of light so that at some point in time the energy will reach the area indicated by wavefront 1 in Figure 1-6. The power density at wavefront 1 is inversely proportional to the square of its distance from its source r in meters, with respect to the originally transmitted power. If wavefront 2 in Figure 1-6 is twice the distance of wavefront 1 from the source, then its power density in watts per unit area is just one-fourth that of the wavefront 1. This is according to the *inverse-square law*, which states that power received is inversely proportional to the square of the distance from the source.

A circuit designed especially to enhance the radiation is called an *antenna*. The field on the other hand, extends outward from the circuit, but it does not actually leave the circuit and travel anywhere. When the current through the circuit stops, the field ceases to exist. It may be that a field causes radiation to a certain extent. The circuit becomes an antenna and radiates the maximum proportion of the applied energy when it is resonant. The resonance depends on the length of the circuit. The simplest antenna is a half-wavelength long. As the frequency decreases with respect to its length, the circuit becomes less as an antenna and more as a transmission line. In the furthest case, the transmission line would conduct all its energy along itself and radiate nothing.

1.9 THE ELECTROMAGNETIC FREQUENCY SPECTRUM

The evolution of the electromagnetic frequency spectrum started from the discoveries of Maxwell, Hertz, and Marconi. The EM spectrum under which devices and systems are working extends from extremely low-frequency (ELF) fields and very low-frequency (VLF) fields to radio frequency radiation (RFR), infrared (IR) radiation, visible light, ultraviolet (UV), X-rays, and gamma-ray frequencies exceeding 10^{24} Hz. The EM spectrum is divided into nonionizing and ionizing parts, as shown in Figure 1-7.

According to the frequency, EM radiation is classified as either *nonionizing* or *ionizing*. Nonionizing radiation is a general term for that part of the EM spectrum with weak photon energy that cannot break atomic bonds on irradiated material, but still has a strong effect, which is heating. To understand this, consider the energy of a quantum of 50 Hz exposure, given by Planck's constant h times the frequency (50 Hz), which is 2×10^{-13} eV. As the energy required for ionization by breaking a chemical bond is typically 1 eV, it is clear that low-frequency fields do not cause ionization.

Ionizing and nonionizing radiation are separated on the EM spectrum. The division between them is generally accepted to be at wavelengths around 1 nm in the far-UV region. Above that frequency is ionizing radiation, which contains enough energy to physically alter the atoms it strikes, changing them into charged particles called *ions*. Below visible light is the nonionizing radiation. All types of EM radiation share the same physical properties of divergence, interference, coherence, and polarization; however, they differ in terms of energy. The frequency range of the EM spectrum that is technically produced and used today covers about 12 powers of ten.

1.9.1 Nonionizing Radiation

Nonionizing radiation is EM radiation that does not have sufficient energy to cause ionization in living systems. Nature's sources of nonionizing radiation are few and extremely weak; the only sources are the sun, distant radio stars, other cosmic sources, and the terrestrial sources like lightning, basically in the tropics. With the explosion of electricity applications, the density of man-made EM energy around us is much higher than natural levels.

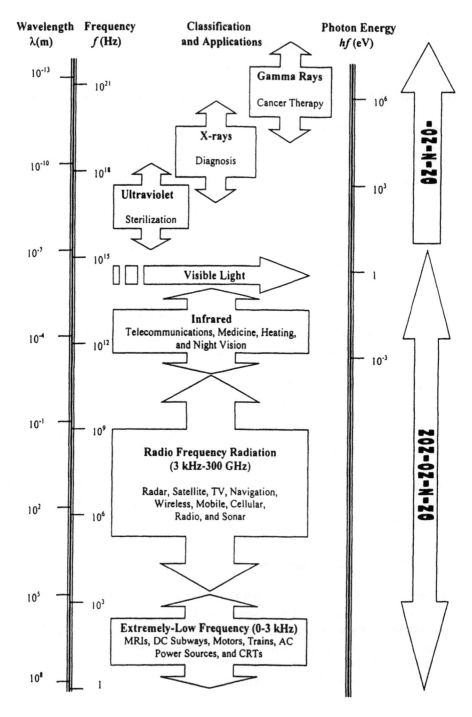

Figure 1-7 The electromagnetic spectrum.

In general, the nonionizing part of the EM spectrum is divided into three main ranges: extremely low-frequency (ELF) fields, radio frequency radiation (RFR) and noncoherent light.

ELF Electric and Magnetic Fields (0-3 kHz)

Extremely low-frequency (ELF) fields are defined as those having frequencies up to 3 kHz. At these frequencies, the wavelengths in air are very long (6000 km at 50 Hz and 5000 km at 60 Hz). Electric and magnetic fields at this range act independently of one another and are measured independently. Since the 6000/5000-km wavelength of 50/60 Hz radiation is much larger than the relevant distances from the source of field, the nonradiative, near-field terms are considerably larger than the radiative terms. Practically, only 1 mW is radiated from a 10-km section of 60 Hz, 500-MW power line, which represents a small fraction of the transmitted power.

ELF fields are generally useful for power utilities (transmission, distribution, and applications) and for strategic global communications with submarines submerged in conducting seawater. ELF fields are produced by a wide variety of products in the home and in the workplace as well, such as copiers, power lines, transformers, household appliances, electric trains, and computers. ELFs are not suitable for telecommunications because of the extremely severe bandwidth limitation and the difficulties of generating energy at these levels of frequency from any reasonably sized antenna. Yet, if these waves are transmitted, the field strength tends to be constant around the earth, since the earth is only 133 wavelengths in circumference at 1 kHz.

RFR (3 kHz-300 GHz)

Radio frequency radiation (RFR) is a general term applying to the use of EM waves for radio and television, radar, and other RF/microwave communication applications. RFR is composed of moving waves, which lie in the frequency range of 3 kHz to 300 GHz.

The lower portion of the RFR range is called the low-frequency (LF) band. It extends from 30 to about 500 kHz. It is primarily used for marine and aeronautical radio navigation beacons. The medium frequency (MF) band is assigned for wavelengths shorter than 200 meters and is left to experiments and radio amateurs. The high-frequency (HF) band extends from 3 to 30 MHz. This is a band used for traditional worldwide communications. Satellite services are gradually replacing the HF services.

Interesting bands of frequency with wide applications especially in wireless, mobile, cellular, personal, and satellite communications are the VHF and UHF

(30 MHz-3 GHz). Propagation above 30 MHz is basically a straight line (line of sight) with probability of scattering. Frequencies of special interest for cellular communications are in the range of 800-900 MHz, while personal communications band extends from 1700-2200 MHz.

The 2.45 GHz is reserved for industrial, scientific, and medical (ISM) applications, mainly microwave ovens. Frequencies above 3 GHz may be divided into the super high-frequency band (3-30 GHz) and extra high-frequency band (30-300 GHz). These frequencies are mainly used for radar, mobile radio, and satellite-based services.

Noncoherent Optical Radiation

An obvious division between the noncoherent optical radiation region and RFR region occurs at wavelengths of approximately 1 mm. The optical radiation is the other part of the EM spectrum to which human eyes respond. It is mainly divided into UV and infrared (IR) radiation.

UV rays (5 to 380-400 nm) are present in sunlight. Also, they arise from various man-made sources. It is well known that UV rays can initiate photochemical reactions and may burn the human skin if doses are large enough, although small doses have beneficial effects. Their main advantage is the production of vitamin D_3, which is necessary for the avoidance of rickets. Most of these rays are blocked by the ozone layer in the earth's upper atmosphere.

The UV region is divided into three regions due to their wavelengths and biological effects: UVA (400-315 nm) where fluorescence can be induced in many substances; UVB (315-280 nm) which is considered the most harmful UV reaching the surface of earth from the sun; and UVC (< 280 nm), which occurs in the radiation emitted by welding arcs, but not in the sunlight reaching the earth because it is absorbed by air.

Visible light (400-740 nm) covers a very narrow range of frequencies. Our eyes receive the light and produce electrical impulses, which are interpreted as vision by the brain [4]. The rainbow of colors we see in the sky is a portion of the visible light.

IR radiation (750 nm-1 mm) is the region of the EM spectrum that extends from the visible region to about one millimeter. IR waves include thermal radiation. For example, burning charcoal may not give off light, but it does emit IR, which is felt as heat. Most sources that emit UV or visible light will probably emit infrared. Such sources can be classified as either artificial or natural sources. Artificial sources include fluorescent and discharge lamps, flames, and heaters. The most known natural source for IR is the sun.

The IR region is subdivided into three bands according to their biological effects: IRA (0.78-1.4 µm), IRB (1.4-3 µm), and IRC (3-1000 µm) [5]. IR can be measured using electronic detectors and has applications in telecommunications, medicine, and in finding heat leaks from houses.

1.9.2 Ionizing Radiation

Ionizing radiation is radiation that has sufficient energy to remove electrons from atoms. One source of ionizing radiation is the nuclei of unstable atoms. For these radioactive atoms to become more stable, the nuclei eject or emit subatomic particles and high-energy photons. Included in this part are X-rays, gamma rays, and cosmic rays. This high-frequency radiation ($f > 10^{15}$ Hz) is characterized by short wavelengths and high energy. Ionizing radiation can cause changes in the chemical balance of cells, which results in damage to genetic material.

Ionizing radiation contains so much energy in its individual quanta of energy (for example, 12 eV and above) that it is able to expel electrons from their orbits in the atom shells as illustrated in Figure 1-8. This creates free radicals in living matter, increasing the risk of chromosomal damage and fatal abnormalities, which may lead to cancer.

Atoms of all elements may become ionized, however, only gamma rays, X-rays, alpha particles, and beta particles have enough energy to create ions. Because ions are charged particles, they are chemically more active than their electrically neutral forms. Chemical changes that occur in biological systems may be cumulative and detrimental or even fatal.

X-rays (10^{-9}-10^{-11} m)

X-rays are high-energy waves, which have large penetrating power. They are produced when energetic electrons in a vacuum tube strike heavy metal atoms (usually tungsten). X-rays have the ability to penetrate tissues and reasonably thick metals. They are used extensively in medical applications and in inspecting welds. Also, stars, including the sun, produce X-rays, particularly in their corona. X-ray images of the sun may yield important clues to solar flares and other changes on the sun that can affect space weather.

Gamma Rays (10^{-10}-10^{-14} m)

Gamma rays have the smallest wavelengths and the most energy of any other wave in the EM spectrum. They are generated by radioactive atoms and in nuclear explosions. Man-made sources include plutonium-239 and cesium-137. Gamma rays can kill living cells, a fact which medicine uses to its benefit, using gamma rays to kill cancerous cells. They travel across enormous distances of the

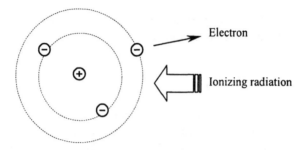

Figure 1-8 An electron being expelled from an atom.

universe. They are more penetrating than X-rays. Gamma rays can pass completely through the human body or be absorbed by tissue, therefore causing a radiation hazard for the entire body. Images of our universe taken in gamma rays have yielded important information on the life and death of stars, and other violent processes in the universe.

1.10 BIOLOGICAL MATERIALS

It is important to know some of the characteristics of cells and tissues in human body in order to appreciate the associated interaction mechanisms. In this section, very little will be said about anatomical configurations—the interest here is primarily in tissues and cellular structures.

1.10.1 Cells

Each human being is a collection of billions of living cells, which group together as an organ to perform essential functions. Cells come in all sizes and shapes, and are commonly several microns in diameter. For example, muscle cells may be a few millimeters long and nerve cells over a meter long. The entire characteristics of a cell include a thin *membrane* that holds the cell together, *cytoplasm*, which is a gel-like material within a membrane, and usually a *nucleus*. However, not all cells have a nucleus: some muscle cells have several, but red blood cells have none. Within the cytoplasm, there are several types of smaller structures called *organelles*, which perform certain metabolic functions. Vesicles partition the cell interior so that materials can be separated and compartmentalized for specific reactions. Organelle sizes vary from fractions of a micron up to a micron, and are therefore close in size to very short wavelengths.

  Biological cells are complex structures rich with complicated charged surfaces. Cells are stuffed with highly charged atoms and molecules that can change their orientation and movement when exposed to force as illustrated in Figure 1-9. A cell with distribution of charges is shown in Figure 1-9 (a), while the alignment of positive charges in the direction of the **E** field is shown in Figure 1-9 (b) [6].

EM interactions with biological systems may be realized through cells. They are categorized according to the cell structure [7]:

1. Interactions with the cell membrane.
2. Interactions with the cytoplasm.
3. Interactions with the nucleus.

The details of EM interaction with biological systems will be discussed in chapters 3 and 8 for ELF fields and RFR, respectively.

The cell nucleus contains most of the body's hereditary information in the chromosomes and the genes arranged in strands along the chromosomes. Genes are usually composed of double strands of *deoxyribonucleic acid* (DNA) arranged in a twisted helix. A cell reproducing itself uses a blueprint stored in genetic material in the nucleus. The genetic material is encoded as a long sequence of different organic molecules that bind together in DNA. The DNA controls most cellular activities by synthesizing protein. It uses single-strand *ribonucleic acids* (RNA) molecules, which the DNA synthesizes, to transfer information across the cell's cytoplasm. There are various phases of RNA: the formation of messenger RNA from DNA, which is called *transcription*; the synthesis of protein by messenger RNA, which is called *translation*; and the duplication of DNA, which is called *replication*.

Cells grow, change, and reproduce in a continuous process called *mitosis*. It starts in the nucleus through duplication and equal distribution of the chromosomes. Cells without nuclei, such as mammalian red blood cells, cannot divide, while other cells undergo mitosis often, for instance, the embryo. This is why exposure to EM fields is of special concern during the pregnancy.

The process of mitosis has four phases: *prophase*, *metaphase*, *anaphase*, and *telophase*. The period between divisions is called the *resting phase*. In the prophase, chromosomes appear out of the DNA. The membrane around the nucleus disappears. In the metaphase, the chromosomes line up along the equatorial plate at mid-center. In the anaphase, the chromosomes separate. During the last stage, telophase, the cell pinches in until two daughter cells have formed. It is evident that there are several processes during the mitosis that may be affected by being exposed to an external force, like EM fields. It is a potential area for research to study the effect of EM fields on various activities of the chromosomes during the four phases of mitosis.

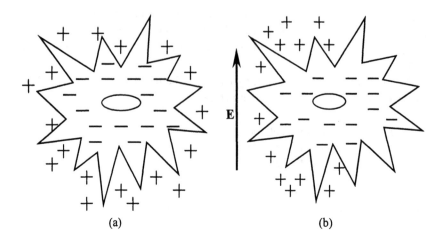

Figure 1-9 (a) A resting cell. (b) A cell under the influence of an electric field.

1.10.2 Tissues

Cells are grouped and combined with other materials to form several characteristic types of materials called *tissues*. There are four basic types of tissues: *epithelial, connective, muscular,* and *nervous*. Epithelial tissues consist of cells in single or multilayered membranes. They perform the functions of protection and regulation of secretion and absorption of materials.

Connective tissues consist of cells and nonliving materials such as fibers and gelatinous substances, which support and connect cellular tissues to the skeleton. Connective tissues comprise much of the intercellular substances that perform the important function of transporting materials between cells. Examples of such tissues are bone and cartilage. Subdermal connective tissues contain collagen and elastic fibers, which give the skin its properties of toughness and elasticity.

Muscle tissues consist of cells that are 1-40 mm in length and up to 40 µm in diameter. Muscles contain an extensive blood supply, and are hence filled with blood vessels and capillaries with their attendant connective tissue. A large group of muscle fibers are commonly bound together in a sheath. Skeletal muscle has a regular internal striated fine structure due to an ordered array of protein filaments.

Nervous tissues are used to sense, control, and govern body activity. They consist of nerve cells called *neurons*. Neurons have long projections called *axons*, which are analogous to transmission lines. Neurons are located in every protein of the body, sending information to the central nervous system (CNS) from different information receptors and from the CNS to muscles, organs, glands, etc.

1.11   DO EM FIELDS POSE A RISK TO OUR HEALTH?

It seems there is no one answer to this question! EM fields and their hazard to humans are a controversial scientific, technical, and often public, issue. This is an example of a product of technology that must be used in everyday life despite the unknown risk. However, people's conception about the risk of technology changes widely due to their technical knowledge and the role of the media. The conception, fear, and concern regularly turn the discussion into a heated controversy. The argument over such issues in today's society is often one of risk versus essential advantage. It is more an issue of calculating whether any chance for damage is justified by the advantages we get from the technology.

In our daily life, we are assaulted by the amount of information, often conflicting, by the media on hazards from power utilities and communication radiators. The widespread use of electricity means that in all residences and workplaces, there are levels of fields that would be considered normal. A controversy is flaming everywhere over whether field emissions from such sources might lead to cancer or other human diseases. This controversy is polarized along the same lines as many other issues in society. There are those who believe and protest about EM bioeffects. They are usually cautious about their health and may be categorized as conservationists. On the other hand, we have the developers and the industrialists, who do not believe in the EM scare. So the controversy is polarized on both sides and it is quite possible that there is a big debate coming. The only group that lies outside the area of argument is the scientists who are working in good faith to find facts. The main problem is that reliable results are not forthcoming.

Since the earliest investigations into the EM bioeffects, scientists, engineers, technicians, and physicians have worried about their potential health hazards. Public concerns are raised whenever issues in which words like field, radiation, and cancer appear in the media. The public anxiety is swinging between ELF fields and RFR. But the public concern constantly changes: the focus on ELF fields may increase, while concern about possible hazards of RFR decreases, or vice versa, due to the widely publicized claims of these issues in the media.

During the past few decades people were especially concerned about the safety of radar equipment at the workplace and microwave ovens at homes. Currently, it is wireless communication equipment; especially those fancy pieces of telecommunications (e.g., cellular phones) that are considered sources of concern. It is now accepted that modern microwave ovens are harmless, at least when properly used, whereas a number of investigations on radar operators has identified some thermal effects that lead to safety precautions minimizing the hazards.

While cellular communications are advancing, the idea of health effects from cellular phones is quickly becoming the focus of much research. There have been few scientific studies of this new service and there is limited information on whether the radiation emitted by cellular equipment poses a risk to human health. For many researchers, the findings are confirming the observations made over the years of the effects of low-level energy on living systems: They believe that small amounts of energy when delivered in the right way can have the same effect as a massive dose of chemicals. Others just do not see the threat.

The permanent problem in the controversy of risk is the limited knowledge about the fact that very specific fields interacting with our bodies can have critical effects on our health. These effects vary throughout populations as some are affected to a greater degree than others. This is related to our physical and biochemical differences.

It is still clear that this is the largest question looming in the minds of people, and it is striking how much the answers they receive depend on who are providing the answers and why. The average person is flooded with information and misinformation, which come from both sides of the debate. It is supported by claims and counter-claims so that this circumstance of scientific uncertainty has created a condition of suspicion in the community. The more we read about the work of scientists, the more we know, the more fearful we turn, and the more we feel a need to protect ourselves. This is just one part of the controversy. Meanwhile, we find assurances of safety and denial of harmful effects pioneered by people in government, industry, and health agencies. Between both sides remains only one thing that is our confusion! The various interests of governments, manufacturers, consumers, scientists, courts, and controversy-seeking news media only add to the confusion.

Finally, the government should be responsible for managing risks, especially when the risk factors are matters of public controversy.

1.12 RISK MANAGEMENT POLICIES

Evaluation of any health risk due to exposure to EM fields relies on the results of a well-established body of research based on experimental data from biological systems, epidemiological and human studies, as well as on understanding the various mechanisms of interaction. Sometimes, the evaluation of risk could be an unreliable process, so the resulting confusion remains that the results can be provoked even without deceiving conclusions based on solid evidences. Therefore, there is an apparent need for involvement of governments, manufacturers, scientists, and consumers in risk management decisions and fortunately there is a movement in risk management toward this end.

There has been an increasing movement to adopt *precautionary approaches* for management of health risk in the face of scientific uncertainty. Several risk management policies promoting caution have been developed to address the public concerns in the face of uncertainty. These include [8]:

1.   Precautionary principle
2.   Prudent avoidance
3.   ALARA (as low as reasonably achievable)

The precautionary principle reflects the need to take action at reasonable expense and with reasonable consequences for a potentially serious risk without awaiting the results of scientific research.

Drs. Morgan, Florig, and Nair initially developed the prudent avoidance as a risk management strategy for the power frequency EMF at Carnegie Mellon University. In their 1989 report to the U.S. Office of Technology Assessment these authors defined prudent avoidance as, "taking steps to keep people out of fields by rerouting facilities and redesigning electrical systems and appliances." It has been adopted as policy in a few parts of the world. This policy refers to taking certain steps to reduce exposure that may be done with minimal cost, until more is known about the possible health effects. Also the policy encourages the adoption of individual or societal actions to avoid unnecessary exposures to electromagnetic fields that entail little or no cost.

ALARA is a policy used to minimize known risks, by keeping exposures as low as reasonably possible, taking into consideration costs, technology, benefits, safety and other societal and economic concerns.

The above policies and other cautionary policies regarding EM exposure are popular among citizens, who feel that they offer further protection against scientifically unproven risks. They could be at least a possible solution.

1.13   AUTHORITATIVE RESOURCES

It is not a difficult task for the reader to find information about EM bioeffects. Gathering of comprehensive information on the subject is only time consuming and to a certain extent an expensive duty. Such a task has already been done by a number of highly qualified individuals, scientific groups, and various organizations. A large body of research has been conducted over the past few decades, with more currently underway. Research programs, committees, and working groups have been initiated at various parts of the world. Meetings, workshops, and symposia are held continuously to discuss and present recent work done in this field. Still, information, which provides the public with enough understanding of RF exposure and effect-related issues, is rarely available.

The literature is diverse. Journal, magazine, and monograph literature contains numerous reviews of this field, which vary in scope and viewpoint, with conflicting and even confusing results. It has been estimated that there are some 20,000 scientific reports in the literature. A few hundred are included in the reference sections related to each chapter of this book. Many literature reviews have been produced by in the last ten years with vastly different conclusions and have served to heighten the controversy surrounding the issue. Given the degree of uncertainty as to whether exposure levels below those permitted by recognized protection guidelines could result in adverse health effects, the majority of conclusions stressed the importance of additional research.

What adds to the difficulty of gathering reliable information is that many clinical-oriented papers on bioeffects of low-power ELF fields, RFR, and modulated (mixed frequency) fields on humans and other living systems have been missed because they were not published in medical journals. Some of the reports appear in journals relating, not essentially to the research results, but to the methodologies involved, e.g., appearing in electronics, physics, communications, life sciences, and unclear specialty publications. Review articles appear in magazines and newspapers with less in-depth treatment for the subject and occasionally not based on scientific facts; however, a few valuable reviews appear from time to time.

Table 1-2 lists a wide variety of journals and newsletters covering research and advances in the field.

Over the years, a good number of books containing comprehensive coverage of the biological and physical aspects of electromagnetic fields have been published [9-38].

Also, during the last few years many Web sites have been on the Internet. The list of Web sites focusing on EM bioeffects and safety continues to grow every year. Table 1-3 lists many of the popular Web sites in this field.

Table 1-2   Journals and Magazines Covering EM Bioeffect Research

Journals and Magazines	Newsletters
Advances in Electromagnetic Fields in Living Systems	Bioelectromagnetics Newsletter
American Journal of Epidemiology	Electromagnetic Forum
American Journal of Public Health	EMF Health and Safety Digest
Annals of Biomedical Engineering	EMF Health Report
Bioelectromagnetics	EMF Keeptrack
Biomedical Radioelectronics	EMF News
Biophysical Journal	EMF Update
British Medical Journal	EMRAA Newsletter
Cancer Causes and Control	Environews
Compliance Engineering	IRPA Bulletin
Computers in Biology and Medicine	Microwave News
Electromagnetic Forum	Powerwatch
Epidemiology	RF Safety Bulletins
EPRI Journal	The EMR Alliance
Health Physics	
IEEE Engineering in Medicine and Biology Magazine	
IEEE Transactions on Antenna and Propagation	
IEEE Transactions on Biomedical Engineering	
IEEE Transactions on Electromagnetic Compatibility	
IEEE Transactions on Microwave Theory and Techniques	
International Journal of Radiation Biology	
Journal of Biological Chemistry	
Journal of Comparative Physiology	
Journal of Microwave Power	
Journal of the American Medical Association	
Journal of Theoretical Biology	
Nature	
New England Journal of Medicine	
Physical Review	
Physics Today	
Proceedings of the National Academy of Sciences	
Public Health	
Radiation Research	
Science	
The Cancer Journal	
Transmission and Distribution World	
Wirelesseurope	

Table 1-3   List of a Few Useful Web Site Resources

Organization	Address	Web Site
California EMF Program	USA	www.dnai.com/~emf/
Coghill Research Laboratories Ltd	UK	www.cogreslab.demon.co.uk/
Electric Words	Australia	www.electric-words.com/
EM Bioprotection	USA	www.emxgroup.com/
EMFacts Consultancy	Australia	www.tassie.net.au/emfacts/
EMF Effects	USA	www.thwww.com/mrwizard/wizardEMF.HTM
EMF Guru	USA	www.emfguru.com/
EMF/RFR Bioeffects and Public Policy	USA	www.wave-guide.org/
F.A.C.T.S	USA	www.flipag.net/nopoles/
FEB	Sweden	www.feb.se/
Frequently Asked Questions on Cell Phone Antennas and Human Health	USA	www.mcw.edu/gcrc/cop/cell-phone-health-FAQ/toc.html
Frequently Asked Questions on Power Lines and Cancer	USA	www.mcw.edu/gcrc/cop/powerlines-cancer-FAQ/toc.html
Frequently Asked Questions on Static Electromagnetic Fields and Cancer	USA	www.mcw.edu/gcrc/cop/static-fields-cancer-FAQ/toc.html
International EMF Project	Switzerland	www.who.ch/emf/
Less EMF	USA	www.lessemf.com/emf-news.html
Microwave News	USA	www.microwavenews.com/
NEFTA	USA	kato.theramp.net/nefta/
NRPB	UK	www.nrpb.org.uk/
OSHA	USA	www.osha-slc.gov/SLTC/radiofrequencyradiation/
Powerwatch	UK	www.powerwatch.org.uk/
Radiation and Health Physics	USA	www.umich.edu/~radinfo/
RF Safe	USA	www.rfsafe.com/
RF Safety Program	USA	www.fcc.gov/oet/rfsafety/
SAR Data	USA	www.sardata.com/
SARTest	UK	www.sartest.com/

REFERENCES

[1]   Karus, J. D., and K. R. Carver, *Electromagnetics*, McGraw Hill, Kogakusha, Japan, 1973.

[2]   Jackson, J. D., *Classical Electrodynamics*, John Wiley & Sons, New York, NY, 1975.

[3]   Wangsness, R. K., *Electromagnetic Fields*, John Wiley & Sons, New York, NY, 1986.

[4]   Cheng, D. K., *Field and Wave Electromagnetics*, Addison-Wesley, USA, 1989.

[5]   International Lighting Vocabulary, International Commission on Illumination,

Publication No. 17 (E-1.1), Paris, France, 1970.

[6] Magnussen, T., Electromagnetic Fields, EMX Corporation, 1999.

[7] Meyer, R., *In Vitro* Experiments Dealing with the Biological Effects of RF Fields at Low Energies, COST 244 bis Project, *Forum on Future European Research on Mobile Communications and Health*, pp. 39-47, 19-20 April 1999.

[8] Electromagnetic Field and Public Health: Cautionary Policies, World Health Organization Report, Geneva, Switzerland, 2000.

[9] Barnothy, M. F., (ed.), *Biological Effects of Magnetic Fields*, Plenum Press, New York, NY, 1969.

[10] Marha, K., J. Musil, and H. Tuha, *Electromagnetic Fields and Life Environment*, San Francisco, CA, 1971.

[11] Sheppard, A. R., and M. Eisenbud, *Biological Effects of Electric and Magnetic Fields of Extremely Low Frequency*, New York University Press, New York, NY, 1977.

[12] Becker, R. O., and A. A. Marino, *Electromagnetism and Life*, State University of New York Press, Albany, NY, 1982.

[13] Dutta, S. K., and R. M. Millis, *Biological Effects of Electropollution: Brain Tumors and Experimental Models*, Information Ventures, 1986.

[14] Michaelson, S. M., and J. C. Lin, *Biological Effects and Health Implications of Radio Frequency Radiation*, Plenum Publishing, New York, NY, 1987.

[15] Gandhi, O. P., (ed.), *Biological Effects and Medical Applications of Electromagnetic Fields*, Prentice-Hall, Englewood Cliffs, NJ, 1990.

[16] Carpenter, D. O., (ed.), *Biologic Effects of Electric and Magnetic Fields*, Academic Press, Orlando, FL, 1992.

[17] Foster, K. R., D. E. Bernstein, and P. W. Huber, (eds.), *Phantom Risk: Scientific Inference and the Law*, The MIT Press, Cambridge, MA, 1993.

[18] Lin, J. C., *Advances in Electromagnetic Fields in Living Systems*, Vol. 1, Plenum Press, pp. 196, New York, NY, 1994.

[19] Brodeur, P., *The Great Power-Line Cover-Up: How the Utilities and the Government are Trying to Hide the Cancer Hazard Posed by Electromagnetic Fields*, Little Brown and Co., New York, NY, 1994.

[20] Milburn, M., and M. Oelbermann, *Electromagnetic Fields and Your Health*, New Star Books, Vancouver, BC, 1994.

[21] Tarkan, L., *Electromagnetic Fields: What You Need to Know to Protect Your Health*, Bantam Books, New York, NY, 1994.

[22] Brodeur, P., *The Great Power-Line Cover-Up: How the Utilities and the Government are Trying to Hide the Cancer Hazards Posed by Electromagnetic Fields*, Little Brown & Co., Boston, MA, 1995.

[23] Grant, L., *The Electrical Sensitivity Handbook: How Electromagnetic Fields (EMFs) are Making People Sick*, Weldon Owen Publishing, Sydney, Australia, 1995.

[24] Hitchcock, R. T., (ed.), *Radio Frequency and ELF Electromagnetic Energies: A Handbook for Health Professionals*, Van Nostrand Reinhold, New York, NY, 1995.

[25] Horton, W. F., and S. Goldberg, (eds.), *Power Frequency Magnetic Fields and Public Health*, CRC Press, Boca Raton, FL, 1995.

[26] Levitt, B. B., *Electromagnetic Fields: A Consumer's Guide to the Issues and How to Protect Ourselves*, Harcourt Brace & Company, New York, NY, 1995.

[27] Morgan, M. G., *Fields from Electric Power, Department of Engineering and Public Policy*, Carnegie Mellon University, Pittsburgh, PA, 1995.
[28] Malmivuo, J., and R. Plonsey, *Principles and Applications of Bioelectric and Biomagnetic Fields*, Oxford University Press, New York, NY, 1995.
[29] Pinsky, M. A., *The EMF Book: What You Should Know About Electromagnetic Fields, Electromagnetic Radiation and Your Health*, Warner Books, Somerville, MA, 1995.
[30] Polk, C., and E. Postow, (eds.), *Handbook of Biological Effects of Electromagnetic Fields*, CRC Press, Boca Raton, FL, 1996.
[31] Sagan, L. A., *Electric and Magnetic Fields: Invisible Risks*, Gordon and Breach, Amsterdam, NL, 1996.
[32] Stevens, R., B. Wilson, and L. Anderson, (eds.), *The Melatonin Hypothesis: Breast Cancer and Use of Electric Power*, Battelle Press, Columbus, OH, 1996.
[33] Foster, K., D. Bernstein, and P. Huber, (eds.), *Phantom Risk: Scientific Interpretation and the Law*, The MIT Press, Cambridge, MA, 1996.
[34] Kuster, N., Q. Balzano, and J. Lin, (eds.), *Mobile Communications Safety*, Chapman & Hall, London, UK, 1997.
[35] Lin, J. C., *Advances in Electromagnetic Fields in Living Systems* 2, Plenum Press, New York, NY, 1997.
[36] Ramel, C., and B. Norden, (eds.), *Interaction Mechanisms of Low-Level Electromagnetic Fields in Living Systems*, Oxford University Press, Oxford, UK, 1998.
[37] Sugarman, E., *Warning: The Electricity Around You May Be Hazardous to Your Health*, The Miriam Press, Miami Beach, FL, 1998.
[38] Bersani, F., (ed.), *Electricity and Magnetism in Biology and Medicine*, Kluwer Academic/Plenum, New York, NY, 1999.

Part I
Extremely Low-Frequency Fields

Chapter 2
Sources of Electric and Magnetic Fields

Chapter 3
Bioeffects of ELF Fields

Chapter 4
Epidemiological Assessment Studies

Chapter 5
Regulatory Activities and Safety Trends

2

Sources of Electric and Magnetic Fields

2.1 INTRODUCTION

Electricity is the most common source of power throughout the world because it is easily generated and transmitted to where it is needed. Since the beginning of the twentieth century, electricity-based industry and related technologies have become an integral part of our society, and consequently electric and magnetic fields are widespread as electricity moves through wires and machines.

A lot of developments were observed since the birth of the electrical power industry. From a moderate beginning in New York in 1882, the industry began the orderly electrification that resulted in a regular growth of power network construction and in the proliferation of devices and appliances that they serve.

The power grids of nations consist of electrical generation, transmission, and distribution facilities. With increasing availability of electrical energy, there arose the opportunity for accidents. The early kind of accidents was electrical shock, which results in injury if a very low current flows through the human body. High current causes loss of human life.

Because electricity use is prevalent and plays a vital role in society's economic and environmental well being, the possibility of harm from electric and magnetic fields to electric utility customers and workers is a matter that needs attention. Along with the above growth, a number of issues related to considerable public concerns over adverse health hazards due to exposures to ELF (0-3 kHz) fields have been surveyed and investigated, but mostly at levels above those encountered in the environment.

Electric and magnetic fields at ELF range are commonly found around our homes and workplaces. In homes, the immediate sources of fields include electric blankets, electric waterbed heaters, hairdryers, electric shavers, television sets,

35

video display terminals (VDTs), stereo systems, air conditioners, fluorescent lights, refrigerators, blenders, portable heaters, clothes washers and dryers, coffee makers, vacuum cleaners, toasters, and other appliances. In the workplace, sources of ELF fields include computers, fax machines, copy machines, fluorescent lights, printers, scanners, telephone (PBX) switching systems, motors, and other electrical devices. The above sources have been present in our environment for only about one hundred years.

As stated in Chapter 1, an EM field is composed of two components, electric and magnetic fields. The discussion in this chapter focuses primarily on magnetic fields; however, it covers electric fields when possible because of their close association with electric power systems. The source of magnetic field that we are concerned about from the health effect standpoint is alternating current (AC), or time-varying fields whose strength and direction change regularly with time. These fields arise particularly from the presence of man-made sources, specifically electric power utilities, electrical appliances, and communication systems.

As a matter of comparison, the earth's strong natural steady-state magnetic field is often cited as a potential source for attention, but this comparison is not considerable since the influence on matter is quite different between time-varying fields and static (non-time-varying) fields. Naturally occurring geomagnetic disturbances, associated with geological and meteorological phenomena, do exist and can be disruptive, but are not considered harmful.

Much of the public concern focuses on the proximity of power utilities to residential areas, workplaces, and schools. Currently, worries are about lower levels of fields that might have health effects based on certain epidemiological studies tracking large groups of people. However, definitive physical or biological evidence for a possible link between ELF fields and diseases does not exclusively support these results. Although no such evidence has emerged to entirely establish a high priority for research into the possible connection of ELF fields and cancer, as well as other illnesses, intense public interest and international research efforts are in progress. Some of the efforts have just been gathered, even throughout conflicting research results, in order to establish sets of protection guidelines for exposure to fields.

So how well prepared are the governments, industry, and the public to deal with this sort of conflict? The picture is complex and mixed. Are the efforts along with the existing evidences and assigned sets of protection guidelines going to justify the drastic and expensive measures to mitigate harm done, if any, by ELF exposure? Or the other way, are these steps going to answer all the public concerns over the suspected health effects? Certainly, behind this and that is just a big question mark.

2.2 SOURCES OF ELF FIELDS

Human exposure to ELF electric and magnetic fields is primarily associated with the generation, transmission, and use of electrical energy. Varieties of ELF sources are found in the community, home, and workplace. These sources are categorized into two main types: DC and AC.

2.2.1 DC Sources

A direct current (DC) field is sometimes referred to as a static field or static electricity, which means not changing over time. DC lies at the far end of the electromagnetic spectrum, to a frequency of zero; therefore its wavelength is infinite. In such case, any circuit automatically becomes a complete transmission line that conducts all and radiates nothing. Consequently, there will be only field and no radiation. Since the field is static, not changing with time, there is no excitement of nearby molecules and of course, no heating. DC field might be experienced as a tingling sensation when standing near a very high voltage source or as hair stands on end. Scooting the feet across a carpet may sometimes generate a static field on the body. Lightning, which is a transient high current discharge that occurs when an area of the atmosphere attains electric charges sufficient to produce an electric field strong enough to break down the insulation provided by the air certainly causes serious health problems due to conduction currents.

Magnetosphere

The earth is composed of four main layers: *inner core, outer core, mantle,* and *crust.* The core is solid and composed mostly of iron (Fe) and is so hot that the outer core is molten, with about 10% sulphur (S). Most of the earth's mass is in the mantle, which is composed of iron (Fe), magnesium (Mg), aluminum (Al), silicon (Si), and oxygen (O) silicate compounds at over $1000^{\circ}C$. The crust is relatively cold and thin, and is composed of the least dense calcium (Ca) and sodium (Na) aluminum-silicate minerals.

Earth produces field, which is largely static. The earth's static electric field is about 120 V/m near ground level [1, 2], while the earth's magnetic field has a magnitude of about 50 µT (0.5 G) over most of the world and is oriented toward the magnetic north [3]. Earth can be thought of as a dipole (2-pole) magnet as shown in Figure 2-1. Magnetic field lines emerge between Earth's North and South Poles just as they do between the poles of a bar magnet. Yet, the earth's magnetic field lines are not as symmetrical as those of the bar magnet are.

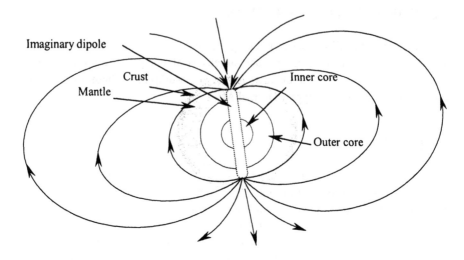

Figure 2-1 Earth may be thought of as a dipole magnet.

In the upper (northern) half of the earth, the magnetic field is directed toward the earth; in the lower (southern) half, the field is directed away from the earth.

Charged particles become trapped on these field lines (just as the iron filings are trapped on a piece of paper that is placed directly over a dipole bar magnet), forming the *magnetosphere*, which is the region in space close to Earth, just above the ionosphere. Earth's magnetosphere is a dynamic belt of flowing plasma guided by magnetic field, which at times connects into the sun's magnetic field. The magnetosphere extends into the vacuum of space from approximately 80 to 60,000 km on the side toward the sun, and trails out more than 300,000 km away from the sun [4]. Within Earth's magnetosphere are found cold plasma from the earth's ionosphere, hot plasma from the sun's outer atmosphere, and even hotter plasma accelerated to huge speeds, which can light up like a neon tube on Earth's upper atmosphere creating mysterious *aurora* in both the Northern and Southern Hemispheres. The magnetosphere itself has several components, occasionally diverting the sunrays away from Earth and occasionally absorbing them. The geomagnetic intensification effect implies that so-called radiation cancers should be more common in industrial nations at high geomagnetic latitudes.

The force of the solar wind pushes on the magnetosphere, squeezing in the sunward side and stretching the night side into a long tail. This phenomenon is called *magnetotail*, which extends hundreds of thousands of kilometers into space. The impact of the solar wind causes the lines facing sunward to compress, while the field lines facing away from the sun stream back [5]. The solar activity causes *geomagnetically induced currents* (GICs), which may flow into and out of the electric power grid through various ground points. The driving force is the voltage induced in the transmission lines both by the ionospheric current and by the earth current. The frequency of the GIC is very low (below 1 Hz); therefore, it can be categorized as a quasi-direct current. Currents have been measured in a single transformer neutral in excess of 184 A in North America and 200 A in Finland [6].

Magnetic Resonance Imaging

Magnetic resonance imaging has become a significant diagnostic procedure because of its high resolution. The magnetic part of the DC field is widely generated by a medical diagnostic tool called a *magnetic resonance imager* (MRI). MRI is an imaging technique used primarily in medical settings to produce high-quality images of the inside of the human body. MRI may subject the human body to up to 2000 mT for a short period of time. It is believed to be harmless for humans, but beyond that level is considered critical, as it may affect the electrical activity of heart.

DC Power Supply System

Though these days DC power supply systems are not common, except at a few locations worldwide, some information about them will be of interest for the reader. The early DC system had a two-wire configuration, with a positive and a negative conductor. The supply voltage varied between 110 V and 250 V. As the need to transmit larger quantities of energy increased, a system of distribution was adopted, the three-wire system. This consists of a generator and two conductors. A third conductor called *neutral* is grounded (zero volt reference for an electrical system through a connection to the ground).

2.2.2 AC Sources

For a long time, the main electrical power supply was DC, however, gradually as the advantages of AC became apparent, there was a changeover to AC. AC fields resulting from the transmission, distribution, and use of electric power allow a good deal of simplification as they vary rather slowly over time. The frequency of ELF fields depends on the source of exposure. Although the power frequency (50/60 Hz) is the predominant fundamental frequency, humans are mostly exposed to a mixture of frequencies, and much higher frequencies may arise. For example, frequencies from certain electronic equipment like televisions and VDTs may extend up to 50 kHz. In addition, switching events may generate abrupt spikes in voltage and current waveforms, leading to high-frequency transients that might extend into RFR above several megahertz. Nonlinear characteristics in electrical devices generate harmonics at integer multiples of the fundamental frequency extending up to several kilohertz [1, 7].

   Electric and magnetic fields are the main components of EM fields. Electric fields are generated when electric appliances are plugged in but not necessarily turned on. They are relatively easy to shield or alter by most commonly available materials. However, current produces magnetic fields when appliances are turned on. Magnetic fields completely pass through Earth, humans, and most building materials. They are difficult to be magnetically shielded with a conduit or enclosure using any material including highly permeable sheets or highly conductive copper and aluminum materials.

   The magnetic field strength from an ELF source decreases with distance from the source. For example, for a single current-carrying conductor source the magnetic field strength is directly proportional to the inverse of the distance from the source ($1/r$). The field levels close to these sources are relatively high. The magnetic field strength varies inversely, as the square of the distance ($1/r^2$) for a multiple conductor source, and as the cube of the distance ($1/r^3$) for a loop or coil. Such relationships are significant while implementing magnetic field mitigation schemes. For further details, we will consider the following four types of AC sources.

Single-Conductor Source

A straight single conductor of current is considered as a basic source of field. It is possible to determine the magnetic flux density B at all points in a region about a long current-carrying conductor. Experiments show that for a homogeneous medium, B is related to the current I. Thus

$$B = \frac{\mu I}{2\pi r} = \mu H \tag{2.1}$$

where r is the distance in meters from the source. The direction of the magnetic field due to moving charges depends on the *right-hand rule*, which states that if the right thumb points in the direction of conventional current, the fingers of the right hand curl around the wire in the direction of the magnetic field. Typical line sources are multiconductor cables, long-wire conductors, plumbing and net currents, electrically powered subway, rail, and trolley bus systems. Magnetic fields from a single conductor are circularly emanating out from the center as shown in Figure 1-2.

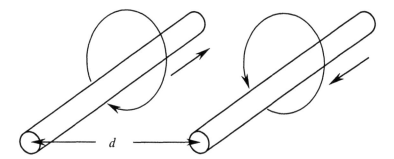

Figure 2-2 Magnetic field for an opposing current pair of dual conductors.

Dual-Conductor Source

The magnetic field for an opposing current pair of dual conductors separated by a small distance d relative to the distance from the pair r diminishes at a nonlinear $1/r^2$ distance rate (because of the inverse-square law), as illustrated in Figure 2-2. This is defined as

$$B = \frac{2Id}{r^2} \qquad\qquad (2.2)$$

Basically, by doubling the distance r for a fixed spacing d and current I, the magnetic flux density reduces by a factor of four. Electrical appliance cords transmission and distribution lines commonly fall into this category.

Loop Source

A single loop can be considered as another typical source of field. It exists in AC motors, transformers, computers, power supplies, electric stoves, and microwave ovens. Using again the right-hand rule, a magnetic dipole has a dipole moment M whose direction is in the direction of the thumb as the finger of the right hand follows the direction of the current. The magnitude is equal to the product of the loop current I and the enclosed loop area S, defined as

$$M = I \times S \qquad\qquad (2.3)$$

The magnetic dipole produces magnetic field that diminishes at a $1/r^3$, as illustrated by Figure 2-3. This is,

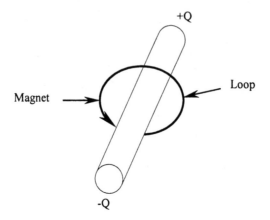

Figure 2-3 Magnetic field of a loop.

$$B = \frac{\mu_o M}{4\pi r^3} \tag{2.4}$$

As seen from Equation (2.4), the radiation effect is sharply reduced by a slight increase in distance.

Three-Phase Source

Electric power is generated and distributed via three-phase AC transmission, distribution, and service feeder lines to commercial and industrial buildings. Each of the three-balanced phase voltages and currents are ideally represented as magnitude and angle 120 degrees apart. The magnetic field for balanced three-phase circuits of three horizontally or vertically arrayed conductors separated by equal distances d diminishes at a nonlinear $1/r^2$ distance rate according to

$$B = \frac{3.46Id}{r^2} \tag{2.5}$$

However, if the three-phase circuit is unbalanced and/or there are significant net, ground, and plumbing currents on the service feeder neutral, then the dominant magnetic field becomes

$$B = \frac{2I}{r} \tag{2.6}$$

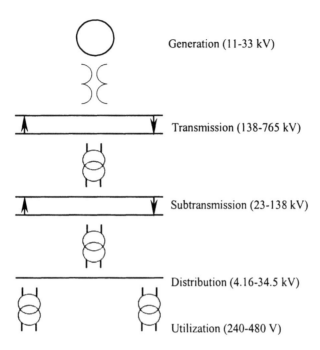

Figure 2-4 Electricity generation, transmission, distribution, and utilization.

where I is the sum of the net, ground, and plumbing currents. Furthermore, magnetic fields produced by three-phase lines are generally elliptically polarized. This means a rotating vector that traces an ellipse for every cycle of the conductor current can represent the magnetic field.

2.3 ELECTRIC UTILITY SYSTEM

In North America, power systems operate at a frequency of 60 Hz. However, power companies in Europe, Asia, and many other places in the world supply residential users with 50 Hz electrical powers. Aircraft electrical systems use 400 Hz power. Some electric trains use DC. Some high-speed electric trains use 16.67 Hz power. Electric commuter trains use 25 Hz electric powers and may have fields as high as 0.5 G.

The electric power network is operated at several voltage levels. Figure 2-4 shows a simple power system with typical voltage levels from generation to consumption. The method by which electricity is generated in any country or region reflects the energy resources available in that country or region. Electricity is typically generated at voltage levels ranging from 11 to 33 kV for three-phase synchronous generators. The output voltage of the generator is stepped up to transmission levels in the generating plant substation. Usually, power is transferred on transmission lines at a very high voltage in order to reduce energy losses along the way (the higher the voltage, the lower the losses). Transmission voltages typically range from 138 to 765 kV. Currently available are higher voltage overhead transmission lines for up to 1100 kV.

The subtransmission network receives power from the transmission network at various transmission substations. Typical voltage levels for the subtransmission network range from 23 to 138 kV. The distribution system is to distribute power on a local level. Common voltage levels for distribution are 4.16 to 34.5 kV. Utilization voltage supplies residential and industrial facilities with levels range from 240 to 480 V. This part of the grid is classified as *low-voltage system* [8].

The electric power system is arranged in a series of segments, with power lines connecting generating stations via a network of transmission lines, intermediate substation, and switching points to the local distribution lines, and then to utility customers. The voltage in a given portion of the system remains nearly constant, namely the high-voltage transmission lines. These voltages are stepped down at substations by transformers to produce voltages for the primary distribution lines. Transformers at the other points to a correspondingly lower voltage and higher current for residential or commercial use further reduce the primary distribution lines.

The power delivery in each segment of the electric system is the product of the voltage and current load. Creating high voltage at moderate current in the transmission segments and transforming it into high current at moderate voltage for residential distribution deliver the power. The three-phase four-wire standard system is common for AC supply. The supply is standard at 50/60 Hz. There are three live conductors, each called the *phase* or *line*. The phase means the relationship of two waveforms with respect to time. The voltage between any of these three phases is usually 415 V. If a neutral conductor is grounded, then the voltage between any phase conductor and the neutral will be 240 V. Supplies to premises are always connected to different phases to balance the load.

If the user is a small one, a house for example, the supply cable will have two conductors, live and neutral. The supply voltage is usually 240/120 V, and such configuration is known as single-phase two-wire system. The single-phase supply is the most common supply for domestic premises and other single-occupier premises where the demand for energy is relatively small. Larger consumers receive three-phase four-wire supplies. The higher voltage is generally used for motors and heavy loads. Other small loads are connected across the outers and the neutral in such a way that when the whole installation is operating, the load across the three phases is reasonably balanced.

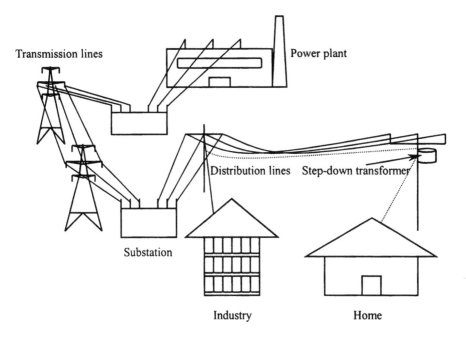

Figure 2-5 Actual electric utility system.

The conclusion is that transmission lines, which carry currents, are the main source of electric fields, because of the high line voltage. Nevertheless, the commercial and residential distribution systems are a significant source of magnetic fields, but are usually not a significant source of large electric fields. Figure 2-5 illustrates the actual electric utility system.

2.4 ELF FIELDS IN THE ENVIRONMENT

We are exposed to ELF electric and magnetic fields from many sources: transmission lines carrying electricity from generating plants to communities; distribution lines and cables that bring electricity to homes, schools, and workplaces; substations; transformers; wiring in homes and buildings; transportation; and various electrical appliances.

2.4.1 Overhead Power Lines

Transmission and distribution lines may be collectively referred to as *power lines*. Although the term transmission line includes all structures that serve to transfer energy or information between two points, we shall concentrate our discussion in

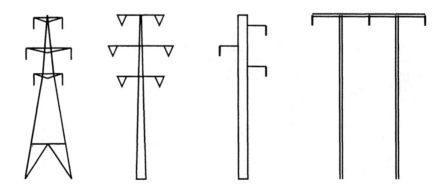

Figure 2-6 Common configurations of transmission and distribution line towers.

Part I of this book on transmission lines used for transfer of energy.

Overhead power lines are the cheapest method of carrying electrical power. They are usually constructed as parallel wires, which conduct lots of power very efficiently, but radiate very little. The field between the wires is quite intense, but usually contained between the wires. Magnetic field levels emanating from power lines are determined by the amount of current flowing through the lines, the proximity of the lines themselves with respect to each other, the height of the lines above the ground, and the proximity of the lines to other power lines.

Power lines include transmission lines (mounted on large metal towers) and distribution lines (mounted on concrete or wood poles placed on the road reserve). Many sizes and shapes of towers and poles are utilized depending on the voltage driving the current. The higher the voltage, the taller the tower, and the wider apart the wires must be placed. Figure 2-6 illustrates common configurations of power transmission and distribution line towers. Transmission lines carry electricity over long distances and operate at different amounts of voltages and currents, usually above 100 kV.

Distribution lines operate at lower voltages and bring power from substations to businesses and homes. The distribution network is divided into primary lines and secondary lines. Primary lines are mounted at the top of the poles and serve an entire region. They carry currents to *step-down* transformers, which may be pole mounted. The step-down transformers reduce the voltage of the primary lines to values, which are suitable for domestic wiring. Secondary lines are placed slightly lower on the poles. They carry currents driven by voltage in the range 240/120 V. In fact, these are the lines that supply us with electricity in the home.

There are huge transmission and distribution networks worldwide. This means that almost every population is exposed to fields from various components of these networks. The difference is only in the degree of exposure. In general, fields from both transmission and distribution lines will vary, depending on the time of day, the day of week, the time of year and the ambient temperature. Transmission lines generate both strong electric and magnetic fields. Distribution lines generate weak electric fields, but can generate strong magnetic fields, depending on the number of houses they supply.

Corona (an effect that occurs on insulators and wires) or electrical discharges into the air are produced around high-voltage power lines. They are sometimes visible on humid nights or during rainy days. Corona may produce noise and *ozone*, a colorless gas having a pungent smell. Virtually all these power lines carry three-phase circuits. They produce fields, which peak underneath the conductors and fall rapidly with distance on either side.

The strongest fields are normally encountered beneath high-voltage transmission lines; however, fields depend on the current flowing. Directly below overhead power lines, the maximum magnetic fields at ground level depend on the line voltage. For example, magnetic field ranges between 40 to 1 µT for line voltages ranging from 400 kV to 415 V.

Zaffanella [9] estimated the fields from transmission lines and certain types of distribution lines. The *median* ranged from 0.09 to 0.38 µT for transmission lines, although the number of residences exposed to these fields was small. Several types of primary distribution lines produced lower median fields (ranging from 0.01 to 0.02 µT).

The actual field produced by power lines depends on many factors such as current, clearance, spacing, and relative phasing of circuits [1, 5]:

Current

Today's largest power lines in use have a rating of over 4 kA per circuit, but the average current in a typical circuit is more like 700 A. Knowledge of the current (amplitude and phase) is essential to calculate the induced magnetic field. Generally, it is not easy to determine the current. It is known that voltage throughout the power system can be reasonably calculated where it does not vary significantly with time, but the current varies with time, day, and season depending on electricity use. This occurs because the demand for power (approximately proportional to current) follows daily and annual cycles. The daily variation occurs because of work and home activity figures in an area served by certain line, while the annual cycles follow climatic changes, which result in different heating, air conditioning, and lighting needs. Since currents are impractical to predict, it is difficult to exactly predict the associated magnetic fields due to the continuous change in current. A possible way to estimate the magnetic field, is to calculate the probability distribution of the magnetic field using data available about current unbalance and timely current variation.

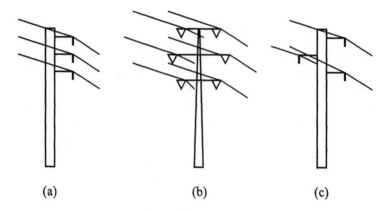

Figure 2-7 Wiring settings for power lines.

Clearance

The strength of magnetic fields from a power line depends on the power line's height. For example, the minimum ground clearance of a 400 kV overhead power line is 7.6 meters, but it is rare for such lines to be this low. In addition, the ground level field falls rapidly with the height of the line above ground.

Spacing

The strength of magnetic fields from power lines depends also on the way the wires are distanced from each other. The higher the current the more apart the wires are spaced. The 50/60 Hz magnetic field observable from a transmission or distribution line is proportional to the inductance of that segment of line. Usually, designers wish to keep the inductance as low as possible because the inductance causes voltage drop that limits the usable length of the line. Low inductance is achievable by mounting the opposing conductors of a circuit close to each other. However, conductors must be separated far enough apart in order to avoid possible contact and minimize chances of corona formation.

Wiring

Power lines are configured according to three wiring settings: first, *single-configuration* three-phase circuits [Figure 2-7 (a)], which produce high magnetic fields. Second is the *double-configuration* three-phase circuit [Figure 2-7 (b)], which produce lower magnetic fields; these are lines with three vertically stacked wires on both sides of a tower. Third is the *delta configuration* [Figure 2-7 (c)], which is the best style for reducing magnetic fields.

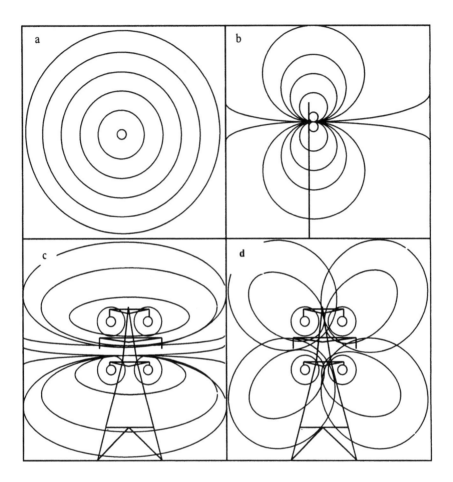

Figure 2-8   Magnetic field lines. (a) Single line. (b) Three-phase low voltage line. (c) Double circuit (untransposed phasing). (d) Double circuit (transposed phasing). (Adapted from [1].)

Relative Phasing of Circuits

As illustrated in Figure 2-8, a few power lines have *untransposed* phasing, with phases in the same order from top to bottom on the two sides of the tower. The magnetic field falls off as the inverse square of distance r from the line. However, most power lines have *transposed* phasing, with opposite order of the phases on one side to the other. This brings additional symmetry and cancellation between fields from equal currents on the two sides. The resulting field falls as the inverse cube of distance, producing lower fields at further distance from the line.

2.4.2 Underground Cables

A cable is defined as a length of insulated conductor, or more such conductors, each provided with its own insulation, which are laid up together. There are many types of cables ranging from heavy lead-sheathed and armored paper-insulated power cables to the domestic and workshop flexible cables used with ordinary appliances. In this part of the book, we are concerned with power cables, which are heavy, generally lead-sheathed and armored. These cables are usually used under the ground to transmit power from place to place within the power network.

A significant percentage of the high-voltage network worldwide is underground, mainly in urban areas or areas where there is a visual objection to the usage of overhead power lines, or where it is not convenient to use these lines. With underground cables, the individual conductors can be closer together, leading to greater cancellation and accordingly lower fields. Unless they are buried very deeply, they may lead to higher fields. Ground-level magnetic fields from cables fall much more rapidly with distance than those from the corresponding overhead lines, but can actually be higher at small distances from the cables. Occasionally, burying electric power lines reduce fields, but this is not necessarily the case, as magnetic fields travel through mud, sand, rocks, and cement. Unless the underground cables are configured to reduce fields, simply hiding the cables out of sight may create a false sense of safety. If the underground service is just a single-phase wire, radiation levels on the ground directly over the wire will be higher than from overhead lines because of the proximity to the source. Still, some underground cables have several circuits, which may be balanced to cancel the magnetic field.

The presence of underground cables near and in homes contributes to the exposure levels. Zaffanella [9] estimated the magnetic fields from underground distribution lines at homes with a median of 0.03 μT and with 5% exceeding 0.13 μT (roughly 75% of the median for all homes).

2.4.3 Substations

Substations are main components in the power transmission system, which adjust levels of electricity and thereby provide a link with the electricity supply. They are often located very close to residences and schools; therefore, substations are considered potential sources of electric and magnetic fields. They serve many functions in controlling and transferring power on electric systems. Several substation layouts are used by electric utilities to achieve reliable system operation. Some of these layouts are used in large commercial and industrial power systems. Figure 2-9 shows a typical layout of a substation.

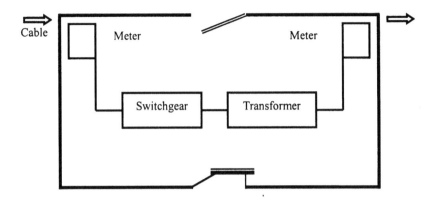

Figure 2-9 Typical layout of a substation.

A substation is an assemblage of circuit breakers, disconnecting switches, and transformers designed to change and regulate the voltage of electricity. Power lines carrying high voltages bring the current from the power plant to the substation, where transformers reduce it to lower voltages. Transformers give off magnetic fields because they principally depend upon magnetic fields to operate. Worsening the problem of field exposure is the incoming and outgoing currents at the substation, which are generally unbalanced.

Fields produced by substation equipment quickly diminish in strength a short distance away (at a rate of $1/r^3$) and do not extend beyond the substation limits. However, magnetic fields near substations are stronger than in other parts of the neighborhood since power lines drop down closer to the ground as they go in and out of the substation. This brings magnetic fields closer to people on the ground. The approximate magnetic fields normally encountered at perimeter fence around substations depend on the level of voltage: 10 μT for a 275-400 kV substation and 1.6 μT for an 11-kV substation.

2.4.4 Transformers

Transformers are electrical devices commonly used to adjust the voltage-current relationship of an electrical power circuit for best efficiency during transmission and distribution of power. They are essentially found in industrial applications.

The core of the transformer is built up from thin sheets or laminations of special steel. To reduce eddy-current losses, the laminations are insulated from one another by means of paper, china clay, or a coating of phosphate. The windings of the transformer are either copper or aluminum conductors in wire or strip form. The primary and secondary windings are regularly arranged concentrically. Each turn of the windings is insulated from adjacent turns by a thin layer of enamel, paper, or woven-glass insulation [10]. Power flows from the primary to the secondary windings by means of the magnetization of the transformer's ferromagnetic core. The power the transformer is transferring to the secondary windings is equal to the product of the secondary current times the voltage.

Basically, transformers are either step-up or step-down. Step-up transformers are used at the power generating station to raise the voltage so the power can be economically delivered over transmission lines. The magnetic fields from this type of transformer are high but localized and do not travel beyond the bounds of the substation. Step-down transformers are used to reduce line voltages of the primary distribution lines so that electricity will be usable at homes and workplace. Pole-mounted transformers are used where distribution lines are overhead while pad-mounted transformers are used where distribution lines are underground.

Frequently in urban situations, transformers are located within buildings. Such transformers reduce the voltage to 240/120 V, which is needed by nearby homes. Since transformers are seen in almost every neighborhood, they are certainly a source of popular concern. ELF fields near a transformer can be high, but due to its small structure, the field strength diminishes rapidly with distance, as it does from a loop source. Measurements at street level directly underneath a power-pole transformer are no greater than underneath the overhead power lines. Noise in the form of a buzzing or humming sound may be heard around transformers or high-voltage power lines producing corona.

2.4.5 Wiring Systems

The distribution of electrical energy on consumers' premises starts at the supply intake position. The latter may take various forms depending on the type of the premises. It could be a simple single-phase arrangement in homes to a large substation supplying an industry. Whatever, the size of the premises, however, certain wiring system must be adopted.

A wiring system is an assembly of various parts used in the formation of one or more electric circuits. It consists of conductors, together with certain wiring accessories for fixing the system, and joining and terminating the conductors. These include sheathing materials, conduits, ducts, switches, socket-outlets and plugs, grounding, etc. The main function of the wiring system is to divide and subdivide the total load at the consumer's premises into a small individual load, which is protected and controlled by certain devices and loads. The wiring system is another source of ELF fields similar to transmission and distribution lines, substations, transformers, and electric appliances, but at a different level.

Home Wiring

The electricity, which we receive at home, comes from a distant power plant. A generator in that power plant produces a substantial electric current of medium-high voltage. This current is AC, and it flows through transmission lines, substations, distribution lines, and transformers. When it reaches our home, a network of cables takes it from room to room and from floor to floor. The way in which power is distributed at homes varies from one wiring system to another. There are many wiring systems on the electrical installation market today. Each is designed to perform its duty in a specific way. One system is to use cables, which take power from a main panel box. Each cable will serve a number of rooms with limited capacity. Another system is called the *ring circuit*. This is generally used for power supplies where socket outlets are connected in a certain area to one continuous circuit, using a loop of cable that runs from the main panel box through all the socket outlets, returning to the same point on the main panel box.

Home electrical wiring produces electric fields from the voltage and magnetic fields from the current. Electric fields are usually attenuated by most building materials. AC current flowing through household wiring generates magnetic fields. They are generated either because of the loads or from unbalanced circuits. More currents produce higher magnetic fields. The greater the separation of the conductors, the less cancellation of the fields and therefore greater magnetic fields over greater distances. A few homes have 415-V distribution with separated-phase overhead wiring. With separated phases, magnetic fields may arise from the load currents on the conductors, just as with transmission lines.

Usually, modern homes have standard electrical outlets with three holes (2-pin-and-ground type) made in different sizes: 2 A, 5 A, 15 A and 30 A. The right hole is for the live wire (black in the United States, brown in Europe), left is for the neutral wire (white in the United States, blue in Europe). The neutral is the return for the live wire from the circuit. The difference in voltage between the neutral and live propels current through electric appliances. The neutral is solidly connected (bonded) to the home's ground system at the first disconnect at the main panel box to the grounding conductor so that any stray current will go to ground. This keeps large voltage differences from developing between the neutral and ground. The bonding also provides the proper path for lightning. The safety ground (green in the United States, green/yellow in Europe) is wired to the bottom. It is important that the safety ground wires and neutral wire be kept separate and run back to the main panel box, where they are grounded. The neutral or safety ground wire should not be grounded to the plumbing or any other ground except at the main panel box.

Electric current needs to flow through a closed path in order to work. This closed path is referred to as a circuit. To understand how the current is supposed to flow in a correctly wired circuit, we will consider a circuit used to power a sewing machine. The electricity flows from the main panel box through the live wire to the sewing machine, where it turns the motor. The electricity then flows back through the neutral wire to the main panel box. In such case, the field is canceled out because the live and neutral wires are close together. A ground wire runs from the main panel box to the sewing machine, but if everything is wired correctly then the ground carries no current.

Grounding is necessary for safety purposes, otherwise, every time the user touches a live wire, for instance, his/her body may complete the circuit and could receive a fatal shock. The ground connection allows any extra current to flow to the ground easily so that if a huge current is drawn out of the main panel box, it causes the fuse or circuit breaker in that panel box to break the connection. Also, grounding helps to disperse into the earth the surplus electricity from a lightning strike or an accidental power surge. In addition, it keeps the whole electrical system steady at 240/120 volts.

If the neutral has been grounded to the plumbing system instead of running back to the main panel box, the house is wired incorrectly, and this might result in a significant magnetic field. In this case, the electric current, which comes from the main panel box to the powered sewing machine, will run to the neutral and, if wired incorrectly, through the plumbing where it is grounded. Since it is no longer paired with the live wire, the magnetic field will not cancel out. Instead, there will be a magnetic field around the live wire that is connected to the sewing machine, and another field may surround all the plumbing system. In such circumstances, just one incorrectly grounded appliance may send electricity through all water pipes, and produce a magnetic field around the entire house. Plumbing currents may move from the water pipes into metal-conduit system and grounded equipment housings emanating magnetic fields everywhere.

Usually, magnetic fields in homes far away from power lines and substations are very low. The median value for homes in major towns or cities is approximately 0.1 µT. The values in smaller towns and rural areas are approximately half this value. In metropolitan regions, about 10% of homes have at least one room with a magnetic field exceeding 0.2 µT. Adjacent to power lines and substations levels of magnetic field are higher. Right underneath a power line, the level is usually the highest. It is estimated that 0.5% of housing has a magnetic field exceeding 0.2 µT, due to the proximity of power lines and substations.

Commercial and Industrial Buildings

The complexity of an electrical system depends on the function of a building or buildings. Multitenanted office blocks or apartments require detailed planning for the provision of adequate socket outlets for main-operated equipment, and right locations for indoor and outdoor lighting. Separate metering for different tenants may also have to be considered.

The idea of how fields are distributed throughout a building structure is illustrated in the simplified drawing of the electrical wiring of a building shown in Figure 2-10. A strong magnetic field is usually noticed near the switch panels. This is often the case because of the fact that all the electrical power for the facility normally enters the building through a single electrical room, typically in the basement, and is distributed to other parts of the building through heavy-duty switch panels. The switch panels produce highly complex magnetic fields due to the geometry of internal busbars and conductors, which travel asymmetrically in all directions within the interior of the panels. Although often similar to each other, service entrance panels may vary severely in design and construction by manufacturer, date of manufacturing, and load capacity. The characteristics of magnetic fields produced by panels, therefore, vary from panel to panel.

While the incoming utility power is contained within cables, the individual current carrying conductors are generally spread apart on the interior of the switch apparatus leading to considerably stronger fields due to less phase cancellation. A common scenario is for outside utility power to enter the bottom of the switch panels from beneath and to exit the panel from the top, where it is distributed via either cable contained within large electrical conduits or via busbars. It is interesting to note that busbars usually lead to greater magnetic fields in their vicinity than cables carrying the same currents because of the greater separation of the conductors. Phase cancellation afforded by busbars is less than that provided by tightly configured bundled cables.

In commercial buildings, transformers and network protectors are placed in secured vaults commonly located within the buildings; whereas, suburban utilities mount the transformers on outside pads. High-current, low-voltage feeders supply the main switch panels rates between 1000 and 4000 A per phase. In multistory buildings, substations, electrical rooms, and high current (1000-2500 A) busway risers are necessary for every few floors. Usually, areas above, below, and adjacent to the substations and busway risers are subject to very high (10-1000 mG) and extremely high (1000-100000 mG) magnetic fields.

In addition to current load, conductor spacing is another critical factor affecting field levels. Closely stacked, solid busbars, and busways minimize phase conductor spacing, thereby promoting self-cancellation and lower field levels. If a four-wire three-phase system is unbalanced by more than 15% or the neutral has excessive net, ground, or plumbing currents, then the magnetic field becomes highly elevated and a serious electromagnetic interference (EMI) threat will occur. Stray grounding currents in the building steel, ducts, and conduits plus plumbing currents on the water pipes also create elevated magnetic fields.

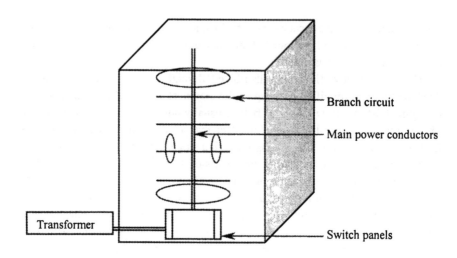

Figure 2-10   A simplified model of the electrical wiring of a building.

Raised levels of magnetic fields in commercial buildings are often caused by net-current conditions present on conduits and other distribution circuits. In multigrounded, four-wire industrial and commercial building wiring systems, some portion of the neutral current may return to the source transformer via building grounds. Meanwhile, neutrals of different circuits may be tied together thus allowing current from one neutral to return to the transformer via alternate neutral conductors. In such instances, the vector sums of the currents for any given circuit might not add up to zero. When the vector sum of the phase, neutral, and parallel ground wire (if present) for a given circuit does not equal zero, a net-current condition is present. This circuit condition creates net-current magnetic fields that decay at a $1/r$ rate versus the $1/r^2$ rate normally associated with magnetic fields supposed emanating from such distribution circuits [11].

2.4.6 Transportation Sources

Inside a car, the dominant sources of ELF fields are those people pass by, or under, as they drive, such as power lines. Car batteries are the main source of DC fields. Also, car phones, which are battery-powered equipment, are another source of DC, although they transmit and receive signals in the RF range. Some car components, such as alternators, might create alternating fields but not necessarily in the 50/60-Hz power-frequency fields.

Electric trains and trams are a source of exposure to both static and ELF fields. Some trains run on AC while others use DC. Near the floor within the passenger compartment, static fields might reach 0.2 mT, and the magnetic field

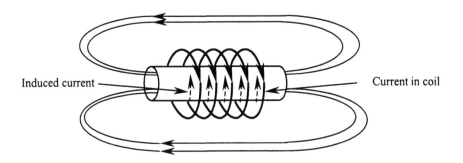

Figure 2-11 Layout of an induction heater.

can be several hundred µT, with lower values (tens of µT) at the seat level and elsewhere in the compartment. Sometimes, electric fields may reach 300 V/m.

Actual exposure levels are very dependent on equipment design and location within the train. Train motors and traction devices are usually located underneath the floor of passenger cars. They create very intense fields in the regions of the floor just above the motors. In addition, train passengers are exposed to magnetic fields from sources the train passes on its route.

2.4.7 Induction Heaters

Induction heating is a method of providing fast and consistent heat for manufacturing applications, which include bonding or changing the properties of conductive materials. The process relies on electrical currents within the material to produce heat.

The basic components of an induction heating system are an AC power supply, induction coil, and material to be heated or treated. High-frequency currents typically in the kilohertz are passed through coils (normally made of copper) that surround conductive materials to be heated or treated. Strong eddy currents are produced in the target material generating precise amounts of localized heat without any physical contact between the coil and the material. Figure 2-11 shows a typical layout for an induction heater.

While dielectric heat sealers are predominately electric field sources, induction heaters produce very strong magnetic fields. Stray magnetic fields in the vicinity of the coils may exceed applicable limits for exposure in some cases.

Although magnetic fields are the most prominent feature of the induction heating process, strong electric fields might also be encountered near the power leads that extend from the power supply cabinet to the heating coils. However, with the low frequencies involved, there may be a remarkable coupling between the user's body and the electric fields resulting in significant induced currents.

2.4.8   Electric Appliances

Main-powered appliances produce magnetic fields whenever they draw current. Such fields generally fall as the inverse cube of distance ($1/r^3$), and thus are significant only within short distances from the appliances. In typical homes, people probably receive about a third of their time-averaged exposure from appliances and the remainder from net currents in the current distribution system. Table 2-1 shows a list of common appliances and their associated magnetic fields.

Many workers receive more exposure at work than at home, despite less time spent there. Fields in the workplace tend to be higher than in the home, partly because of the greater concentration of appliances. Electrical devices such as photocopiers are common high-intensity sources and can emit high magnetic fields when in standby and double than that when making copies. Photocopiers or other devices using high voltage to operate may also produce ozone. Electrical discharges in the air convert oxygen molecules into ozone, which can be smelled easily by users.

Certain industries have particular equipment, which involve high currents and produce high magnetic fields. In the electricity supply industry, examples are generator busbars in power stations and some reactive-compensation plants in substations. In other industries, certain welding, heating and electrolytic processes can produce high fields that may affect only specific workers.

2.4.9   Video Display Terminals

The application of computers and the accompanying use of VDTs are revolutionizing living and working lifestyles. Since the introduction of personal computers (PCs), their usage has grown from a few million during the 1980s to a few hundred million in use today. Companies and individual users of computers are certainly aware of the benefits generated from these high-tech devices. Yet, too few users are aware of the real or suspected dangers derived from the exposure to emissions from VDTs.

What is a VDT?

A VDT is part of the computer system. It is a television-like screen commonly called the monitor. The operator types information on a keyboard and the computer displays the information on the VDT. VDTs serve as a suitable way for people to interact with computer systems. Certain techniques are used to generate and move an electron beam that illuminates the screen of a cathode ray tube (CRT).

Table 2-1   Common Electric Appliances and Their Associated Magnetic Fields [12-18]

Source	Magnetic Field in μT (Distance = 30 cm)	Magnetic Field in μT (Distance = 90 cm)
Office Appliances		
Computer monitor	0.02-13.00	0.001-0.9
Copy machine	0.005-1.80	0.00-0.2.0
Fax machine	0.00-0.016	0.00-0.003
Fluorescent light	0.50-2.00	0.02-0.25
Printer	0.07-4.30	0.02-0.25
Scanner	0.20-2.60	0.009-0.3
Workshop Appliances		
Electric drill	0.02-3.3	0.003-0.80
Band saw	0.05-1.4	0.005-0.075
Kitchen Appliances		
Can opener	0.70-16.30	0.10-0.60
Coffee maker	0.009-0.70	0.00-0.06
Dishwasher	0.50-0.80	0.08-0.16
Electric oven	0.15-0.50	0.01-0.04
Garbage disposal	0.27-0.78	0.02-0.15
Microwave oven	0.05-5.00	0.011-0.45
Mixer	0.05-4.00	0.009-0.40
Refrigerator	0.01-0.30	0.001-0.06
Toaster	0.03-0.45	0.001-0.05
Multiroom Appliances		
Analog clock	0.18-4.10	0.003-0.32
Digital clock	0.03-0.57	0.00-0.13
Portable radio	0.04-0.40	0.003-0.10
Vacuum cleaner	0.70-2.20	0.05-0.13
Bathroom Appliances		
Electric shaver	0.01-10.00	0.01-0.30
Hair dryer	0.01-7.00	0.01-0.03
Living Room Appliances		
Fan	0.04-8.50	0.03-0.30
Color TV	0.02-1.20	0.007-0.11
Utility Room Appliances		
Clothes iron	0.15-0.30	0.025-0.035
Portable heater	0.011-1.90	0.00-0.14
Washing machine	0.15-3.00	0.01-0.15

These displays are used in television receivers, computers, automated teller machines, video games, and other devices. Different technologies, such as transistor displays and liquid crystal displays (LCDs), are used in laptop computers and do not have the same characteristics as CRTs. All relevant health concerns of VDTs pertain to CRTs.

Emission from VDTs

Most VDTs currently in use are based on CRT technology. VDTs can have emission in the entire EM spectrum. Emission is not bound to the VDT screen— they occur in all directions as shown in Figure 2-12. Scientific investigations focus on the following parameters relative to VDTs [19]:

1. X-rays and ultraviolet (UV) light (wavelengths below 400 nm).
2. Visible light at the frequency range $4.3-7.5 \times 10^{14}$ Hz generated due to the interaction of electrons with the phosphor layer inside the CRT causes the emission of visible radiation from the screen.
3. Infrared (IR) radiation from heat generated by the electronics circuitry.
4. RFR generated by the electrical pulses, oscillator, and digital circuits.
5. VLF electric and magnetic fields generated by the horizontal deflection system on the CRT and the high-voltage flyback transformer.
6. ELF electric and magnetic fields generated by the power supply, vertical deflection system, transformer, and electrons impinging on the screen.
7. Static electric fields associated with high voltages applied to the internal surface of the cathode screen.
8. Ion depletion in air environment.
9. Chemical gases from hardware materials.

CRTs are built so that the lead glass in the tube will absorb the low-energy X-rays and UV rays and only visible light is transmitted. IR radiation may cause temperature increase in the working environment. X-rays, UV, visible light, and IR are considerably below the safety standards for ordinary CRT screens.

Contrary to popular belief, most of fields do not extend from the front of the screen but from inductive components located near the inside rear or sides of the equipment. Currently, manufacturers have been required to add internal shielding to the high-voltage transformer used in TVs and VDTs, which limit the amount of interference and emission produced by such appliances.

However, LCDs do not emit electrostatic fields and X-rays. They are driven by low power, which imply low emission of electric and magnetic fields. Also low levels of VLF fields are emitted by LCDs due to the operation of backlight and power supply.

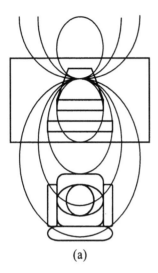 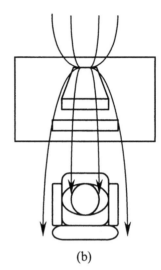

(a)   (b)

Figure 2-12 Exposures produced by a computer monitor. (a) Magnetic fields. (b) Electric fields.

Description of Operation

The CRT is an evacuated glass tube, which has a source of electrons at one end and an internally coated screen with phosphor at the other end. When high voltage is applied to the CRT, a focused beam of electrons is produced, which is scanned across the screen. The beam is switched on and off in order to generate the display.

The electron beam in the CRT moves across the screen in a series of horizontal lines starting at the top left and moving down left-to-right. In turn lines are displaced vertically in order to cover the screen from top to bottom. The horizontal and vertical steering of the electron beam is done by fast-changing magnetic fields at the neck of the tube. For each horizontal line the beam must be swept constantly across the screen by an increasing magnetic field while the electron beam is turned on. Once the beam reaches the right-hand edge of the screen, the electron beam is turned off and retraced to the left side of the screen by a rapidly decreasing magnetic field. This combination of slow- and fast-changing magnetic fields produces a sawtooth-shaped waveform. Figure 2-13 shows the process of a screen scanning.

For a typical video graphics array (VGA)-mode computer monitor, about 31,500 horizontal lines are painted each second. This requires 31.5-kHz magnetic field aligned, or polarized, in the vertical direction.

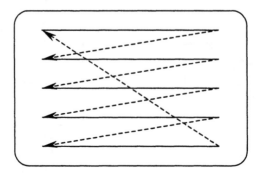

Figure 2-13 Scanning of a screen.

The circuit that controls the horizontal movement of the beam is called the horizontal deflection system, which operates at a frequency of 15-100 kHz. It is the major source of VLF electric and magnetic fields in the VDT. While, the circuit that controls the vertical movement of the beam is called the vertical deflection system. This circuit operates at a frequency of 50 to 80 Hz in the majority of VDTs and is the major source of ELF fields.

Additionally, the high static positive voltages on the inside of the front of the CRT generate a charge on the front of the CRT surface that depends on factors such as humidity, clothing worn by the user, and the floor covering material.

Because electric and magnetic fields come from the internal components, its levels on the back and sides of a VDT are higher than in front, often by a factor of 2. Accordingly, the most dangerous area is believed to be at the back of the VDT near the deflection yoke. In addition, there is always that worry about the front of the picture tube emitting X-rays. This means distance between the operator and screen should be extended further (preferably 70 cm) in order to achieve the same level of exposure. Smaller VDTs are not necessarily better, either. A 12-inch VDT might well generate a stronger magnetic field than a 19-inch one, because the field strength depends mainly on the internal design of the deflection system and electronic circuitry than on the screen size. Monochrome displays typically produce 1/2 to 1/5 the levels of fields than color displays, although this is not always the case.

2.5 EFFECT OF ELF FIELDS ON EQUIPMENT

In addition to their effect on human body, electric and magnetic fields affect several types of equipment. Yet, fields required are usually rather higher than those commonly encountered [1].

Devices that have information encoded on a magnetic strip are subject to being affected by exposure to ELF fields. They may be corrupted by magnetic fields above about 10 mT. Such fields almost never occur at 50/60 Hz, but the problem may arise with static fields, such as those produced from magnetic catches on handbags.

It has been observed that vehicles with electronic control systems are more likely to be susceptible to interference from magnetic fields at levels above about 2 mT. This tends to be a serious problem at higher frequencies.

Quartz watches with analog dials (not digital quartz watches), which use a tiny stepper motor to drive the hands, are also sensitive to ELF fields. The stepper motor can be driven by a suitably oriented external magnetic field of about 1 mT or greater, causing the hands of the watch to rotate many times faster than normal. Although analog watches may gain time, lose time, or even stop under the influence of powerful magnetic fields, they will usually return to normal time keeping as soon as they leave the source of ELF exposure.

Strong ELF fields cause EMI in cardiac pacemakers or other implanted electromedical devices. Individuals using these devices should contact their doctor to determine their susceptibility to these effects. Interference has been related in certain models of implanted cardiac pacemaker with electric fields above about 20 µT at 50 Hz. This may affects only certain models of pacemaker and is generally not regarded as a health hazard.

It is also common to see image movement on the screen of computer terminals, especially at spaces of high magnetic fields such as offices at commercial buildings. It generally becomes noticeable at about 1 µT and a serious problem at about 10 µT. This may cause interference with the electrons producing the image on the screen. Technically, the electron beam can be deflected by an external magnetic field. This effect is known as *wobble*.

REFERENCES

[1] Swanson, J., and D. C. Renew, Power-Frequency Fields and People, *Engineering Science and Education Journal*, pp. 71-79, 1994.
[2] Bennet, W. R., Jr., Cancer and Power Lines, *Physics Today* 47, pp. 23-29, 1994.
[3] Lou, V., EMF Fundamentals, Presentation to the New York Interagency Engineering Council, New York, NY, 1995.
[4] Sadiku, M. N. O., *Elements of Electromagnetics*, Oxford University Press, Oxford, UK, 2000.
[5] Levitt, B. B., *Electromagnetic Fields: A Consumer's Guide to the Issues and How to Protect Ourselves*, A Harvest Original Harcourt Brace & Company, San Diego, CA, 1995.
[6] Molinski, T. S., W. E. Feero, and B. L. Damsky, Shielding Grids from Solar Storms, *IEEE Spectrum* 37 (11), pp. 55-60, 2000.

[7] Habash, R. W. Y., N. M. Abdul Kadir, and A. H. Abu Bakar, Power Frequency 50 Hz Fields and People: In Search of Answers, *The Conference on Electricity Power Supply Industry (CEPSI)*, pp. 47-57, Kuala Lumpur, Malaysia, 1996.

[8] Bosela, T. R., *Introduction to Electrical Power System Technology*, Prentice Hall, New Jersey, NJ, 1997.

[9] Zaffanella, L., Survey of Residential Magnetic Field Sources, Volume 1: Goals, Results and Conclusions, Volume 2: Protocol, Data Analysis, and Management, TR-102759-V1, TR-102759-V2, EPRI, Palo Alto, CA, 1993.

[10] Thompson, F. G., *Electrical Installation and Workshop Technology*, Longman, 1978.

[11] Munderloh, J. W., K- L. Griffing, M. L. Hiles, and K. C. Holte, Reduction of ELF Magnetic Fields Emanating from Circuits with Net Current Conditions by Cancellation Techniques, *Annual Review of Bioeffects Research*, Tucson, AZ, 1998.

[12] Gauger, J. R., Household Appliance Magnetic Field Survey, Technical Report EO6549-3, IIT Research Institute, Chicago, IL, 1984.

[13] Survey of Residential Magnetic Field Sources, Interim Report of Electrical Power Research Institute, TR-100194, Project 2942-06, EPRI, Palo Alto, CA, 1992.

[14] EMF in Your Environment, EPA Document No. 402-R-92-008, 1992.

[15] Sawicki, D. S., 60 Hertz Electromagnetic Field (EMF) Exposure, Internet Document at http://members.aol.com/cemf/, 1997.

[16] Preece, A. W., W. T. Kaune, P. Grainger, and J. Golding, Magnetic Fields from Domestic Appliances in the UK, *Physics in Medicine and Biology* 42, pp. 67-76, 1997.

[17] Questions and Answers About EMF Electric and Magnetic Fields Associated with the Use of Electric Power, National Institute of Environmental Health Sciences (NIEHS), National Institutes of Health, Internet Document at http://www.niehs.nih.gov/oc/factsheets/emf/emf.htm, 1998.

[18] Short Factsheet on EMF, California EMF Program, California Electric and Magnetic Field Program, CA, 2000.

[19] Hamnerius, Y., Exposure from VDT, *6th COST 24 bis Workshop: Exposure Systems and their Dosimetry*, pp. 26-30, Zurich, Switzerland, 15 February 1999.

3

Bioeffects of ELF Fields

3.1 INTRODUCTION

A biological effect occurs when exposure to EM fields causes some noticeable or detectable physiological change in a living system. Such an effect may sometimes, but not always, lead to an adverse health effect, which means a physiological change that exceeds normal range for a brief period of time. It occurs when the biological effect is outside the normal range for the body to compensate, and therefore leads to some detrimental health condition. Health effects are often the result of biological effects that accumulate over time and depend on exposure dose. Therefore, detailed knowledge of the biological effects is important to understand the generated health risks.

Let us consider the example of exposure to sunlight as one of the most familiar forms of nonionizing radiation [1]. The sun delivers light and heat, which may lead to sunburn when the amount of exposure exceeds what, can be protected against by the skin's melanin (a pigment which gives skin and hair its color and provides protection against UV and visible light). We control its effect on us with sunglasses, shades, hats, clothes and sunscreens. Some effects due to sunlight exposure may be harmless, such as the body's reaction of increasing blood flow in the skin in response to greater heating from the sun. Other effects may be advantageous, for instance, the feeling of warmth due to exposure to sun on a cool day. It may even lead to positive health effects where sunlight exposure assists the human body to produce vitamin D, which helps the body absorb calcium for stronger bones. However, extensive exposure to sunlight might lead to severe health effects, such as sunburn or even skin cancer.

We are exposed to extremely low-frequency (ELF) fields from many sources, including transmission lines, distribution lines, substations, and various electrical appliances. Usually, exposure to ELF fields occurs at distances much shorter than the wavelength of ELF radiation. This has important implications, because under such conditions, electric and magnetic fields are treated as independent components. This is different from radio frequency radiation (RFR), in which the electric and magnetic fields are inextricably linked. For this reason, researchers have separately focused on the interaction of either electric or magnetic fields with the living system in order to identify their possible health risk.

Over the years, scientists have attempted to prove the ELF interaction theories. Although the photon energy at the ELF band of the spectrum is smaller than that needed to break even the weakest chemical bond, well established mechanisms exist by which electric and magnetic fields could produce biological effects without breaking chemical bonds. Electric fields can apply forces on charged and uncharged molecules or cellular structures within living systems. These forces can cause movement of charged particles, orient or distort cellular structures, orient dipolar molecules, or induce voltages across cell membranes. Magnetic fields can also apply forces on cellular structures, but since biological materials are largely nonmagnetic, these forces are usually very weak. Also, magnetic fields may induce electric fields in the body.

Although electric and magnetic fields often occur together, most concerns while dealing with these fields have focused on the potential health effects of magnetic fields only. The argument is that magnetic fields are difficult to shield, and easily penetrate buildings and people, contrary to electric fields, which have very little ability to penetrate buildings or even human skin.

3.2 INTERACTION MECHANISMS

Scientists with decades of practical experience are actively working to explain how EM fields interact with biological systems, particularly when the applied EM energy is not sufficient to damage biomolecules or induce heating. Perhaps, the explanation may go beyond the belief that EM properties of cells and tissues are prime pillars of EM interaction mechanisms by considering models for the scientific apprehension of life processes in biological systems.

The basics of EM interaction with materials were elucidated over a century ago and stated as the well-known Maxwell's equations. The application of these basics to biological systems, however, is very difficult because of the extreme complexity and multiple levels of organization in living organisms, in addition to the wide range of electrical properties of biological tissues. The above difficulty has slowed the progress of understanding the EM bioeffects. Yet, knowledge of the interaction mechanisms could be utilized to identify appropriate dosimetry, to predict dose-response relationships, to design better experiments, and to assist in determining whether harmful effects are likely at specific levels of exposure.

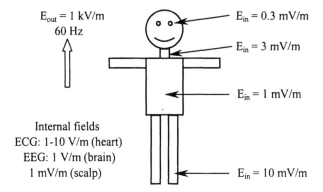

Figure 3-1 Electric fields in a human model exposed to incident electric field of 1 kV/m at 60 Hz [2].

There are several proposed mechanisms for the interaction of EM fields with living systems. Before discussing these mechanisms, one must understand the relationship between electric and magnetic fields outside and inside biological systems (a process called *coupling*), which varies greatly with frequency. Electric fields are greatly diminished by many orders of magnitude inside biological tissues from their values in air external to the tissues. This is because boundary conditions on Maxwell's equations require current density inside the biological system to approximately equal the displacement current density outside the system.

Biological tissues are nonmagnetic materials, which means the magnetic field inside the human body is same to those outside it. Most of the debate going on over acceptable exposure limits of ELF fields is expressed in terms of magnetic fields. Meanwhile, the case is not same for electric fields. Consider a case of a human body under electric field exposure, as illustrated in Figure 3-1 [2]. Electrically, the coupling is too poor to the external field. For example, an external field of 1 kV/m may induce an electric field within the body of about 1 mV/m. It is observed that electric fields induced inside the bodies of humans and animals are generally less than about 10^{-7} of the field outside the body and rarely exceed about 10^{-4} of the external field. This is the typical strength at ground level beneath a high-voltage power line. Also, those low-level electric fields produce currents, which are orders of magnitude weaker than the currents induced naturally from the function of heart, nerves, and muscle [2-4]. Meanwhile, the highest field strength to which the human may be exposed (those associated with electrical appliances) might produce electric fields within a small region of the body that are comparable to or may be larger than the naturally occurring fields. Still, the magnitude of such large locally induced fields is not accurately known.

EM interaction mechanisms have been proposed but are not well established.

Valberg et al. [5] have reviewed several mechanisms by which electric and magnetic fields at 50/60 Hz might influence biology, e.g., energy transfer, force, resonance, and magnetic moments including signal averaging.

Fundamentally, proposed mechanisms include induced electric currents, direct effect on magnetic biological materials, effects on free radicals, and excitation of cell membranes.

3.2.1 Induced Currents

At ELF range, a biological material is regarded as a conducting medium. At the microscopic level, all tissues are composed of cells and extracellular fluids. As discussed in 1.10.1, a cell has two distinct parts: the outer, insulating membrane and the inner cytoplasm and nucleus, which like the extracellular fluid, has high conductivity. Because of the membrane, cells appear to be insulators and almost all the currents induced in tissues by low-frequency electric fields flow around the cells. The insulating membrane, which completely surrounds the conducting core, makes the cell itself a series combination of the membrane capacitance and the cytoplasmic resistance. The thickness of the insulating portion of the membrane is less than 10 nm. Therefore, the membrane capacitance is very large. Usually, below 100 Hz, the impedance of biological materials is generally resistive. In most cases, contribution of the capacitive component is in the order of 10%, but it increases with frequency.

A possible effect of EM fields on living systems has been theorized to involve the ability, through magnetic induction, to stimulate eddy currents at cell membranes and in tissue fluids, which circulate in a closed loop that lies in a plane normal to the direction of the magnetic field. However, secondary magnetic fields produced by such currents may be neglected. The above current can be calculated using only Faraday's law and Laplace's equations, without simultaneously solving Maxwell's equations. Hence, both current and electric fields are induced inside living systems by external ELF magnetic fields [6-8]. Such induced current may cause a kind of effect in the biological system. In the ELF range, the variation in surface charge density is very slow so that the current and field generated inside the object are very small.

Accurate calculation of the induced current in a human body is only possible using numerical simulations, but if the body has a homogeneous and isotropic conductivity, the current distribution in different organs, e.g., the head, could be expressed analytically. The current density in a circular path perpendicular to a sinusoidal magnetic field is derived from Faraday's law of induction [9]

$$J = \pi \sigma r B f \qquad (3.1)$$

where J is the current density in amperes/meter^2 (A/m^2), σ is the conductivity of the medium in siemens/meter (S/m), r is the radius of the loop for induction of current in meters (m), B is the magnetic flux density in teslas (T) or webers/meter^2 (Wb/m^2), and f is the frequency in Hz.

If the properties of the biological system are constant, the induced current is directly proportional to the frequency of the applied field. However, the value of current based on Equation (3.1) is limited. Currents usually interface between different layers in a heterogeneous object and are quite different from that predicted analytically.

Xi and Stuchly [10] made calculations based on anatomically and electrically refined models resulted in a maximum current densities exceeding 2 mA/m^2 for 100-μT field at 60 Hz.

Kaune et al. [11] numerically analyzed currents induced in a rat by linearly- and circularly-polarized magnetic fields of 50 Hz. Special focus was placed on pineal gland and retina of rats since these organs were often associated with the changes of melatonin synthesis. Induced currents in two MRI-based rat models with resolutions of up to 0.125 mm^3 were calculated by using the *impedance method*. Calculated current densities were extremely small, i.e., $< 30\ \mu$A/m^2 for both polarized fields of 1.41 μT (peak). There were no significant differences in amplitude nor polarization of induced currents in the pineal gland between the linearly and the circularly polarized fields when the polarization was in a vertical plane. In contrast, magnetic fields rotating in the horizontal plane produced most circularly polarized currents both in the pineal gland and in the retina.

At very high frequencies (above 100 kHz), induced currents heat the exposed biological system, causing thermal damage. At ELF fields, tissue heating is not a problem, but if the induced current is too strong, there is a risk of stimulating electrically excitable cells such as neurons. At frequencies below approximately 100 kHz, currents necessary to heat biological systems are greater than currents necessary to stimulate neurons and other electrically excitable cells.

3.2.2 Magnetic Biosubstances

All living organisms are essentially made of diamagnetic organic compounds, but some paramagnetic molecules (e.g., O_2), and ferromagnetic microstructures (hemoglobin core, magnetite) are also present. Biological magnetites are usually found in single domain units, covered with thin membranes called *magnetosomes* (Fe_3O_4). These microstructures behave like small magnets and are influenced by external fields changing their energy content. They are usually found in bacteria and other small biological elements. It is believed also that the human brain contains magnetosomes. Such bacteria and biological elements orient with the applied magnetic fields. Magnetosomes exist in the interior of cells bound to cell bodies through cytoskeleton. In such gathering, torque generated by the action of the magnetic field acts to rotate the whole cell through forces on the individual magnetosomes that are magnetically lined up. The impedance of the surrounding environment restrains the movement of these composite systems, induced by fields. Magnetosomes, which are not rigidly bound to the whole cell structure, may rotate in the cell in such a way to create biological effects.

ELF fields might create biological effect by acting on such particles [12-16]. But the effect occurs only with strong magnetic fields. Calculations show that these effects require at least 2-5 μT [12-14].

3.2.3   Free Radicals

Free radicals are atoms or molecules with at least one unpaired electron. Unpaired electrons are very unnatural, unstable, and hazardous because electrons normally come in pairs. These odd, unpaired electrons in free radicals cause them to collide with other molecules so they can steal electrons from them, which change the structure of other molecules and cause them to also become free radicals. This can create a self-perpetuating chain reaction in which the structure of millions of molecules is altered in a matter of nanoseconds reeking havoc with DNA, protein molecules, enzymes, and cells [17].

Free radicals are remarkably reactive. They just exist for very short periods (typically less than 1 ns), but their effect is extreme in terms of cell aging and various kinds of cancer because of the damage they do to DNA, cells, and tissues. Radical pairs exist in either singlet (reactive) or triplet (diffusive) states, depending on whether their unpaired spins are antiparallel or parallel to the applied field.

Static magnetic fields may influence the response rate of chemical reactions involving free-radical pairs [18-23]. Since the lifetime of these free radicals is so short compared to the cycle time of the ELF fields in general and power frequency (50/60-Hz) fields in particular, the applied fields act like static fields during the time scale over which these reactions occur. Biological effects due to fields less than 50 μT are not significant because any effect of field would be additive with a 30-70-μT geomagnetic field.

Brocklehurst and McLauchlan [22] discussed the effects of environmental magnetic field on radical pair reactions. They anticipated that such effects are theoretically conceivable down to fields of geomagnetic strength, with effects at static fields as low as 0.1 mT. The effect seen at 0.1 mT was very small (1% increase in free radical concentrations). The body possesses sophisticated defense mechanisms to cope with these radicals under normal conditions.

3.2.4 Cell Membrane and the Chemical Link

According to Foster [2], "low-frequency electric fields can excite membranes, causing shock or other effects. At power line frequencies, the threshold current density required to produce shock is around 10 A/m^2, which corresponds to electric field of 100 V/m in the tissue. However, electric fields can create pores in cell membranes by inducing electric breakdown. This requires potential differences across the membranes at levels between 0.1-1 V, which, in turn, requires electric field in the medium surrounding the cell of at least 10^5 V/m."

Many life scientists through series of findings [4, 23-29] believe the cell membrane plays a principal role in the EM interaction mechanisms with biological systems. Indications point to cell membrane receptors as the probable site of initial tissue interactions with EM fields for many neurotransmitters, growth-regulating enzyme expressions, and cancer-promoting chemicals.

Scientists theorizing this mechanism conclude that biological cells are bioelectrochemical structures, which interact with their environment in various ways, including physically, chemically, biochemically, and electrically. According to Dr. William Ross Adey at the University of California, Riverside [30], "the ions, especially calcium ions could play the role of a chemical link between EM fields and life processes. The electrical properties and ion distribution around cells are perfect for establishing effects with external steady oscillating EM fields." He presented a three-step model involving calcium ions, which could explain observed EM-induced bioeffects. Key to the model is the activation of intracellular messenger systems (adenylate cyclase and protein kinase) by calcium in a stimulus amplification process across the cell membrane.

The impact of ELF fields may also be understood in terms of amplification and/or the cooperative sensing associated with simultaneous stimulation of all membrane receptors. Dr. Litovitz and his team at the Catholic University of America (CUA) [25], hypothesized that oscillating EM fields needs to be steady for certain period of time (approximately 1 second) for a biological response to occur. This allows cells to discriminate external fields from thermal noise fields, even though they might be smaller than the noise fields.

3.2.5 Summary of Interaction Mechanisms

It is concluded from the three biophysical mechanisms (induced electric currents, direct effect on magnetic biological materials, and effects on free radicals) that high field strength is needed to produce noticeable biological effects in living systems. These strengths are usually much higher that the typical environmental exposures. However, to understand the bioelectrochemical mechanism, we need to emphasize on how ELF fields affect life processes. A concept, according which most life scientists believe that only the chemical processes is involved in growth and healing in the living system. A clear distinction between this mechanism and the previous three biophysical mechanisms is summarized in Adair's comment [28], "any biological effect of weak ELF fields on the cellular level must be found outside the scope of conventional physics."

3.3   ELF FIELDS AND CANCER

Various health effects from electric and magnetic fields have been discussed in the literature, but most of the attention has focused on possible relationship with the initiation or promotion of cancer. Attention is partially derived from the concept of cancer as a dread disease. The rest of the attention is connected with the epidemiological data, which suggests a possible involvement of such weak fields in the incidences of leukemia and other types of cancer. This issue has raised significant interest in the interactions of ELF fields with living organisms.

3.3.1   Cancer Mechanisms

Cancer is a term applied to describe at least 200 different diseases, all of which involve uncontrolled cell growth. Cancer is a case of uncontrolled mitosis in which cells randomly divide and grow after escaping the body's normal control condition. As a primary disorder of cellular growth and differentiation, cancer is essentially a genetic disorder at the cellular level. With cancer, the fault is in the cell itself rather than in the overall body. Causes of most cases of cancer are unknown, but factors that influence the risk of cancer are many. Each of the known risk factors such as smoking, alcohol, diets, ionizing radiation, or others contributes to specific types of cancer.

Cancer risk is related to many causes. The risk with asbestos is related to fiber length and toughness. The risk from particles in air pollution is related to their size and propensity to settle in the lung. Ionizing radiation has sufficient energy to directly initiate cancer. Visible light breaks bonds in the process of photosynthesis but is not usually suspected of causing cancer. Radiation of solar origin, like UV (especially UVB) is associated with skin cancer and malignant melanoma. However, the photon energy from 50/60 Hz fields (2.5×10^{-13} eV) is insufficient to directly break chemical bonds.

In general, cancers potentially associated with exposure to EM fields are leukemia, brain and breast cancers. Leukemia and lymphoma (lymphoma is a cancer that arises in the lymphoid tissues) are complex of malignant diseases of the hematopoietic system.

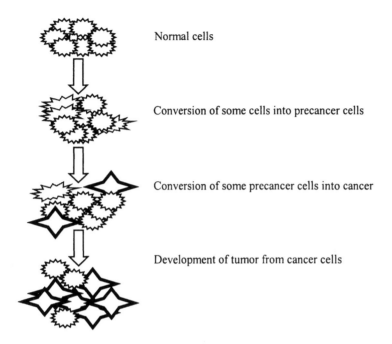

Normal cells

Conversion of some cells into precancer cells

Conversion of some precancer cells into cancer

Development of tumor from cancer cells

Figure 3-2 The multistep carcinogenesis model [31].

3.3.2 Carcinogenesis

Transformation of healthy cells to malignant cells is a complex process, which includes at least three distinct stages driven by a series of injuries to the genetic material of cells. This process is referred to as the *multistep carcinogenesis* (cancer-producing) model [31], as illustrated in Figure 3-2. This model may replace an earlier model, called the *initiation-promotion model*, which proposed that carcinogenesis was a two-step process, with the first step being a genotoxic injury (initiation). This is an irreversible step in which some agent causes genetic mutations. The second step is a nongenotoxic process (promotion) that enhances the proliferation of already damaged cells.

Human cancer is the result of the accumulation of various genetic and epigenetic changes in a given population of cells. Cancer is initiated by damage to the DNA. An agent causing such injury is called a *genotoxin*. It is extremely unlikely that a single genetic injury to the cell will result in cancer; rather it appears that a series of genetic injuries are required. The genotoxin may affect various types of cells, and may cause more than one kind of cancer. An epigenetic agent is something that increases the probability of causing cancer by a genotoxic agent. There are no standard assays for epigenetic activity and hence, there is no easy method to predict that an agent has such activity.

Consequently, the sign for genotoxicity of an agent at any exposure level, in any recognized test for genotoxicity, is likely to assess carcinogenic potential in humans [32-34]. There are various ways to assess genotoxicity. Among the approaches is the whole-organism exposure, which may be used to know whether an exposure to fields causes cancer, mutations, or chromosomal damage. Usually, cellular studies are used to detect DNA or chromosomal damage.

The genotoxic effects of ELF fields have been extensively reviewed by McCann et al. [35, 36] and Moulder [37]. So far, no significant cellular genotoxic effects have been confirmed under most of ELF exposure conditions [38-58]. These studies showed that ELF fields do not cause DNA damage, chromosome aberrations, mutations, cell transformations, micronucleus formation assays, or mutagenesis assays under exposure levels comparable to those available in the environment.

Only a few studies [59-61] reported genotoxicity from animal experimental systems, but most lacked the similarity of environmental exposure or have not been replicated. Other studies have indicated that ELF fields might have some epigenetic activity [25, 62, 63].

The main drawbacks in the majority of the experimental findings are that most of the studies have not been replicated, where replication could be the only way for verification. Also, these findings need supporting confirmed mechanisms, which are yet clearly not available.

From the large number of studies conducted in this field, it is concluded that electric and magnetic field exposures delivered at field strengths similar to those measured for typical exposure below 0.1 mT do not produce any significant cellular effects such as genotoxic or epigenetic activity. However few studies have shown some evidence of epigenetic activity. Also, evidences of possible effects could be available for magnetic field strengths above 0.1 mT [64].

In addition, few of the positive reports have also used exposure conditions (e.g., spark discharges, pulsed fields, or very high fields) that are largely unlike those encountered in the real-world exposure conditions.

3.3.3 Hypothesis of Melatonin

One possible interaction hypothesis under investigation is that exposure to electric and magnetic fields suppresses the production of *melatonin*, which is a hormone produced by the pineal gland, a small pinecone-shaped gland located deep near the center of the brain. Melatonin is produced mainly at night and released into the blood stream to be dispersed throughout the body. It surges into almost every cell in the human body, destroying the free radicals and helping cell division to take place with undamaged DNA. Melatonin also assists in regulating

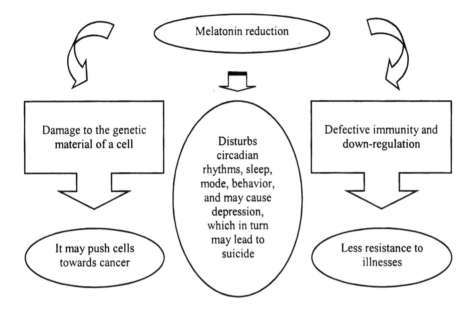

Figure 3-3 Biological consequences of melatonin reduction.

the female menstrual cycle and circadian rhythms. Melatonin secretion decreases over a lifetime, peaking in childhood and gradually lessening after puberty. Usually, people over sixty secrete far less than they do when young. Also, melatonin regulates sleep, mood, behavior, and gene expressions. It reduces secretion of tumor-promoting hormones. It has the ability to increase cytotoxicity of the immune system's killer lymphocytes; therefore, its production is essential for the immune system, which protects the body from infection and cancer cells. Various cancers might proliferate if melatonin is lowered in the body. Decreased melatonin levels have been implicated in breast cancer, prostate cancer, and ovarian malignancies. In brief, Figure 3-3 illustrates the consequences of the melatonin reduction.

It is known that melatonin is affected by light. This is evident from the fact that blind women typically have higher levels of it than do sighted women. Also the incidence of breast cancer is much less in blind women. Frequencies other than those of light may have influence on the production of melatonin in humans and animals. Scientists are interested in melatonin because it could help explain results of some epidemiological studies.

Baldwin et al. [65] have extensively discussed the hypothesis of melatonin and its mechanism of action. It has been shown to attenuate estrogen-induced proliferation of breast cancer cells.

Several laboratories have found melatonin reduction in cells, animals, and humans exposed to ELF fields. The effect varies according to the period of exposure and strength of ELF fields. In 1987, Stevens [66] found reductions in the melatonin production by the pineal gland and therefore suppression in the development of breast cancer due to ELF field exposure.

In 1993, Blask et al. [67] first reported that physiological levels of melatonin reduce MCF-7 human breast cancer cell growth.

Liburdy et al. [68] indicated that melatonin reduces the growth rate of human breast cancer cells in culture, but a 12-mG (60 Hz) magnetic field can block the ability of melatonin to inhibit breast cancer cell growth.

Selmaoui and Touitou [69] conducted a study on rats exposed to 50 Hz fields at 1, 10, and 100 µT for 12 hours, or for 30 days at 18 hours/day. Decreased melatonin was observed for 30-day exposures at 10 and 100 µT (about 40% decrease), and 12-hour exposure at 100 µT (about 20% decrease). No effects were observed at 1 µT.

Harland et al. [70] defined the parameters by which a 12 mG 60-Hz magnetic field blocks the inhibitory action of melatonin. They found that a 12-mG field could reduce the growth inhibitory action of melatonin on human breast cancer cells in culture.

Results from five cellular studies, conducted in three major laboratories, using human breast cancer cell cultures, have shown that low-level power-line frequency magnetic fields in the order of 12 mG can block melatonin's ability to suppress breast cancer cells [71].

In contrast, Rogers et al. [72, 73] exposed baboons to 60 Hz fields at 6 kV/m plus 50 µT or at 30 kV/m and 100 µT (12 hours per day for 6 weeks). They noticed no evidence of any effect on melatonin levels.

Löscher et al. [74] studied the ability of a 100-µT (50 Hz) magnetic field to reduce nocturnal production of melatonin after various exposure periods ranging from 1 day to 13 weeks. No consistent effect of ELF exposure was found.

John et al. [75] exposed groups of eight adult male rats to a 1-mT linearly-polarized 60 Hz magnetic field for 20 hours per day for 10 days, or to 1 mT intermittently (1 minute on, 1 minute off) of a linearly-polarized 60-Hz magnetic field for 20 hours per day beginning 1 hour before darkness for two days. Urine was collected at 2-hour intervals. The circadian profile of urinary 6-sulfatoxymelatonin was examined before, during, and after exposure. No significant effect on excretion was observed during the exposure.

In 2000, Graham et al. [76] found no effects on melatonin levels among young men volunteers exposed on 4 continuous nights to 60-Hz fields at 28.3 µT.

3.4   CELLULAR STUDIES

Laboratory research on cultured cell systems, referred to as *in vitro* (literally in cell culture or "in glass") is defined as experimental or theoretical studies of the effects of EM fields on individual cells or explanted tissues, exposed and assayed outside of human or animal bodies. It is often useful in establishing the response of certain cell type to a suspected toxic or mutagenic agent, and in elucidating the molecular mechanism by which an effect may occur.

Although cellular studies are not related to immediate application of EM fields to human health, they may assist in understanding the possible bioeffects. They are most likely to lead to theories on field-cell or field-tissue interactions, which are subject to experimental judgment. A major advantage of *in vitro* exposure studies is their potential for large sample size and accuracy, since the geometry and physical properties of exposure parameters are well controlled. That allows for comparability of findings across various laboratories.

In general, the number of cellular studies is large due to the large number of cellular processes and systems that may probably be affected by ELF fields.

3.4.1   Effects Relevant to Cancer

From the various studies referred to, it appears that ELF fields may have some effects relevant to cancer. These effects are illustrated in Figure 3-4. A brief list is given below for possible general observations.

Genetic Material

The human *genome*, which is a chemical sequence that contains the basic information for building and running a human body, consists of tightly coiled threads of DNA and associated protein molecules. It is organized into structures called chromosomes. The DNA is a double-stranded molecule held together by weak bonds between base pairs of nucleotides. Each strand is a linear arrangement of repeating similar units called *nucleotides*, which are each composed of one sugar, one phosphate, and a nitrogenous base. Weak bonds between the bases on each strand hold the two DNA strands together. Each time a cell divides into two daughter cells, its full genome is duplicated; for humans and other complex organisms, this duplication occurs in the nucleus.

Each DNA molecule contains many *genes*, the fundamental physical and functional unit of heredity. A gene is an ordered sequence of nucleotides located in a certain position on a specific chromosome that encodes a particular functional product. We can think of genes as information in a computer; they are

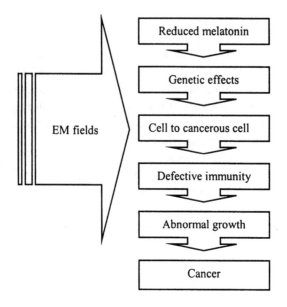

Figure 3-4 Effects that may lead to cancer due to EM exposure.

a bit like files. Genes are units of information in the DNA that are used to build proteins, among other things in the human body.

The human genome is estimated to comprise at least 100,000 genes. The nucleus of most human cells contains 2 sets of chromosomes, 1 set given by each parent. Each set has 23 single chromosomes, 22 autosomes, and an X or Y sex chromosome (normal female will have a pair of X chromosomes; a male will have an X and Y pair). Chromosomes contain roughly equal parts of protein and DNA.

Substantial investigation has been carried out to find out if ELF exposure can damage DNA or induce mutations. Generally, it is believed that the energy associated with ELF fields is not enough to cause direct damage to DNA; however, it is understood that indirect effects might be possible by ELF changing processes within cells that could lead to DNA breakage. Meanwhile, ELF fields well above environmental field intensities might enhance DNA synthesis, change the molecular weight distribution during protein synthesis, delay the mitotic cell cycle, and induce chromosome aberrations.

Preston-Martin et al. [77] observed a significant increase in DNA synthesis. An increase in cell division and transcriptional activity was also reported [78, 79].

In 1997, Lai and Singh [80] at the University of Washington, Seattle, assayed levels of DNA single-strand break in brain cells from rats being exposed to a 60-Hz magnetic field (flux densities 0.1, 0.25, and 0.5 mT). An increase in single-strand DNA breaks was observed after exposure to magnetic fields of 0.1, 0.25, and 0.5 mT, whereas an increase in double-strand DNA breaks was observed at 0.25 and 0.5 mT. It is evident that DNA strand breaks may affect cellular functions and lead to carcinogenesis and cell death.

In 1998, Wu et al. [81] reported carcinogenic effects and adverse pregnancy outcomes due to exposure to ELF and LF fields. They investigated the effect of both 50-Hz and 15.6-kHz magnetic fields on DNA damage/repair in the normal human amniotic FL cell.

Investigators considered the capability of ELF exposure to differ the repair of DNA strand breaks caused by hydrogen peroxide or radiation, but no effect with exposure to either magnetic or electric fields were reported [82, 83].

Chromosomal aberrations were reported by Khalil et al. [58] using pulsed magnetic fields, but the exposures tried were within the range of exposures reported in other studies with negative effects.

In contrast to the above study, ELF fields are, according to a number of *in vitro* studies [84-87], unable to induce chromosomal aberrations even under relatively strong magnetic field exposure.

Regarding chromosomal damage, Dr. Neil Cherry of Lincoln University, New Zealand [88], has summarized a number of studies associating EM exposure with effects on chromosomes.

Few studies investigated the relationship between exposure to ELF fields and genetic mutations. Enhanced mutagenicity was reported by Miyakoshi et al. [89], but at higher field strength (400,000 μT, 50 Hz).

Dr. Reba Goodman and her team at Columbia University, New York [90, 91], found that EM fields change the transcription of proto-oncogenes (*c-mys*, for example), which gene factors are believed to be linked to cancer.

Yet, no damage at exposure levels less than 1000 μT was reported by two studies using bacteria or yeast cells [92, 93].

Calcium Transport

Calcium ions are charged particles that have a vital role in various cellular processes. Calcium is one of the key messenger ions, a critical component of intercellular communication in the body and a regulator of cell growth. It is essential for many cellular functions, especially for transmission of extracellular signals, regulation of intracellular transport of compounds, release of secretion products, bone metabolism, muscle contraction, etc. Maintaining an optimal cellular calcium concentration is therefore very important. Calcium is released when hormones transmit instructions to the receptors, which are located at the surface of the cell.

The phenomenon of Ca^{++} efflux (release of calcium ions from a sample into a surrounding solution) from cells due to EM exposure is well known, especially in brain and lymphatic cells. Raised levels of calcium are found with low-level and with high-level exposures in animal studies and in cell cultures. Ca^{++} efflux may also have a synergistic role with chemical cancer promoters (toxic substances). The excess of Ca^{++} may directly disturb external hormonal activity. Many scientists underestimate the role of Ca^{++} efflux in cancer or leukemia, although it is known that cells secrete the calcium ion and carry it to the surrounding cells as a messenger to block cell development.

Earlier investigations [94, 95] have shown that ELF fields influence the calcium efflux. However, the calcium effect is windowed (effects found within bands of frequency or intensity separated by bands without effect) in frequency.

In 1979, Dr. Carl Blackman [96], a prominent biologist and biophysicist at the U.S. Environmental Protection Agency's Health Effects Research Laboratory, found that the ham radio frequency of 50 MHz, modulated at 16 Hz, would increase calcium ion release from chick brain tissue in a cell culture.

In the following years, Blackman et al. [97, 98] reported frequency windows at 15, 16, 45, 75, 105, and 135 Hz, and some much weaker reactions at 30, 60, and 90 Hz. The effect turned off at 30 Hz and at other frequencies under certain circumstances.

Cell Proliferation and Differentiation

The biology of cell division and differentiation is similar in both normal and cancer cells. A cancer cell differs from a normal cell in that it is deviously regulated. Cancer cells contain the full complement of biomolecules that are essential for survival, proliferation, differentiation, and expression of many cell-type-specific functions. Failure to regulate these functions efficiently, however, results in an altered phenotype and cancer.

Cell proliferation is a complex, genetically regulated process, which is under the control of cellular signal transduction pathways. Cell differentiation is also a very complex process in which the expression of cell specific genes is induced.

Altered proliferation of cells *in vitro* due to ELF field exposure has been observed in a number of studies [99-102].

Enzyme Activity

Just like other proteins, enzymes consist of long chains of amino acids held together by peptide bonds. They are present in all living cells, where they perform an important function by controlling the metabolic processes.

Ornithine decarboxylase (ODC) is an important enzyme for the role it plays in regulating cell growth through synthesis of polyamines necessary for protein and DNA synthesis. ODC is an enzyme activated during carcinogenesis. Increased

ODC activity is an indication for cancer.

Studies were carried out to investigate whether there were effects on ODC due to ELF exposure. An early study [25] found increased ODC activity in three cell lines in response to a sinusoidal 60-Hz electric field (10 mV/cm).

Litovitz et al. [26] indicated increased ODC activity in mouse lymphoma cells exposed to 10-μT 60-Hz magnetic fields. Still, attempts to reproduce the same finding under the same environments did not succeed [103].

Byus et al. [104] and Penafiel et al. [105] reported stimulation in the activity of ODC in cultured cells by RFR with ELF modulation. The results depended upon the type of modulation employed. These effects were noted only for certain modulations of the carrier wave, again portraying the window effect.

Activation of ODC as a response to ELF field exposure was also reported by Litovitz et al. [106]. The researchers worked for more than ten years on the effects of EM fields on the activity of ODC. They found EM-induced changers in the ODC activity, and EM-induced increase in the rate of fetal abnormalities in developing chicken embryos.

Meanwhile, Byus et al. [107] noted reduction in the activity of messenger enzymes, the protein kinases, in human leukocytes when exposed to a 450-MHz field modulated at 16 Hz.

Hormones

Hormones are chemical substances, formed in one organ or part of the body and carried in the blood to another organ or part where it alters the functional activity and sometimes the structure of one or more organs in a specific manner. As discussed in 3.3.3, many studies demonstrated that a decrease in melatonin synthesis and its secretion by the pineal gland due to ELF exposure is associated with increased cancer risk.

Immune System

The immune system is a protection mechanism composed of many interdependent cell types that jointly defend the living body against bacterial, microbes, toxins, parasitic, fungal, viral infections, and the growth of tumor cells. Cells of the immune system are initially derived from the bone marrow.

The immune system does not appear to be affected by ELF fields at low strengths. Several studies [108-112] reported no effect of exposure at very low field strength in mice or rats. However, a study in mice found some effects on immune parameters after 6 weeks of exposure in the 200- and 2000-μT groups, but no significant effects were seen at 2 or 20 μT [113].

Intercellular Communications

Intercellular interactions and signal transductions play a primary role in the development of the nervous system of all organisms. Electrical and chemical signals through membranes are responsible for intercellular communications. It has been suggested that EM fields in general and ELF fields in particular can change the properties of cell membranes [114], modify cell functions and interfere with the intercellular information transfer [115], which also explains the existence of a window effect.

3.4.2   Noncancerous Effects

Noncancerous effects of ELF electric and magnetic fields on living systems have been investigated in various laboratories. In this section, few significant cellular effects are considered for evaluating the contribution of *in vitro* research in understanding the effects of ELF fields on human health.

Effects on cell division and growth appeared at field strength of the order of tenths of a V/m or tenths of a mT in the medium [116]. But, electrical cell rotation and fusion appeared at higher strength (10-100 kV/m) [117].

Berman et al. [118] estimated the developmental effects associated with embryonic exposure to electric and magnetic fields. The importance of this study was derived from being an international collaboration involving six laboratories in four countries. Each laboratory used two identical egg incubators equipped to produce a 500-ms pulse of 1 μT with a 2-ms rise-and-fall time. The pulse was repeated at a frequency of 100 Hz. As a result from the combined investigation was a 6% increase in the number of abnormal embryos.

3.5   ANIMAL STUDIES

Studies of animals referred to as *in vivo* aim to determine the biological effects of electric and magnetic fields on whole animals. Research studies of animals exposed to suspect toxic agents are important in predicting potential toxicity to humans and in confirming an effect indicated by epidemiological studies. They also provide valuable information for estimating the level at which toxicity may occur. For this reason, animal experiments are more likely to reveal indirect effects that might be relevant to human health. The usual process is to expose animals to electric or magnetic fields to observe whether they develop certain health risks such as cancer or other diseases. Such experiments by themselves are inadequate because the animals might not exhibit the same response and sensitivities as humans to the parameters of the exposure.

Animal studies are very important because they can provide a reliable model in which to look at exactly how ELF field characteristics cause the risk. They also provide critical confirmation for results obtained through studies in humans. Animal studies have produced interesting results, but these results neither confirm nor contradict the increased health risk incidence reported in many epidemiological studies.

Current interest is mainly oriented toward a possible relation between ELF exposure and cancer. While the epidemiological studies that have stimulated this interest are not conclusive, they do suggest that research on animal models, especially for leukemia and other types of cancer, is needed. Perhaps, without the support of animal experiments, the scientific community will maintain the belief that reported EM health effects in humans are not real and must be the result of a false correlation with some unknown health risk factors. Meanwhile, the search for an ideal animal model is not an easy task since it is never clear if the animal used in the experiment is the most likely to show health risk.

3.5.1 Animal Cancer Studies

There has been no absolute evidence in any study that low-level ELF fields alone can cause cancer in animals. This is supported by the findings of many studies conducted during the last few years [119-132].

A study of animals treated with a known chemical initiator have shown greater numbers of tumors, or greater tumor mass, in those animals subsequently or concurrently exposed to magnetic fields at moderate to high exposure levels [133].

An initial study [134] showed that magnetic fields promoted mammary tumors development in rodents.

A series of studies on ELF exposure and mammary tumor initiation and promotion in the rodent model were conducted [135-137]. The first study [135] provided evidence that magnetic fields of low-flux density (100 µT) promoted growth and size of mammary tumors but did not affect tumor incidence. The same laboratory repeated this work through other studies at various field densities [138, 139]. They examined the question of whether a dose-response relationship exists with field intensity. Over the exposure range of 10 to 100 µT (50 Hz), more tumors were found in the exposed groups.

On the basis of evaluating the published studies, it is possible to conclude that there is no convincing evidence linking exposure to electric and magnetic fields at the environmental levels to cancer in animals. One area with some laboratory evidence of health-related effects is that animals treated with carcinogens show a positive relationship between intense magnetic field exposure and incidences of cancer.

3.5.2 Animal Studies—Noncancer

A number of noncancer studies were investigated for possible adverse effects of ELF field exposure. House et al. [140] carried out investigations in mice and rats to measure body weight, cellularity and lymphocyte subtypes in spleen, functional activity, and host resistance of the immune system *in vivo*. Mice and rats were exposed to 2, 200, and 1000 μT (60 Hz) continuously. No significant change in the distribution of lymphocyte subsets in the spleens of exposed mice was observed when compared with controls. They concluded that exposure of mice to linearly polarized, sinusoidal 60 Hz magnetic fields at field strengths up to 1000 μT for up to 3 months did not significantly affect a broad range of immune effect or functions. Also, the exposure had no effect on the ability of mice to resist a bacterial infection. The above results showed no evidence to support the idea that ELF magnetic fields alter immune responses. Tremblay et al. [141] also found no or inconsistent effects of ELF fields exposure on immune system indices and function.

There is insufficient evidence that exposure to ELF field causes behavioral changes of animals. Coelho et al. [142] reported that exposure to electric fields at 30 kV/m (60 Hz) increased the occurrence of three out of ten categories of social behavior of baboons during a six-week exposure, compared with equivalent rates observed in six-week pre- and post–exposure periods. Trzeciak et al. [143] noted that exposure to magnetic fields (50 Hz, 18 mT) had no effect on open-field behavior of 10-12 adult male and female Wistar rats. But the investigators recommended the need for further studies to fully determine conditions under which an effect can be observed. Meanwhile, Sienkiewicz et al. [144] reported that short-term, repeated exposure to intense magnetic fields might affect the behavior of mice. Mice were exposed each day to a 50-Hz magnetic field before being tested in a radial arm maze, a standard behavioral test of the ability of mice to learn a procedure for seeking food. Likewise, similar effects have been reported from a study of ELF exposure of rats [145].

There is weak evidence that occupational exposure to ELF fields affects cardiovascular functions, but those functions assessed by measuring blood pressure and heart rate by performing electrocardiogram (ECG) appear to be relatively affected by exposure to ELF electric or magnetic field. Cerretelli and Malagutti [146] observed transient increases in blood pressure in dogs exposed to electric field strengths greater than 10 kV/m. Also, magnetic field exposure caused stimulation of the heart of dogs in the diastolic phase of ectopic beats in the ECG [147].

There is no evidence for the reproductive or developmental effects of exposure to magnetic fields in experimental animals. Ryan et al. [148] studied the effect of magnetic field (2, 200, and 1000 μT continuous exposure and 1000 μT intermittent exposure) on fetal development and reproductive toxicity in the rodent. There was no evidence of any maternal or fetal toxicity or malformation.

3.6 HUMAN STUDIES

ELF effects might be studied safely and effectively in the laboratory with human volunteers in spite of limitations to the duration of exposure and types of tests that are performed. The focus in human studies is usually on effects that occur within a time frame of minutes, hours, days, or perhaps weeks. Longer-term studies in which exposure is controlled enough are difficult, if not impossible, to carry out with human volunteers in laboratory settings. The selection of physiological mechanisms for study is also limited to those that can be measured by noninvasive or minimally invasive procedures.

Laboratory studies on humans have certain advantages. They focus directly on the "right" species, thus avoiding the problem of extrapolation from data obtained in other species. Even negative results can be of immediate use in addressing public concerns. Such studies may also be used to directly evaluate the effects of exposure on "real-life" functions, such as memory, attention, and information processing. Controlled laboratory testing with human volunteers may help to define dosimetry and response categories for epidemiological studies, and might guide animal research to areas in which more invasive mechanistic investigations are valuable. Like animal studies, human laboratory studies allow separate testing of the risk to determine whether the observed effects are related to specific characteristics of the EM exposure situation or to their interactions.

Various health effects are claimed by people due to exposure to ELF fields, including headache, cardiovascular changes, behavioral changes, confusion, depression, difficulty in concentrating, sleep disturbances, decreased libido, poor digestion, etc. The main sources of information in this field are surveys of people and workers living close to potential sources of ELF fields, laboratory tests, and epidemiological data.

3.6.1 Behavioral Effects

The central nervous system (CNS) is a potential site of interaction with ELF fields because of the electrical sensitivity of the tissues. The CNS consists of the peripheral nerves, the spinal cord, and the brain. It is the system that controls the transfer of information between the environment and organisms. It also controls the internal processes.

The possibility that exposure to ELF fields affects the brain and nervous system and may cause adverse effects on normal behavior or cognitive abilities of humans have been a persistent concern. Some anecdotal evidence would suggest that memory loss, lack of attention, depression and other symptoms may be associated with exposure to ELF electric and magnetic fields, although scientific evidence indicates that acute exposure to low-intensity fields tends to cause a few robust, consistent or reproducible effects on behavior of animals.

In the early studies of occupational exposure to ELF fields reported by Asanova and Rakov [149] and Sazonova [150], switch yard workers in the former Soviet Union who differed in the duration and intensity of their exposure to 50 Hz fields suffered from an abnormally high incidence of neurophysiological complaints. A recent review study on behavioral effects of electric and magnetic fields was conducted by Zenon [151].

3.6.2 Cardiovascular System

The heart is a bioelectrical organ. The ECG is a basic monitoring apparatus of cardiologists in diagnosing the condition of the heart muscle. Heart rate, blood pressure, and the performance of ECG may assess cardiovascular functions. Current densities of about 0.1 A/m^2 can stimulate excitable tissues, while current densities above about 1 A/m^2 interfere with the action of the heart by causing ventricular fibrillation, as well as producing heat.

Sazonova [150] observed that the pulse rates of people among workers with an average exposure of 12-16 kV/m for more than 5 hours per day were lower by 2-5 beats/minute at the end of the day, although they had been equivalent at the start of the day.

According to a review by Stuchly [152], exposure of healthy male volunteers to 20-μT electric and magnetic fields at 60 Hz has been linked to a statistically significant slowing of the heart rate and to changes in a small fraction of the tested behavioral indicators.

Korpinen et al. [153] used ambulatory recording techniques to carry out an extensive study on the effects of EM occupational exposure on heart rate. No field-related changes in mean heart rate were found as a result of exposure to 50 Hz fields directly under power lines ranging in intensity from 110 to 400 kV.

Sastre et al. [154] noted a slowing in the low spectral band among men exposed to magnetic fields that cycle on and off every 15 seconds for an hour.

3.6.3 Chronic Fatigue Syndrome (CFS)

Chronic Fatigue Syndrome (CFS), also known as Chronic Fatigue and Immune Dysfunction Syndrome (CFIDS), is a general term used to describe an emerging illness characterized by debilitating fatigue, neurological problems, and a variety of flu like symptoms. One feature of the disorder is a depressed immune system. It affects adults, children, and adolescents. Within the past few years, various abnormalities have been found in the immune system of CFS patients. These include alterations in the activity and cell surface structure of two important types of white blood cells: natural killer cells and T-lymphocytes. In some patients subtle changes have been found in the levels of neuroendocrine hormones in the brain. Evidences indicate that CFS is associated with a persistent, low-level impairment of the immune system.

Exposure to ELF fields may be an immune system stressor with a potential to cause hormone disruption and changes at a cellular level. ELF exposure might be evaluated as a potential risk factor for people suffering from disorders with the common feature of unexplained chronic fatigue [155].

3.6.4 Electrical Sensitivity

Electrical sensitivity (ES), also known as *electromagnetic hypersensitivity* or *electrosensitivity* is a disorder whereby neurological and allergic-type symptoms are brought on through exposure to EM fields. It is a serious public health concern and its incidences are growing. Individuals with ES are primarily sensitive to certain frequencies and there is a wide range of sensitivity exhibited by those affected. They react or intensify when placed near EM sources. ES includes repeated feelings of stress or illness when seated near EM sources, even if the person affected has no evident illness when exposed.

Symptoms of ES include headache, eye irritation, dizziness, nausea, skin rash, facial swelling, weakness, fatigue, lack of concentration, pain in joints and/or muscles, buzzing/ringing in ears, skin numbness, abdominal pressure and pain, breathing difficulty, irregular heartbeat, paralysis, balance problems, confusion, depression, difficulty in concentrating, sleep disturbances, and memory difficulties. ES patients fear negative influences, mainly from EM fields, and may become hypersensitive to field levels that normally would not be noticeable to the general public. So far there is no medical treatments for the ES sufferers and no long-term relief for them [156].

A review of the history and peer-reviewed literature on ES was conducted by Liden [157]. The author considers the syndrome most likely a psychosomatic disease and provides a history of previous such syndromes.

3.6.5 Shocks and Microshocks

An established mechanism of interaction between ELF electric fields and living tissues is a direct stimulation of excitable cells and membranes. This proves the capability of the human body to perceive electric currents and the likelihood to produce shocks or microshocks depending on the amount of field. The term microshock refers to cardiac arrhythmias produced by low-intensity current passing through the heart, usually via an intravascular or intracardiac catheter. However, the term *shock* is used to describe all severe injuries from electric current, which often cause loss of consciousness and severe burns, or lead to loss of life. Shock most commonly occurs when a person touches a large conducting object, such as a motor truck or fence, which is insulated from earth.

Bernhart [158] estimated the threshold current density for the stimulation of action potentials in excitable cells as 1 A/m^2. At ELF fields, the threshold current density for producing a shock is roughly 10 A/m, which corresponds to electric field strength of 100 V/m in the human body. The electric field strength needed to produce a shock is comparable to that needed to produce heat. The threshold for shock increases with frequency above 100 Hz. Therefore, at low frequency, a shock is the limiting hazard, while at higher frequencies, heat and burns occur at lower field strength than shock.

Dalziel [159] observed the reaction of the human body after introducing fixed currents. In addition, many investigations have been carried out to estimate values of current densities needed to create shocks [160, 161].

3.6.6 Visual Sensations

Phosphenes are flickering visual sensations caused by nonphotic stimulation such as pressure on the eyes and mechanical shocks. They are caused by induced currents in the retina, where the threshold at 20 Hz (maximum sensitivity occurs between 20 and 30 Hz) is about 20 mA/m^2, a level much higher than endogenous current densities in electrically excitable living tissues [2, 162]. The effect observed in humans at the lowest magnetic field is a kind of visual sensation called a *magnetophosphene*, where a flickering sensation is produced in surrounding vision by 50/60-Hz magnetic fields above about 10 mT. The effect is also connected to biomagnetic particles, which have been reported in the human brain [163]. Induction of magnetophosphenes in humans pertains to DC fields and is sharply frequency dependent. Nevertheless, magnetophosphenese are not considered hazardous.

3.7 CONCLUDING REMARKS

Overall, the literature testifies that while some bioeffects of exposure to ELF electric and magnetic fields take place, there are no subsequent adverse health effects from these exposures. This could mean that public concerns about exposure to ELF fields are not supported by scientifically established proof, yet such proof; is very difficult. Public concerns are expressed well before the proof is reached, with good reason. There are rational grounds for suspicion of associated health risks. The lack of connection between experimental data (cellular and animal), human data, and interaction mechanisms severely complicates the interpretation of outcomes. Given the complexity of living organisms, it is difficult to apply and correlate knowledge from these sources.

Unlike human studies, experimental investigations are applied in the "non-right" species and tied to "non-real-life" exposures; however, they show some correspondence that is hard to ignore. Cellular studies provide an understanding of the potential physiological alterations at the basic cellular level due to exposure and other effects and are necessary in the assessment of the human health effects of chronic or long-term ELF exposure. However, there is some uncertainty about the ability to extrapolate evidences from animal studies across species, but it is widely accepted that the demonstration of an effect in one species increases the plausibility of a similar effect in another species. Animal studies, however, are not able to address many human exposure factors that are sociologically or geographically based, such as personal use of appliances.

Many of the laboratory evidences in the experimental work moderately support a causal relationship between exposure to ELF environmental levels and changes in biological function. The lack of consistent, positive findings in experimental studies, however, weakens the belief that this association is actually due to ELF fields. Therefore, it is not possible for the experimental studies to prove there is risk. It is only possible to prove, under certain exposure conditions, that an effect does exist.

In order to achieve possible proof, there is a need for better ELF exposure assessments, including considering transients, increased animal studies that better simulate the effect on realistic humans, and increased human and laboratory studies with direct significance to effects that could lead to adverse health outcomes.

REFERENCES

[1] Electromagnetic Fields and Public Health: Physical Properties and Effects on Biological Systems, Fact Sheets 182, World Health Organization, 1998.

[2] Foster, K. R., Electromagnetic Field Effects and Mechanisms, *IEEE Engineering in Medicine and Biology* 15, pp. 50-56, 1996.

[3] King, R. W. P., The Interaction of Power Line Electromagnetic Fields with the Human Body, *IEEE Engineering in Medicine and Biology* 17, pp. 67-78, 1998.

[4] Magnussen, T., Electromagnetic Fields, EMX Corporation, 1999.

[5] Valberg, P. A., R. Kavet, and C. N. Rafferty, Can Low-Level 50/60 Hz Electric and

Magnetic Fields Cause Biological Effects? *Radiation Research* 148, pp. 2-21, 1997.

[6] Moulder, J. E., Biological Studies of Power-Frequency Fields and Carcinogenesis, *IEEE Engineering in Medicine and Biology* 15, pp. 31-40, 1996.

[7] Tenforde, T. S., Biological Interactions and Potential Health Effects of Extremely Low Frequency Magnetic Fields from Power Lines and Other Common Sources, *Annual Review of Public Health* 13, pp. 173-196, 1992.

[8] Anderson, L. E., and W. T. Kaune, Electric and Magnetic Fields at Extremely Low Frequencies, In *Nonionizing Radiation Protection* (eds. Suess, M. J., and D. A. Benwell-Morison), World Health Organization Regional Publications, European Series 25, pp. 175-243, 1989.

[9] Reilly, J. P., Peripheral Nerve Simulation by Induced Electric Currents: Exposure to Time-Varying Magnetic Fields, *Medical and Biological Engineering and Computing* 3, pp. 101-109, 1989.

[10] Xi, W., and M. A. Stuchly, High Spatial Resolution Analysis of Electric Currents Induced in Men by ELF Magnetic Fields, *Applied Computational Electromagnetic Society Journal* 9, pp. 127-134, 1994.

[11] Kaune, W. T., and M. F. Gillis, General Properties of the Interaction between Animals and ELF Electric Fields, *Bioelectromagnetics* 2, pp. 1-11, 1981.

[12] Kirschvink, J. L., A. Kobayashi-Kirschvink, J. C. Diaz-Rioci, and S. J. Kirschvink, Magnetite in Human Tissue: A Mechanisms for the Biological Effect of Weak ELF Magnetic Fields, *Bioelectromagnetics* 13 suppl. 1, pp. 101-113, 1992.

[13] Adair, P. K., Constraints of Thermal Noise on the Effects of Weak 60 Hz Magnetic Fields Acting on Biological Magnetite, *Proceedings of the National Academy of Sciences of the United States of America* 91, pp. 2925-2929, 1994.

[14] Moulder, J. E., and K. R. Foster, Biological Effects of Power-Frequency Fields as they Relate to Carcinogenesis, *Proceedings of the Society for Experimental Biology and Medicine* 209, pp. 309-324, 1995.

[15] Vaughan, T. E., and J. C. Weaver, Energetic Constraints on the Creation of Cell Membrane Pores by Magnetic Particles, *Biophysical Journal* 71, pp. 616-622, 1996.

[16] Vaughan, T. E., and J. C. Weaver, Molecular Change Due to Biomagnetic Stimulation and Transient Magnetic Fields: Mechanical Interference Constraints on Possible Effects by Cell Membrane Pore Creation Via Magnetic Particles, *Bioelectrochemistry and Bioenergetics* 46, pp.121-128, 1998.

[17] Dye, M., What are Free Radicals, Internet Document at http://www.mindspring.com/~staywell/freerad.html, 1996.

[18] Blankenship, R. E., T. J. Schaafsma, and W. W. Parson, Magnetic Field Effects on Radical Pair Intermediates in Bacterial Photosynthesis, *Biochimica et Biophysica Acta* 461, pp. 297-305, 1977.

[19] Cozens, F. L., and J. C. Scaiano, A Comparative Study of Magnetic Field Effects on the Dynamics of Geminate and Random Radical Pair Processes in Micelles, *Journal of the American Chemical Society* 115, pp. 5204-5211, 1993.

[20] Scaiano, J. C., N. Mohtat, F. L. Cozens, J. McLean, and A. Thansandote, Application of the Radical Pair Mechanism to Free Radicals in Organized Systems: Can the Effect of 60 Hz be Predicted from Studies Under Static Fields? *Bioelectromagnetics* 15, pp. 549-554, 1994.

[21] Walleczek, J., Magnetokinetic Effects on Radical Pairs: A Paradigm for Magnetic

Field Interactions with Biological Systems at Lower Than Thermal Energy, In *Advances in Chemistry Series: Electromagnetic Fields* (ed. Blank, M.), Biological Interactions and Mechanisms, pp. 395-420, Washington, American Chemical Society, 1995.

[22] Brocklehurst, B., and K. A. McLauchlan, Free Radical Mechanism for the Effects of Environmental Electromagnetic Fields on Biological Systems, *International Journal of Radiation Biology* 69, pp. 3-24, 1996.

[23] Adair, R. K., Effects on Radical Pair Reformation of Very Weak Magnetic Fields, *The Annual Review of Research on Biological Effects of Electric and Magnetic Fields from the Generation, Delivery & Use of Electricity*, pp. 20-22, San Diego, CA 1997.

[24] Byus, C. V., S. E. Pieper, and W. R. Adey, The Effects of Low-Energy 60 Hz Environmental Electromagnetic Fields upon the Growth-Related Enzyme Ornithine Decarboxylase, *Carcinogenesis* 8, pp. 1385-1389, 1987.

[25] Litovitz, T. A., D. Krause, and J. M. Mullins, Effect of Coherence Time of the Applied Magnetic Field on Ornithine Decarboxylase Activity, *Biochemical and Biophysical Research Communication* 178, pp. 862-865, 1991.

[26] Adair, P. K., Constraints on Biological Effects of Weak Extremely Low frequency Electromagnetic Fields, *Physical Review Letters* A 43, pp. 1039-1048, 1991.

[27] Cain, C. D., D. L. Thomas, and W. R. Adey, 60-Hz Magnetic Field Acts as Co-Promoter in Focus Formation of C3H10T1/2 Cells, *Carcinogenesis* 14, pp. 955-960, 1993.

[28] Kolomytkin, O., M. Yurinska, S. Zharikov, V. Kuznetsov, and A. Zharikova, Response of Brain Receptor Systems to Microwave Energy Exposure, In *Nature of Electromagnetic Field Interactions with Biological Systems* (ed. Frey, A. H.), pp. 195-206, R. G. Landes, Austin, Texas, 1994.

[29] Eichwald, C., and J. Walleczek, Magnetic Field Perturbations as a Tool for Controlling Enzyme-Regulated and Oscillatory Biochemical Reactions, *Biophysical Chemistry* 74, pp. 209-224, 1998.

[30] Adey, W. R., Cell Membranes: The Electromagnetic Environment and Cancer Promotion, *Neurochemical Research* 13, pp. 671-677, 1988.

[31] Moulder, J. E., Power Lines and Cancer FAQs, Electromagnetic Fields and Human Health, Medical College of Wisconsin, 1999.

[32] Butterworth, B. E., R. B. Conolly, and K. T. Morgan, A Strategy for Establishing Mode of Action of Chemical Carcinogens as a Guide for Approaches to Risk Assessments, *Cancer Letters* 93, pp. 129-146, 1995.

[33] Moulder, J. E., Power-Frequency Fields and Cancer, *Critical Reviews in Biomedical Engineering* 26, pp. 1-116, 1998.

[34] McCann, J., L. I. Kheifets, and C. N. Rafferty, Cancer Risk Assessment of Extremely Low Frequency Electric and Magnetic Fields: A Critical Review of Methodology, *Environmental Health Perspectives* 106, pp. 701-717, 1998.

[35] McCann, J., F. Dietrich, C. Rafferty, and A. O. Martin, A Critical Review of the Genotoxic Potential of Electric and Magnetic Fields, *Mutation Research* 297, pp. 61-95, 1993.

[36] McCann, J., F. Dietrich, and C. Rafferty, The Genotoxic Potential of Electric and Magnetic Fields-An Update, *Mutation Research* 7481, 1998.

[37] Moulder, J. E., Power-Frequency Fields and Cancer, *Critical Reviews in Biomedical Engineering* 26, pp. 1-116, 1998.

[38] Juutilainen, J., and A. Liimatainen, Mutation Frequency in Salmonella Exposed to Weak 100-Hż Magnetic Fields, *Hereditas* 104, pp. 145-147, 1986.

[39] Cossarizza, A., D. Monti, G. Moschini, R. Cadossi, F. Bersani, and and C. Franceschi, DNA Repair after Gamma Irradiation in Lymphocytes Exposed to Low-Frequency Pulsed Electromagnetic Fields, *Radiation Research* 118, pp. 161-168, 1989.

[40] Fraizier, M. E., J. A. Reese, J. E. Morris, R. F. Jostes, and D. L. Miller, Exposure of Mammalian Cells to 60-Hz Magnetic and Electric Fields: Analysis of DNA Repair of Induced Single-Strand Breaks, *Bioelectromagnetics* 11, pp. 229-239, 1990.

[41] Scarfi, M. R., F. Bersani, A. Cossarizza, D. Monti, G. Castellani, R. Cadossi, G. Franceschetti, and C. Franceschi, Spontaneous and Mitomycin-C-Induced Micronuclei in Human Lymphocytes Exposed to Extremely Low Frequency Pulsed Magnetic Fields, *Biochemical and Biophysical Research Communication* 176, pp. 194-200, 1991.

[42] Livingston, G. K., K. L. Witt, O. P. Gandhi, I. Chaterjee, and J. Roti, Reproductive Integrity of Mamalian Cells Exposed to Power Frequency Electromagnetic Fields, *Environmental and Molecular Mutagenesis* 17, pp. 49-58, 1991.

[43] Ager, D. D., and J. A. Radul, Effect of 60-Hz Magnetic Fields on Ultraviolet Light-Induced Mutation and Mitotic Recombination in Saccharomyces Cerevisaie, *Mutation Research* 283, pp. 279-286, 1992.

[44] Hintenlag, D. E., Synergistic Effects of Ionizing Radiation and 60 Hz Magnetic Fields, *Bioelectromagnetics* 14, pp. 545-551, 1993.

[45] Cain, C. D., D. L. Thomas, and W. R. Adey, 60 Hz Magnetic Field Strength Dependency and TPA-Induced Focus Formation in Co-Cultures of C3H/10T/2 Cells, *Annual Review of Research on Biological Effects of Electric and Magnetic Fields*, pp. 55, 1994.

[46] Tofani, S., A. Ferrara, L. Anglesio, and G. Gilli, Evidence for Genotoxic Effect of Resonant ELF Magnetic Fields, *Bioelectrochem. Bioenerg.* 36, pp. 9-13, 1995.

[47] Antonopoulos, A., B. Yang, A. Stamm, W. D. Heller, and G. Obe, Cytological Effects of 50 Hz Electromagnetic Fields on Human Lymphocytes *In Vitro*, *Mutation Research* 346, pp. 151-157, 1995.

[48] Cantoni, O., P. Sestili, M. Fiorani, and M. Dacha, The Effect of 50 Hz Sinusoidal Electric and/or Magnetic Fields on the Rate of Repair of DNA Single/Double Strand Breaks in Oxidatively Injured Cells, *Biochemistry and Molecular Biology International* 37, pp. 681-689, 1995.

[49] Okonogi, H., M. Nakagawa, and Y. Tsuji, The Effects of a 4.7 µT Static Magnetic Field on the Frequency of Micronucleated Cells Induced by Mitomycin C, *Tokushima Journal of Experimental Medicine* 180, pp. 209-215, 1996.

[50] Morandi, M. A., C. M. Pak, R. P. Caren, and L. D. Caren, Lack of an EMF-Induced Genotoxic Effect in the Ames Assay, *Life Science* 59, pp. 263-271, 1996.

[51] Lagroye, I., and J. L. Poncy, The Effect of 50 Hz Electromagnetic Fields on the Formation of Micronuclei in Rodent Cell Lines Exposed to Gamma Radiation, *International Journal of Radiation Biology* 72, pp. 249-254, 1997.

[52] Jacobson-Kram, D., J. Tepper, P. Kuo, R. H. San, P. T. Curry, V. O. Wagner, D. L.

Putman, Evaluation of the Potential Genotoxicity of Pulsed Electric and Electromagnetic Field Used for Bone Growth Stimulation, *Mutation Research* 388, pp. 45-57, 1997.

[53] Scarfi, M. R., M. B. Lioi, M. DellaNoce, O. Zeni, C. Franceschi, D. Monti, and G. Castellani, Exposure to 100 Hz Pulsed Magnetic Fields Increases Micronucleus Frequency and Cell Proliferation in Human Lymphocytes, *Bioelectrochemistry and Bioenergetics* 43, pp. 77-81, 1997.

[54] Balcer-Kubiczek, E. K., X. Zhang, L. Han, G. H. Harrison, C. C. Davis, X. Zhou, V. Loffe, W. A. McCready, J. M. Abraham, and S. J. Meltzer, BIGEL Analysis of Gene Expression in HL60 Cells Exposed to X Rays or 60 Hz Magnetic Fields, *Radiation Research* 150, pp. 663-672, 1998.

[55] Pakhomova, O. N., M. L. Belt, S. P. Mathur J. C. Lee, and Y. Akyel, Ultra-Wide Band Electromagnetic Radiation and Mutagenesis in Yeast, *Bioelectromagnetics* 19, pp. 128-130, 1998.

[56] Rapley, B. I., R. E. Rowland, W. H. Page, and J. V. Podd, Influence of Extremely Low Frequency Magnetic Fields on Chromosomes and the Mitotic Cycle in Vicia Faba L, the Broad Bean, *Bioelectromagnetics* 19, pp. 152-161, 1998.

[57] Yaguchi, H., M. Yoshida, Y. Ejima, and J. Miyakoshi, Effect of High-Density Extremely Low Frequency Magnetic Fields on Sister Chromatic Exchanges in Mouse m5S Cells, *Mutation Research* 440, pp. 189-194, 1999.

[58] Khalil, A. M., and W. Qassem, Cytogenetic Effects of Pulsing Electromagnetic Field on Human Lymphocytes *In Vitro*: Chromosomes Aberrations, Sister Chromatid Exchanges and Cell Kinetics, *Mutation Research* 247, pp. 141-146, 1991.

[59] Fairbairn, D. W., and K. L. O'Neill, The Effect of Electromagnetic Field Exposure on the Formation of DNA Single Strand Breaks in Human Cells, *Cellular and Molecular Biology Letters* 4, pp. 561-567, 1994.

[60] Miyakoshi, J., Y. Mori, N. Yamagishi, K. Yagi, and H. Takebe, Suppression of High-Density Magnetic Field (400 mT at 50 Hz)-Induced Mutations by Wild-Type p53 Expression in Human Osteosarcoma Cells, *Biochemical and Biophysical Research Communications* 243, pp. 579-584, 1998.

[61] Dibirdik, I., D. Kristupaitis, T. Kurosaki, L. Tuel-Ahlgren, A. Chu, D. Pond, D. Tuong, R. Luben, and F. M. Uckun, Stimulation of Src Family Protein Tyrosine Kinases as a Proximal and Mandatory Step for SYK Kinase-Dependent Phospholipase C Gamma 2 activation in lymphoma B-Cells Exposed to Low Energy Electromagnetic Fields, *Journal of Biological Chemistry* 273, pp. 4035-4039, 1998.

[62] Beniashvili, D. S., V. G. Biniashvili, and M. Z. Menabde, Low-Frequency Electromagnetic Radiation Enhances the Induction of Rat Mammary Tumours by Nitrosomethyl Urea, *Cancer Letters* 61, pp. 75-79, 1991.

[63] Löscher, W., M. Mevissen, W. Lehmacher, and A. Stamm, A Tumor Promotion in a Breast Cancer Model by Exposure to a Weak Alternating Magnetic Field, *Cancer Letters* 71, pp. 75-81, 1993.

[64] Health Effects from Exposure to Power-Line Frequency Electric and Magnetic Fields: Prepared in Response to the 1992 Energy Policy Act (PL 102-486, Section 2118), National Institute of Environmental Health Sciences (NIEHS) and National Institutes of Health, 1999.

[65] Baldwin, W. S., and J. C. Barrett, Melatonin: Receptor-Mediated Events that may

Affect Breast and Other Steroid Hormone-Dependent Cancers, *Molecular Carcinogenesis* 21, pp. 149-155, 1998.

[66] Stevens, R. G., Electric Power Use and Breast Cancer: A Hypothesis, *American Journal of Epidemiology* 125, pp. 556–561, 1987.

[67] Blask, D. E., S. T. Wilson, J. D. Saffer, M. A. Wilson, L. E. Anderson, and B. W. Wilson, Culture Conditions Influence the Effects of Weak Magnetic Fields on the Growth-Response of MCF-7 Human Breast Cancer Cells to Melatonin *in Vitro*, *Annual Review of Research on Biological Effects of Electric and Magnetic Fields from the Generation, Delivery and Use of Electricity*, p. 65, U.S. Dept. of Energy, Savannah, GA, 31 October to 4 November 1993.

[68] Liburdy, R. P., T. R. Sloma, R. Sokolic, and P. Yaswen, ELF Magnetic Fields, Breast Cancer and Melatonin: 60 Hz Fields Block Melatonin's Oncostatic Action on ER$^+$ Breast Cancer Cell Proliferation, *Journal of Pineal Research* 14, pp. 89–97, 1993.

[69] Selmaoui, B., and Y. Touitou, Sinusoidal 50-Hz Magnetic Fields Depress Rat Pineal NAT Activity and Serum Melatonin. Role of Duration and Intensity of Exposure, *Life Sciences* 57, pp.1351-1358, 1995.

[70] Harland, J. D., and R. P. Liburdy, ELF Inhibition of Melatonin and Tamoxifen Action on MCF-7 Cell Proliferation: Field Parameters, *The Bioelectromagnetics Society Meeting*, Victoria, British Columbia, Canada, 1996.

[71] Maisch, D., Melatonin, Tamoxifen, 50-60 Hertz Electromagnetic Fields and Breast Cancer: A Discussion Paper, *Australian Senate Hansard*, pp. 1-9, 1997.

[72] Rogers, W. R., R. J. Reiter, L. Barlow-Walden, and H. D. Smith, and J. L. Orr, Regularly Scheduled, Day-Time, Slow-Onset 60 Hz Electric and Magnetic Field Exposure does not Depress Serum Melatonin Concentration in Nonhuman Primates, *Bioelectromagnetics* Suppl. 3, pp. 111-118, 1995.

[73] Rogers, W. R., R. J. Reiter, H. D. Smith, and L. Barlow-Walden, Rapid-Onset/Offset, Variably Scheduled 60 Hz Electric and Magnetic Field Exposure Reduces Nocturnal Serum Melatonin Concentration in Nonhuman Primates, *Bioelectromagnetics* Suppl. 3, pp.119-122, 1995.

[74] Löscher, W., M. Mevissen, and A. Lerchl, Exposure of Female Rats to a 100-μT 50 Hz Magnetic Field Does not Induce Consistent Changes in Nocturnal Levels of Melatonin, *Radiation Research* 150, pp. 557-568, 1998.

[75] John, T. M., G. -Y. Liu, and G. M. Brown, 60 Hz Magnetic Field Exposure and Urinary 6-Sulphatoxymelatonin Levels in the Rat, *Bioelectromagnetics* 19, pp. 172-180, 1998.

[76] Graham, C., M. R. Cook, A. Sastre, D. W. Riffle, and M. Gerkovich, Multi-Night Exposure to 60 Hz Magnetic Fields: Effects on Melatonin and its Enzymatic Metabolite, *Journal of Pineal Research* 28, pp. 1-8, 2000.

[77] Preston-Martin, S., J. M. Peters, M. C. Yu, D. H. Garabrant, and J. D. Bowman, Myelogenous Leukemia and Electric Blanket Use, *Bioelectromagnetics* 9, pp. 207-213, 1988.

[78] Goodman, R., J. Abbott, and A. S. Henderson, Transcriptional Patterns in the X Chromosome of Sciara Coprophila Following Exposure to Magnetic Fields, *Bioelectromagnetics* 8, pp. 1-7, 1989.

[79] Liboff, A. R., T. Jr. Williams, D. M. Strong, and R. Wistar, Jr., Time-Varying

Magnetic Fields: Effect on DNA Synthesis, *Science* 223, pp. 818-820, 1984.

[80] Lai, H., and N. P. Singh, Acute Exposure to a 60 Hz Magnetic Field Increases NA Strand Breaks in Rat Brain Cells, *Bioelectromagnetics* 18, pp. 156-65, 1997.

[81] Wu, R. W., H. Yang, H. Chiang, B. J. Shao, and J. L. Bao, The Effects of Low-Frequency Magnetic Fields on DNA Unscheduled Synthesis Induced by Methylnitro-Nitrosoguanidine *In Vitro, Electro- and Magnetobiology* 17, pp. 57–65, 1998.

[82] Frazier, M. E., J. A. Reese, J. E. Morris, R. F. Jostes, and D. L. Miller, Exposure of Mammalian Cells to 60-Hz Magnetic or Electric Fields: Analysis of DNA Repair of Induced, Single-Strand Breaks, *Bioelectromagnetics* 11, pp. 229-234, 1990.

[83] Cantoni, O., P. Sestili, M. Fiorani, and M. Dacha, The Effect of 50 Hz Sinusoidal Electric and/or Magnetic Fields on the Rate of Repair of DNA Single/Double Strand Breaks in Oxidatively Injured Cells, *Biochemistry and Molecular Biology International* 37, pp. 681-689, 1995.

[84] Cohen, M. M., A. Kunska, J. A. Astemborski, D. McCulloch, and D. Paskewiz, Effect of Low-Level 6O-Hz Electromagnetic Fields on Human Lymphoblastoid Cells. II. Sister-Chromatid Exchanges in Peripheral Blood Lymphocytes and Lymphoblastic Cell Lines, *Mutation Research* 172, pp. 177-184, 1985.

[85] Rosenthal, M., and G. Obe, Effects of 50-Hz Electromagnetic Fields on Proliferation and on Chromosomal Alterations in Human Peripheral Lymphocytes Untreated or Pretreated with Chemical Mutagens, *Mutation Research* 210, pp. 329-335, 1989.

[86] Scarfi, M. R., M. B. Lioi, O. Zeni, G. Franceschetti, C. Franceschi, and F. Bersani, Lack of Chromosomal Aberration and Micronucleus Induction in Human Lymphocytes Exposed to Pulsed Magnetic Fields, *Mutation Research* 306, pp. 129-133, 1994.

[87] Paile, W., K. Jokela, A. Koivistoinen, and S. Salomaa, Effects of 50 Hz Sinusoidal Magnetic Fields and Spark Discharges on Human Lymphocytes *In Vitro, Bioelectrochemistry and Bioenergetics* 36, pp. 15-22, 1995.

[88] Cherry, N., Actual or Potential Effects of ELF and RF/MW Radiation on Accelerating Aging of Human, Animal or Plant Cells, Lincoln University, Auckland, New Zealand, 1998.

[89] Miyakoshi, J., Y. Mori, N. Yamagishi, K. Yagi, and H. Takebe, Suppression of High-Density Magnetic Field (400 mT at 50 Hz)-Induced Mutations by Wild-Type Expression in Human Osteosarcoma Cells, *Biochemical and Biophysical Research Communications* 24, pp. 579-584, 1998.

[90] Goodman, R., M. Blank, H. Lin, L. Soo, D. Weisbrot, and A. Henderson, Increased Levels of hsp70 Transcripts are Induced When Cells are Exposed to Low Frequency Electromagnetic Fields, *The Bioelectromagnetics Society Meeting*, Copenhagen, 1994.

[91] Goodman, R., H. Lin, and A. Henderson, Increased Transcripts for hsp70 and c-myc in Cells Re-Stimulated with Different Exposure Conditions, *The Bioelectromagnetics Society Meeting*, Copenhagen, 1994.

[92] Ager, D. D., and J. A. Radul, Effect of 60-Hz Magnetic Fields on Ultraviolet Light-Induced Mutation and Mitotic Recombination in Saccharomyces Cerevisiae, *Mutation Research* 283, pp. 279-286, 1992.

[93] Morandi, M. A., C. M. Pak, R. P. Caren, and L. D. Caren, Lack of an EMF-Induced

Genotoxic Effect in the Ames Assay, *Life Science* 59, pp. 263-271, 1996.

[94]   Bawin, S. M., L. K. Kaczmarek, and W. R. Adey, Effects of Modulated VHF Fields on the Central Nervous System, *Annals of the New York Academy of Sciences* 247, pp. 74-80, 1975.

[95]   Bawin, S. M., A. Sheppard, and W. Ross Adey, Possible Mechanisms of Weak Electromagnetic Fields Coupling in Brain Tissue, *Bioelectrochemistry and Bio-Energetics* 5, pp. 67-76, 1978.

[96]   Blackman, C. F., J. A. Elder, C. M. Well, S. G. Benane, D. C. Eichinger, and D. E. House, Induction of Calcium-Ion Efflux from Brain Tissue by Radio Frequency Radiation: Effects of Modulation Frequency and Field Strength, *Radio Science* 14, pp. 93-98, 1979.

[97]   Blackman, C. F., S. G. Benane, L. S. Kinney, W. T. Joines, and D. E. House, Effects of ELF Fields on Calcium-Ion Efflux from Brain Tissue *In Vitro*, *Radiation Research* 92, pp. 510-520, 1982.

[98]   Blackman, C. F., S. G. Benane, D. E. House, and W. T Joines, Effects of ELF (1-120 Hz) and Modulated (50 Hz) RF Fields on the Efflux of Calcium Ions from Brain Tissue *In Vitro*, *Bioelectromagnetics* 6, pp. 1-11, 1985.

[99]   West, R. W., W. G. Hinson, D. B. Lyle, and M. L. Swicord, Enhancement of Anchorage-Independent Growth in JB6 Cells Exposed to 60 Hertz Magnetic Fields, *Bioelectrochemistry and Bioenergetics* 34, pp. 39-43, 1994.

[100] Antonopoulos, A., B. Yang, A. Stamm, W. –D. Heller, and G. Obe, Cytological Effects of 50 Hz Electromagnetic Fields on Human Lymphocytes *In Vitro*, *Mutation Research* 346, pp. 151-157, 1995.

[101] Katsir, G., S. Baram, and A. Parola, Effect of Sinusoidally Varying Magnetic Fields on Cell Proliferation and Adenosine Deaminase Specific Activity, *Bioelectromagnetics* 19, pp. 46-52, 1998.

[102] Chen, G., B. L. Upham, W. Sun, C. –C. Chang, E. J. Rothwell, K. –M. Chen, H. Yamasaki, and J. E. Trosko, Effect of Electromagnetic Field Exposure on Chemically Induced Differentiation of Friend Erythroleukemia Cells, *Environmental Health Perspectives* 108, pp. 967-972, 2000.

[103] Azadniv, M., C. M. Klinge, R. Gelein, E. L. Carstensen, C. Cox, A. A. Brayman, and M. W. Miller, A Test of the Hypothesis that a 60-Hz Magnetic Field Affects Ornithine Decarboxylase Activity in Mouse l929 Cells *In Vitro*, *Biochemical and Biophysical Research Communications* 214, pp. 627-631, 1995.

[104] Byus, C. V., K. Kartun, S. Pieper, and W. R. Adey, Increased Ornithine Decarboxylase Activity in Cultured Cells Exposed to Low Energy Modulated Microwave Fields and Phorbol Ester Tumor Promoters, *Cancer Research* 48, pp. 4222-4226, 1988.

[105] Penafiel, M., T. Litovitz, D. Krause, A. Desta, J. M. Mullins, Role of Modulation on the Effect of Microwaves on Ornithine Decarboxylase Activity in L929 Cells, *Bioelectromagnetics* 18, pp. 132-141, 1997.

[106] Litovitz, T., D. Krause, and J. M. Mullins, The Role of Coherence Time in the Effect of Microwaves on Ornithine Decarboxlyase Activity, *Bioelectromagnetics* 14, pp. 395-403, 1993.

[107] Byus, C. V., R. L. Lundak, R. M. Fletcher, and W. R. Adey, Alterations in Protein Kinase Activity Following Exposure of Cultured Lymphocytes to Modulated

Microwave Fields, *Bioelectromagnetics* 5, pp. 341-351, 1984.

[108] Morris, J. E., and H. A. Ragan, Immunological Studies with 60 Hz Electric Fields, In: Biological Effects of Extremely Low Frequency Electromagnetic Fields, *18th Annual Hanford Life Sciences Symposium*, pp. 326-334, Springfield, VA, 16-18 October 1979.

[109] Morris, J. E., and R. D. Phillips, Effects of 60 Hz Electric Fields on Specific Humoral and Cellular Components of the Immune System, *Bioelectromagnetics* 3, pp. 341-348, 1982.

[110] Morris, J. E., and R. D. Phillips, Immunological Studies with 60 Hz on Specific Humoral and Cellular Components of the Immune System, *Bioelectromagnetics* 4, p. 294, 1983.

[111] Murthy, K. K., W. R. Rogers, and H. D. Smith, Initial Studies on the Effects of Combined 60 Hz Electric and Magnetic Field Exposure on the Immune System of Nonhuman Primates, *Bioelectromagnetics* Suppl. 3, pp. 93-102, 1995.

[112] House, R. V., H. V. Ratajczak, J. R. Gauger, T. R. Johnson, P. T. Thomas, and D. L. McCormick, Immune Function and Host Defense in Rodents Exposed to 60-Hz Magnetic Fields, *Fundamental and Applied Toxicology* 34, pp. 228-239, 1996.

[113] Tremblay, L., M. Houde, G. Mercier, J. Gagnon, and R. Mandeville, Differential Modulation of Natural and Adaptive Immunity in Fischer Rats Exposed for 6 Weeks to 60 Hz Linear Sinusoidal Continuous-Wave Magnetic Fields, *Bioelectromagnetics* 17, pp. 373-383, 1996.

[114] Adey, W. R., Tissue Interactions with Non-Ionizing Electromagnetic Fields, *Physiological Reviews* 61, pp. 435-514, 1981.

[115] Frey, A. H., Is a Toxicological Model Appropriate as a Guide for Biological Research with Electromagnetic Fields? *Journal of Bioelectricity* 9, pp. 233-234, 1990.

[116] Inoue, M., Growth Rate and Mitotic Index Analysis of Vicia Faba L. Roots Exposed to 60-Hz Electric Fields, *Bioelectromagnetics* 6, pp. 293-304, 1985.

[117] Pohl, H. A., *Dielectrophoresis: The Behavior of Matter in Non-Uniform Electric Fields*, Cambridge University Press, London, UK, 1978.

[118] Berman, E., L. Chacon, D. House, B. A. Koch, W. E. Koch, J. Leal, S. Lovtrup, E. Mantiply, A. H. Martin, G. I. Martucci, K. H. Mild, J. C. Monahan, M. Sandström, K. Shamsaifar, R. Tell, M. A. Trillo, A. Ubeda, and P. Wagner, Development of Chicken Embryos in a Pulsed Magnetic Field, *Bioelectromagnetics* 11, pp. 169-187, 1990.

[119] Bellosi, A., Effects of Pulsed Magnetic Fields on Leukemia-Prone AKR Mice: No Effect on Mortality through Five Generations, *Leukaemia Research* 15, pp. 899-902, 1991.

[120] McLean, J. R. N., M. A. Stuchly, R. E. J. Mitchel, D. Wilkinson, H. Yang, M. Goddard, D. W. Lecuyer, M. Schunk, E. Callary, and D. Morrison, Cancer Promotion in a Mouse-Skin Model by a 60-Hz Magnetic Field: II. Tumour Development and Immune Response, *Bioelectromagnetics* 12, pp. 273-287, 1991.

[121] Stuchly, M. A., J. R. N. McLean, R. Burnett, M. Goddard, D. W. Lecuyer, and R. E. J. Mitchel, Modification of Tumor Promotion in the Mouse Skin by Exposure to an Alternating Magnetic Field, *Cancer Letters* 65, pp. 1-7, 1992.

[122] Stuchly, M. A., Tumor Co-Promotion Studies by Exposure to Alternating Magnetic

Fields, *Radiation Research* 133, pp. 118-119, 1993.

[123] Kowalczuk, C. I., L. Robbins, J. M. Thomas, and R. D. Saunders, Dominant Lethal Studies in Male Mice After Exposure to a 50 Hz Magnetic Field, *Mutation Research* 328, pp. 229-237, 1995.

[124] McLean, J., A. Thansandote, D. Lecuyer, M. Goddard, L. Tryphonas, J. C. Scaiano, and F. Johnson, A 60-Hz Magnetic Field Increases the Incidence of Squamous Cell Carcinomas in Mice Previously Exposed to Chemical Carcinogens, *Cancer Letters* 92, pp.121-125, 1995.

[125] Yasui, M., K. Takehiko, M. Ogawa, Y. Otaka, M. Tsuchitani, and H. Iwata, Carcinogenicity Test of 50 Hz Sinusoidal Magnetic Field in Rats, *Bioelectromagnetics* 18, pp. 531-540, 1997.

[126] Mandeville, R., E. Franco, S. Sidrac-Ghali, L. Paris-Nadon, N. Rocheleau, G. Mercier, M. Desy, and L. Gaboury, Evaluation of the Potential Carcinogenicity of 60 Hz Linear Sinusoidal Continuous Wave Magnetic Fields in Fischer F344 Rats, *The Federation of American Societies for Experimental Biology Journal* 11, pp. 1127-1136, 1997.

[127] McLean, J. R. N., A. Thansandote, D. Lecuyer, and M. Goddard, The Effect of 60-Hz Magnetic Fields on Co-Promotion of Chemically Induced Skin Tumors on SENCAR Mice: A Discussion of Three Studies, *Environmental Health Perspectives* 105, pp. 94-96, 1997.

[128] Shen, Y. H., B. J. Shao, H. Chiang, Y. D. Fu, and M. Yu, The Effects of 50 Hz Magnetic Field Exposure on Dimethylbenz (Alpha) Anthracene Induced Thymic Lymphoma/Leukemia in Mice, *Bioelectromagnetics* 18, pp. 360-364, 1997.

[129] Sasser, L. B., J. E. Morris, D. L. Miller, C. N. Rafferty, K. L. Ebi, and L. E. Anderson, Lack of a Co-Promoting Effect of a 60 Hz Magnetic Field on Skin Tumorigenesis in SENCAR Mice, *Carcinogenesis* 19, pp.1617-1621, 1998.

[130] Harris, A. W., A. Basten, V. Gebski, D. Noonan, J. Finnie, M. L. Bath, M. I. Bangay, and M. H. Repacholi, A Test of Lymphoma Induction by Long-Term Exposure of Eu-Piml Transgenic Mice to 50 Hz Magnetic Fields, *Radiation Research* 149, pp. 300-307, 1998.

[131] Babbitt, J. T., A. I. Kharazi, J. M. G. Taylor, C. N. Rafferty, R. Kovatch, C. B. Bonds, S. G. Mirell, E. Frumkin, F. Dietrich, D. Zhuang, and T. J. M. Hahn, Leukemia/Lymphoma in Mice Exposed to 60-Hz Magnetic Fields, *Results of the Chronic Exposure Study* TR-110338, EPRI, Los Angeles, 1998.

[132] Boorman, G. A., D. L. McCormick, J. C. Findlay, J. R. Hailey, J. R. Gauger, T. R. Johnson, R. M. Kovatch, R. C. Sills, and J. K. Haseman, Chronic Toxicity/Oncogenicity Evaluation of 60 Hz (Power Frequency) Magnetic Fields in F344/N Rats, *Toxicologic Pathology* 27, pp. 267-278, 1999.

[133] Stuchly, M. A., J. R. N. McLean, R. Burnett, M. Goddard, D. W. Lecuyer, and R. E. J. Mitchel, Modification of Tumor Promotion in the Mouse Skin by Exposure to an Alternating Magnetic Field, *Cancer Letters* 65, pp. 1-7, 1992.

[134] Beniashvili, D. S., V. G. Bilanishvili, and M. Z. Menabde, Low-Frequency Electromagnetic Radiation Enhances the Induction of Rat Mammary Tumors by Nitrosomethyl Urea, *Cancer Letters* 61, pp. 75-79, 1991.

[135] Löscher, W., M. Mevissen, W. Lehmacher, and A. Stamm, Tumor Promotion in a Breast Cancer Model by Exposure to a Weak Alternating Magnetic Field, *Cancer*

Letters 71, pp. 75-81,1993.

[136] Löscher, W., U. Wahnschaffe, M. Mevissen, A. Lerchl, and A. Stamm, Effects of Weak Alternating Magnetic Fields on Nocturnal Melatonin Production and Mammary Carcinogenesis in Rats, *Oncology* 51, pp. 288-295, 1994.

[137] Mevissen, M., A. Stamm, S. Buntenkotter, R. Zwingelberg, U. Wahnschaffe, and W. Löscher, Effects of Magnetic Fields on Mammary Tumor Development Induced by 7,12-Dimethylbenz(a)anthracene in Rats, *Bioelectromagnetics* 14, pp. 131-143, 1993.

[138] Mevissen, M., A. Lerchl, and W. Löscher, Study on Pineal Function and DMBA-Induced Breast Cancer Formation in Rats During Exposure to a 100-mg 50-Hz Magnetic Field, *Journal of Toxicology and Environmental Health* 48, pp. 169-185, 1996.

[139] Mevissen, M., M. Haubler, A. Lerchl, and W. Löscher, Acceleration of Mammary Tumorigenesis by Exposure of 7,12-Dimethylbenz (a) anthracene-100-mt Magnetic Field: Replication Study, *Journal of Toxicology and Environmental Health* 53, pp. 401-418, 1998.

[140] House, R. V., H. V. Ratajczak, J. R. Gauger, T. R. Johnson, P. T. Thomas, and D. L. McCormick, Immune Function and Host Defense in Rodents Exposed to 60 Hz Magnetic Fields, *Fundamental Applied Toxicology* 34, pp. 228-239, 1996.

[141] Tremblay, L., M. Houde, G. Mercier, J. Gagnon, R. Mandeville, Differential Modulation of Natural and Adaptive Immunity in Fischer Rats Exposed for 6 Weeks to 60 Hz Linear Sinusoidal Continuous-Wave Magnetic Fields, *Bioelectromagnetics* 17, pp. 373-383, 1996.

[142] Coelho, A. M. Jr., S. P. Easley, and W. R. Rogers, Effects of Exposure to 30 kV/m, 60 Hz Electric Fields on the Social Behavior of Baboons, *Bioelectromagnetics* 12, pp. 117-135, 1991.

[143] Trzeciak, H. I., J. Grzesik, M. Bortel, R. Kuska, D. Duda, J. Michnik, and A. Maecki, Behavioral Effects of Long-Term Exposure to Magnetic Fields in Rats, *Bioelectromagnetics* 14, pp. 287-297, 1993.

[144] Sienkiewicz, Z. J., R. G. E. Haylock, and R. D. Saunders, Deficits in Spatial Learning After Exposure of Mice to a 50 Hz Magnetic Field, *Bioelectromagnetics* 19, pp. 79-85, 1998.

[145] Lai, H., Spatial Learning Deficit in the Rat After Exposure to a 60 Hz Magnetic Field, *Bioelectromagnetics* 17, pp. 494-497, 1996.

[146] Cerretelli, D. I., and C. R. Malaguti, Research Carried on in Italy by ENEL on the Effects of High Voltage Electric Fields, *Revue Generale De L'Electrcite*, pp. 65-74, 1976.

[147] Ryan, B. M., E. Mallett, T. R. Johnson, J. R. Gauger, and D. L. McCormick, Developmental Toxicity Study of 60 Hz (Power Frequency) Magnetic Fields in Rats, *Teratology* 54, pp. 73-83, 1996.

[148] Ryan, B. M., R. R. Symanski, L. E. Pomeranz, T. R. Johnson, J. R. Gauger, and D. L. McCormick, Multi-Generation Reproductive Toxicity Assessment of 60 Hz Magnetic Fields Using a Continuous Breeding Protocol in Rats, *Teratology* 56, pp. 159-162, 1999.

[149] Asanova, T. P., and A. N. Rakov, The Health Status of People Working in the Electric Field of Open 400-500 KV Switching Structures, *Gigiena Truda I*

Professionalnye Zabolevaniia 10, pp. 50-52, USSR, 1966. (Available from IEEE, Piscataway, NJ, Special Publication Number 10)

[150]   Sazonova, T., A Physiological Assessment of the Work Conditions in 400 kV and 500 kV Open Switch Yards, In *Scientific Publications of the Institute of Labor Protection of the All-Union Central Council of Trade Unions* 46, Profizdat, USSR, 1967. (Available from IEEE, Piscataway, NJ, Special Issue Number 10)

[151]   Zenon, S., Behavioural Effects of EMFs Mechanisms and Consequences of Power Frequency Electromagnetic Field Exposures, *Electromagnetics Meeting*, Bristol, UK, 24-25 September 1998.

[152]   Stuchly, M. A., Human Exposure to Static and Time-Varying Magnetic Fields, *Health Physics* 51, pp. 215-225, 1986.

[153]   Korpinen, L., J. Partanen, and A. Uusitalo, Influence of 50 Hz Electric and Magnetic Fields on the Human Heart, *Bioelectromagnetics* 14, pp. 329-340, 1993.

[154]   Sastre, A., M. R. Cook, and C. Graham, Cell Membrane Lipid Molecular Dynamics in a Solenoid Versus a Magnetically Shielded Room, *Bioelectromagnetics* 19, pp. 107-112, 1998.

[155]   Maisch, D., B. Rapley, R. E. Rowland, and J. Podd, Chronic Fatigue Syndrome-Is Prolonged Exposure to Environmental Level Powerline Frequency Electromagnetic Fields a Co-Factor to Consider in Treatment? EMFacts Consultancy, 1999.

[156]   Grant, L., *The Electrical Sensitivity Handbook: How Electromagnetic Fields (EMFs) are Making People Sick*, Weldon Publishing, Prescott, AZ, 1995.

[157]   Liden, S., Sensitivity to Electricity-A New Environmental Epidemic, *Allergy* 51, pp. 519-524, 1996.

[158]   Bernhardt, J. H., On the Rating of Human Exposition to Electric and Magnetic Fields with Frequencies Below 100 kHz, *Commission of the European Communities*, Joint Research Centre, Ispra, Italy, 1983.

[159]   Dalziel, C. F., Electric Shock Hazard, *IEEE Spectrum* 9, pp. 41-50, 1972.

[160]   Schwan, H. P., Field Interaction with Biological Matter, *Annals of the New York Academy of Sciences* 103, pp. 198-213, 1977.

[161]   Bernhardt, J. H., Assessment of Experimentally Observed Bioeffects in View of their Clinical Relevance and the Exposures at Work Places, *Symposium on Biological Effects of Static and ELF Magnetic Fields*, Munich, MMV Medizin Verlag, 1985.

[162]   Lovsund, P., P. A. Oberg, and S. E. Nilsson, Influence on Vision of Extremely Low Frequency Electromagnetic Fields: Industrial Measurements, Magnetophosphene Studies in Volunteers and Intraretinal Studies in Animals, *Acta Ophthalmologica* (Copenhagen) 57, pp. 812-821, 1979.

[163]   Adair, A. K., Effects of ELF Magnetic Fields on Biological Magnetite, *Bioelectromagnetics* 14, pp. 1-4, 1993.

4

Epidemiological Assessment Studies

4.1 INTRODUCTION

Public concern over human effects of exposure to ELF fields is largely based on a series of key epidemiological assessment studies. Such studies identify the association between diseases and particular environmental characteristics. It may indicate a cause-and-effect relationship, depending upon the strength of the observed association. Epidemiological studies correlate historical biological data for a large population of people. Any biological data is purely statistical in nature; however, people usually fit a particular category based on location or occupation. The results may only show an association with a stimulus (ELF exposure, for example) since there are many factors involved with each person.

Within the setting of this book, epidemiological studies address the observed effects of possibly harmful EM exposures on human health and whether the exposures are related quantitatively to the effects. They are restricted in that they are indirect experiments where EM exposure can only be assessed by different substitute measures. In laboratory (cellular or animal) studies, exposure may be controlled to a greater degree, but it is still necessary to decide what exposure to apply. However, the epidemiologist does not create the exposure and cannot control the cause of the disease in the way the laboratory researcher generally does. Lack of knowledge about how EM fields interact with the living system makes the issue of exposure assessment a main source of uncertainty. Nowadays, state-of-the-art physics and engineering allow precise measurements to be made. Still, they do not tell which exposure characteristics are the most important to measure for identifying hazards. Moreover, they do not tell which exposure characteristics provide the best estimate of prior exposures during the critical period of disease initiation or advance in the population under study [1, 2].

4.2 EPIDEMIOLOGY

Science uses a powerful tool called epidemiology to determine if there is a health risk for a certain reason from an unknown cause. Epidemiology is the study of occurrence and distribution of disease in a population. The first advantage for humans from this science came in 1855. John Snow, a British physician, observed that death rates from cholera were particularly high in areas of London that where supplied with drinking water that had been extracted from the Thames River at points close to sewage outfalls. He proposed that an unknown agent through sewage transmitted the cholera. This assumption led to the proper treatment of sewage systems.

4.2.1 Odds Ratio

Epidemiological studies are consistently case-control studies. In these studies, two groups of people are identified: the *cases*, people with a particular disease being under study, and the *controls*, who are selected from the same population as the cases, similar to them in every respect except that the controls do not have the disease. The exposure of these two groups to the factor being studied is measured. The result of the study is expressed as an odds ratio (OR) [2]:

$$OR = \frac{\text{Odds of being exposed in cases}}{\text{Odds of being exposed in controls}} \tag{4.1}$$

OR is an estimate. It may be defined as a measure of association, which quantifies the relationship between exposure and health outcome from a comparative study. Epidemiologists must calculate, in addition to the OR, the range over which they are confident that this estimate is reliable. Sample size is an important factor in the calculation. The smaller the sample, the less reliable the information. If OR is 1, no difference has been found between the exposure of people with the disease and people without the disease, meaning *negative association* between the disease and exposure. If OR is greater than 1, however, the cases were more likely to have been exposed than the controls, and there is a *positive association* between the disease and exposure.

For example, to study a case of ELF exposure and cancer, two groups of people must be compared: one group, which has in the past been exposed to ELF field and another group (the control group), which has not. The exposed group is usually made up of people who live near an identified source of ELF field like power lines or a substation, while the nonexposed group lives further away. An observation is then made as whether there are more concerns in the exposed group than in the nonexposed one.

Numerically, consider a study of 500 cancer cases and 500 controls. If 130 cases were exposed to ELF field and 370 were not exposed, the odds of being exposed in cases is 130/370 = 0.35. If 130 controls were also exposed, the odds of being exposed in controls is also 0.35. Accordingly, the OR will be 1, which means negative association between ELF field and cancer.

Now, assume that 200 of the total 500 cases were exposed (ratio = 200/300 = 0.66) and 130 controls were exposed (ratio = 0.35). The OR is 0.66/0.35 = 1.88, meaning positive association between ELF field and cancer.

It is agreed that one of the most valuable tools to detect human health risk associated with EM exposure is to study the human population that has actually experienced the exposure. This can largely be achieved through epidemiological studies, which are usually observational rather than experimental studies; the epidemiologist observes and compares groups of people who have had a disease for possibility of being exposed in order to find a possible association.

4.2.2 Exposure Environments

Health and safety regulations arrange EM field conditions and limits in occupational and public environments. In this chapter, occupational and public environments are considered together. Classification of research papers is based on type of effect.

Occupational (Controlled) Environments

Occupational exposure environments are studied in the context of specific industries and workplaces, particularly in the power-utility industry where high exposure to ELF fields is likely. Workers can be exposed to electric and magnetic fields from the electrical system in their building and the equipment they work with. A variety of methods for exposure assessment are applied to studies in occupational settings. These methods range from job classification to modeling techniques based on personal exposure measurements and occupational history.

Occupational history is a collection of data for a study subject, which may contain information on jobs that the subject held during their employment. Such information is obtained through many ways, such as interviews or through various records. The information contains the industry title, company name, and description, and duration of the job. Medical records may also be obtained from clinics or disease registries.

Electrical appliances, tools, and power supplies in buildings are the main sources of field exposure that most people receive at work. People who work near transformers, electrical closets, circuit boxes, or other high-current electrical equipment may have high-field exposures (hundreds of milligauss or even more). In offices, magnetic field levels are often similar to those found at homes, typically 0.5 to 4.0 mG. However, these levels may increase dramatically near certain types of equipment. The literature is rich with more occupational studies investigating exposure of workers to ELF fields at various places using different techniques of evaluation.

Public (Uncontrolled) Environments

Public environments involve all ELF exposures at residences, schools, and transport avenues. The primary sources of residential and school fields are power lines, distribution lines, substations, wiring, grounding systems, and various electrical appliances. Sources of fields in trains and cars are mainly from the power lines feeding trains. Numerous studies have showed that most high fields in houses are produced by nearby power lines. Residential studies address the exposure of children and adults to EM fields either as population-based or case-control cases. Much of the interest concerning public environments to ELF fields has focused on childhood cancer.

4.3   EPIDEMIOLOGICAL STUDIES OF CANCER

During the past few decades, many epidemiological studies showed a positive association between exposure to ELF fields and various types of cancer, especially childhood leukemia, adult leukemia, brain cancer, breast cancer, lung cancer, and other cancers in both occupational and residential environments. On the other hand, several other studies showed negative association.

Becker [3] performed the first epidemiological study that considered the possible health menace of power-line fields in the early 1970s. He found an association between environmental fields and cancer. He interpreted it to generally support the hypothesis regarding the mechanism of field action. A few months earlier, Milton Zaret [4] published a report that linked occupational exposure to electric and magnetic fields and cancer.

In the following years, more epidemiological studies of cancer were conducted, mainly in the United States, Europe, and Australia. Many studies have shown some clear association between ELF exposure and the development of cancer, but in general the results are mixed, with variation in both strength of association and cancer types noted. Evidences indicate that epidemiological studies are unable to provide a clear correlation between ELF exposure and the development of cancers. Yet, these studies are useful, provided they are designed to identify type, duration, and level of exposure.

Hulbert et al. [5] indicated that epidemiological studies are unable to provide a clear correlation between exposure to power-frequency fields and the development of cancers. They summarized studies and reports of major responses to ELF fields. The opening sections discuss quantitative aspects of exposure to fields and the incidences of cancer that have been correlated with such fields. The concluding section considers problems that confront research in this area and suggests feasible strategies.

Moulder and Foster [6] reviewed the evidence bearing on the issue of whether power-frequency electric fields might cause or contribute to cancer. According to the authors, the overall case that power-frequency electric fields are causally linked to human cancer is even weaker than that for magnetic fields, and can reasonably be called nonexistent.

Most work carried out during the 1990s in the United States is a part of what is known as the Research and Public Information Dissemination (RAPID) Program. Mandated by Congress as a part of the Energy Policy Act of 1992, this multiagency program was planned as an effort to determine if exposure to low-level low-frequency EM fields is detrimental to health, and if so, to provide an assessment of risk. The National Institute of Environmental Health Sciences (NIEHS) and Department of Energy (DOE) led the RAPID program. The program included a wide range of research and communications activities designed to provide answers to health questions in the 5-year program lifetime.

As part of the EMF-RAPID Program's assessment, an international panel of 30 scientists met in June 1998 to review and evaluate the weight of the ELF-EM field scientific evidence. Using criteria developed by the International Agency for Research on Cancer, none of the working group considered the evidence strong enough to label ELF fields exposure as a "known human carcinogen" or "probable human carcinogen." However, a majority of the members of this working group concluded that exposure to power-line frequency ELF fields is a "possible human carcinogen." This decision was based largely on limited evidence of an increased risk for childhood leukemia with residential exposure and an increased occurrence of chronic lymphocytic leukemia (CLL) associated with occupational exposure. For other cancers and for noncancer health endpoints, the working group categorized the experimental data as providing much weaker evidence. The NIEHS agrees that the associations reported for childhood leukemia and adult CLL cannot be dismissed easily as random or negative findings. The lack of positive findings in animals or in mechanistic studies weakens the belief that this association is actually due to ELF-EM fields, but cannot completely discount the finding. The NIEHS also agrees with the conclusion that no other cancers or noncancer health outcomes provide sufficient evidence of a risk to warrant concern.

Meanwhile, the NIEHS report released on 15th June 1999 concluded that ELF fields could cause cancer, based on epidemiological studies indicating an association between some types of leukemia and exposure to magnetic fields [7]. Nevertheless, the report said, there has been no consistent explanation of that association, even though all other causes of the epidemiological results have been ruled out. The report said the ELF field exposure "cannot be recognized as entirely safe," but the probability that ELF-EM fields are a health hazard is small at the moment.

In 2001, Dr. Neil Cherry [8] summarized the evidences that ELF fields are hazardous to human health, especially to young children. He concluded that the link between electromagnetic fields and leukemia is overwhelmingly supported by many epidemiological studies.

4.3.1 Childhood Leukemia

Childhood is a critical period of enormous cell growth. Therefore, particular concerns regarding children's safety and exposure to ELF fields arise, such as exposure of children to fields from nearby power lines, their use of computers at home and school, sitting close to television terminals, or using mobile phones.

The word "leukemia," which literally means, "white blood," describes a variety of cancers that arise in the bone marrow where blood cells are formed. It is known by the creation of abnormal white blood cells called *leukocytes*, which, as the disease advances, battle with the healthy white blood cells that the body needs to fight bacterial, viral, and other infections. In addition, red blood cells, bound for oxygen transport throughout the body, and blood platelets necessary for clotting, are also affected.

Leukemia represents less than 4% of all cancer cases in adults. However, leukemia is the most common form of cancer found in children, mainly acute lymphocytic leukemia (ALL). Only few risk factors are known about ALL, although many have been proposed and studied. Children with Down syndrome have a greatly increased risk of ALL, reported to be 10 to 40 times the risk of other children. Other, more rare chromosomal and genetic abnormalities may also increase risk for ALL. Children whose mothers had diagnostic X-rays during pregnancy are more likely to have ALL compared with children whose mothers had no X-rays.

Poole and Ozonoff [9] reviewed epidemiology data on residential exposure to power-line fields and childhood cancer, in search of a "dose-response" relation. Cartwright [10] presented results pertaining to childhood leukemia that are currently available. He reviewed and suggested a few interpretations.

Mechanisms and consequences of EM field exposures had been raised when one of the first epidemiological studies indicating a health risk appeared in 1979 with OR equal to 2.35 [11]. The authors, Dr. Nancy Wertheimer and Ed Leeper, conducted the study at the University of Colorado. An excess of electrical wiring configurations suggestive of high current flow was noted in Denver, Colorado, in 1976-1977 near the homes of children who developed cancer, as compared to the homes of control children. The finding was strongest for children who had spent their entire lives at the same address, and it appeared to be dose-related. They reported two- to threefold increase in cancer deaths among children living near high-current power lines. The investigators used a single measure of AC magnetic field exposure wiring configuration code (type of power lines and distance from the wiring to the residence). Due to this technique, they needed a way of classifying homes with respect to AC magnetic fields that did not require taking measurements or entering homes. The technique was based on estimated thickness of primary and secondary distribution lines, the relation and proximity of these lines to transformers, and the distance of lines from consumers. As a result, they claimed that children had double or triple the chance of developing leukemia or tumors of the nervous system if they live near high-power transmission lines as compared to those who do not. Apart from that, the study was criticized because of inaccurate use of types and layout of transmission and distribution lines.

In a study based in Rhode Island (OR = 1.09) [12], another coding system as an index of exposure for identifying the presence of magnetic fields was used. No link with childhood leukemia was found. The authors seemed to say that their study was relevant to the Werheimer and Leeper study [11], though the chosen endpoint was childhood leukemia, not childhood cancer as in the Werheimer and Leeper study.

Several studies were conducted during the 1980s, but the studies, which confirmed Werheimer and Leeper finding, were published by Savitz et al. [13-15]. They found increased cases of childhood cancer and leukemia associated with magnetic field exposures above 2.5 mG. A better research methodology relating intensified risk of childhood cancer to the presence of certain configurations of power lines was implemented.

The above findings were confirmed by a 1991 study carried out by London et al. [16]. This study is considered one of the largest studies in childhood leukemia. It was conducted in Los Angeles, California, with OR = 2.15. Childhood leukemia was considered in relation to magnetic fields as indexed by the Werheimer and Leeper codes with 24-hour measurements and spot measurements. The study seems best characterized as outstanding, in which the author described a series of actions that led to various kinds of data, followed by expression of opinions regarding the meaning of the data.

Bowman et al. [17] hypothesized that the risk of childhood leukemia is related to specific combinations of static and ELF fields. Childhood leukemia data from the Los Angeles childhood was analyzed on the basis of these combinations. As a result, no association of cancer with measured static or power-frequency fields was found, and point estimates for the selected combinations did not show significant associations.

Three collaborative population-based Nordic studies using calculated fields were conducted in Sweden, Denmark, and Finland [18-20]. In the Swedish study [18], which is considered the largest, the authors defined the population base as all children in Sweden 15 years of age or younger who lived within 800 meters from high-voltage power lines during the years 1960-1985. As a result, only 142 cases (39 leukemia and 33 nervous system cancer) were identified.

The Danish study [19], considered residences within specified distances (25-50 meters) from power lines, substations, and underground cables. The study demonstrated a significantly increased risk of childhood lymphoma in the highest exposure category. Although the study was conducted with a large segment of the Danish population, the final number of children in the exposed and control groups with lymphoma were small (six cases and three controls) making the reliability of the results questionable. Incidences of childhood leukemia, which have been reported to increase with presumed ELF fields exposure in other studies, were not significantly elevated in the Danish study. Further, the study demonstrated the increased risk of lymphatic cancer among children with exposure to magnetic fields from high-voltage lines of 0.1 µT or greater.

In the Finnish study [20], risk of cancer in children living close to overhead power lines with magnetic fields greater than or equal to 0.01 µT was assessed. The study involved 68,300 boys and 66,500 girls aged 0-19 years living during 1970-1989 within 500 meters from overhead 100-400-kV transmission lines. No statistically significant increases in all cancers, leukemia, and lymphoma were found in children at any exposure level. A statistically significant excess of nervous system tumors was found in boys (but not in girls) who were exposed to magnetic fields greater or equal to 0.2 µT or cumulative exposure greater or equal to 0.4 µT. The study, however, concluded that residential magnetic fields of power lines do not constitute a major public health risk regarding childhood cancer.

A Canadian ecological study [21] addressed the incidences in childhood cancer rates using data from Statistics Canada. The authors found that provinces with a high residential electric consumption were found to have higher brain and leukemia cancer rankings when compared to other provinces. The methodology used has limitations due to the type of data collected. This study suggests, but does not prove, associations between cancer and electric consumption.

In 1991 U.S. Congress asked the National Academy of Sciences (NAS) to review and evaluate the existing body of scientific research in order to determine whether the findings were sufficient to assess any health risks. In November 1996, the National Research Council (NRC) of NAS reported on a three-year meta-analysis of eleven epidemiological studies (meta-analysis combines data from a number of studies and inspects them in a new way). The NAS-NRC report [22] concluded that, "An association between residential wiring configurations (wire codes) and childhood leukemia persists in multiple studies, although the causative factor responsible for that association has not been identified. No evidence, which links contemporary measurements of magnetic field levels to childhood leukemia, has been found."

A widely publicized study through collaborative effort by researchers from the National Cancer Institute (NCI) and the Children's Cancer Group (CCG) in the United States found no evidence that links exposure to magnetic fields at homes to the risk of childhood cancer. This case-control study was conducted by Linet et al. [23] to evaluate residential exposure to magnetic fields (629 children with ALL under age 15 and 619 controls). The researchers took actual measurements of fields in various locations around homes involved in the study. They found no overall correlation between the level of field exposure and risk of childhood ALL, regardless of the measure of exposure used. There was a small increase in the risk of ALL for children whose residences measured in the very highest range of magnetic fields. However, the number of children living in such homes was small in this study, making it hard to draw conclusions.

Another study from the NCI/CCG [24], investigated whether use of household electrical appliances by mothers during pregnancy and by their children is associated with increased risk of ALL. Electric appliances included were electric blankets, mattress pads, heating pads, water beds, stereo or other sound systems, television and video games connected to a television, video machines located in arcades, computers, microwave ovens, sewing machines, hair dryers, curling irons, ceiling fans, humidifiers, night lights, and electric clocks. In general, there was no evidence for any association between appliances used during pregnancy and the risk of childhood ALL. No significant association was found with time spent watching TV or distance from TV during pregnancy. Childhood ALL was also not associated with the use of most of the appliances.

A Norwegian study [25] comprised of children who had lived in a census ward crossed by a high-voltage power line during at least one of the years 1960, 1970, 1980, 1985, 1987, or 1989. The cases were diagnosed from 1965 to 1989 and were matched to controls by year of birth, sex, and municipality. Exposure to electric and magnetic fields was calculated by means of computer programs in which power line characteristics and distance were taken into account. No association was found between exposure to magnetic fields and few cancers at all sites. However, this study provides little support for an association between children's exposure to magnetic fields and leukemia.

In Germany, Michaelis et al. [26] found an excess of childhood leukemia associated with residential exposures to magnetic fields. The researchers obtained measurements in two population-based case-control studies on childhood leukemia in the northwestern part of Germany and in Berlin for the period from 1992 to 1996. Exposure assessment comprised residential 24-hour measurements and short-term measurements. They obtained 24-hour measurements for a total of 176 cases and 414 controls. They compared subjects exposed to median 24-hour measurements of 0.2 µT or more with those exposed to lower amounts. Multivariate regression analysis revealed an OR of 2.3. The association was statistically significant for children 4 years of age or less and for median nighttime magnetic field, but not for all children.

A study from Taiwan [27] reported elevated risk of leukemia among children living near high-voltage transmission lines in three urban districts of northern Taiwan. Twenty-eight cases of leukemia among some 120,696 children aged 14 years or less were reported to the National Cancer Registry between 1987 and 1992. It was found that children living in areas within 100 meters of a transmission line had a leukemia rate 2.7 times higher than that of children in the nation as a whole. Their cancer risk was 2.4 times higher than that of other children in the same neighborhoods. The findings suggest that children living near high-voltage power lines tend to experience an elevated risk of leukemia.

Two Canadian studies [28, 29] of power-line exposure were published in 1999. In the first case-control study [28], 399 children residing in five Canadian provinces who were diagnosed at age 0-14 years between 1990 and 1994 were enrolled, along with 399 controls. Exposure assessment included 48-hour personal ELF measurement, wire coding and magnetic field measurements for subjects from conception to diagnosis/reference date, and a 24-hour magnetic field bedroom measurement. Personal magnetic field was not related to risk of leukemia (OR=0.95) or ALL (OR=0.93). There were no clear associations with predicted magnetic field exposure two years before the diagnosis/reference date, over the subject's lifetime, or with personal electric field exposure. A statistically elevated risk of ALL was observed with high-wiring configurations among residences of subjects two years before the diagnosis date (OR=1.72).

In the second Canadian study [29], wire codes and measurements inside the residences showed no significant association with leukemia, while measurements external to the residences were associated with increased leukemia occurrence. The finding did not support an association between leukemia and proximity to power lines with high-current configuration.

4.3.2 Adult Leukemia

A large number of studies with mixed results relating ELF fields to adult leukemia have been carried out worldwide. A study was conducted at Southern California Edison Company [30], among 36,221 electric utility workers in one of the most comprehensive occupational studies to date. It involved a careful measurement of magnetic fields associated with particular types of utility jobs. Although the risk of cancer associated with certain ELF exposure was slightly elevated in a few cases, none were significantly above normal levels.

Researchers at AT&T and Johns Hopkins University studied the occurrence of leukemia in telephone company workers exposed to similar types of ELF fields [31]. Of all the AT&T workers employed for two years or more that died between 1975 and 1980, 124 died with leukemia as the primary diagnosis. These were compared to a control group of current or retired employees. Magnetic field measurements of occupational conditions were used to relate jobs to actual field exposures. The relationship was not perfect because present-day measurements do not always represent past exposure conditions, which may have existed during the critical period of tumor growth. In particular, central office technicians were formerly exposed to rapidly changing magnetic fields from electromechanical switching equipment, which were replaced with electronic switches after the early 1980s. As a result, leukemia mortality was higher than expected for all line-worker job categories except for cable splicers, but none of the differences were statistically significant because of the small number of cases. It was found that workers with lifetime magnetic field exposures above the median for the population studied had a rate of leukemia 2.5 times higher than that of unexposed telephone workers. Line workers who died before age 55 had higher OR of leukemia than did workers of all ages. Six central office technicians and four engineers died of leukemia before age 55. As a result, these two job classifications had the highest risk elevations with rates approximately 3 times higher than expected.

Canadian and French researchers, led by Dr. Gilles Thériault at McGill University in Montreal [32], conducted a study of 223,292 workers at two large utilities in Canada and a national utility in France. The result shows that workers with acute myeloid leukemia (AML) were about three times more likely to be in the half of the workforce with higher cumulative exposure to magnetic fields. In the analysis of median cumulative magnetic field exposure, no significant elevated risks were found for most types of cancer studied. In a separate analysis of 25 different cancers and 7 regroupings among these cancers, an association was found in only three. For these three cancer-type/regroupings, a link with cumulative exposure to magnetic fields was observed for acute non-lymphocytic leukemia (60 cases), including 47 cases of AML and a type of brain tumor known *astrocytoma* (41 cases). Combining all different cancer types, the study did not find any association between the cancer cases analyzed and exposure to ELF fields.

In 1995, Savitz and his group at the University of North Carolina carried out another major study [33]. It involved more than 138,000 utility workers at five electric utilities in the United States during the period 1950-1986, with at least 6 months of work experience. Exposure was estimated by associating individual work histories to data from 2,842 works shift magnetic field measurements. Mortality follow-up identified 20,733 deaths based on 2,656,436 person-years of work experience. Death rates were analyzed in relation to occupational magnetic field exposure history. The researchers found that both total mortality and cancer mortality rose slightly with increasing magnetic field exposure. Meanwhile, leukemia mortality was not associated with indices of magnetic field exposure except for work as an electrician. In conclusion, the results of this study did not support any association between occupational magnetic field exposure and the risk of leukemia. Still, the study does suggest a link to brain cancer.

A significant study to report an association between cancer and magnetic field exposure in a broad range of industries was conducted by Floderus et al. [34] at the Swedish National Institute of Working Life. The study included an assessment of electric and magnetic exposure at 1015 different workplaces in Sweden and involved over 1600 people in 169 different occupations. The researchers reported an association between estimated field exposure and increased risk for chronic lymphocytic leukemia (CLL). In addition, an increased risk of brain tumors was reported for men under the age of 40 whose work involved an average magnetic field exposure of more than 2 mG.

Another case-control study by Feychting et al. [35], in Sweden included approximately 400,000 subjects who had lived within a range of 300 meters of power transmission lines for at least one year during the period between 1960 and 1985. The researchers found that persons who were exposed to magnetic fields both at home and at workplace are nearly 4 times likely to develop leukemia compared to those who were not exposed to magnetic fields.

Johansen and Olsen [36] conducted a study involving 32,006 men and women who had been employed at 99 electric utilities in Denmark. Their obtained employment history goes back to 1909. Cancer incidents were attained from the cancer registry over the same period. The authors predicted that utility workers have slightly more cancer than expected from general population statistics, with no excess of leukemia, brain cancer, or breast cancer.

Most of the above studies concentrated on magnetic field exposures, assuming that they are the more biologically active components of the ELF fields. However, there are studies that indicate that electric field exposures may play a major role in the possible link with cancer. Miller et al. [37] at the University of Toronto looked at the cumulative effects of both magnetic and electric field exposures on the cancer incidence. The study group consisted of electrical utility workers at the Canadian Power Company Ontario Hydro. Miller's team showed a striking increase in leukemia risk. At the highest level of exposure to both magnetic and electric fields, the OR jumped from 3.51 to 11.2 when the researchers included the interaction of the combined effects of electric and magnetic fields. As yet, these are some of the highest leukemia risks ever reported in a study of ELF fields and cancer. The results went even further. First, all leukemia types studied showed a clear increase in risk. Second, there was evidence of a dose-response risk; in other words, the higher the cumulative exposure to electric fields, the higher the leukemia risk (an effect noticeably absent with exposure to magnetic fields alone, both in this and in almost all previous studies).

The elevated risks of leukemia were seen among senior workers who spent the most time in electric fields above certain thresholds, in the range of 10 to 40 V/m. These findings came in a recent study [38] based on data from Miller's 1996 study [37]. "These studies confirm that electric fields are very important, if not dominant," according to Dr. Anthony Miller, a coauthor of the study said.

4.3.3 Brain Cancer

Brain cancer of the central nervous system (CNS) is not very common. The causes of the disease are primarily unknown, although the same reasons for other types of cancer, such as exposure to chemical and ionizing radiation, smoking, diet, and excessive alcohol consumption are associated with brain cancer.

Floderus et al. [39] conducted a large population-based case-control study of occupational exposure to magnetic fields and brain cancers. The study was concerned only with men (20-64 years old in 1980) living in Sweden. Cases of leukemia (426) and brain cancer (424) that occurred during the period 1983-1987 were identified from the National Cancer Registry. Of the leukemia patients, 325 were contacted and 250 agreed to participate. Two controls matched on age were selected for each case from the 1980 census. The response rates were 77% for leukemia patients and 72% for controls. Measurements were taken using a person whose job was most similar to that of the person in the study. Overall, a rise in incidences was found for leukemia, but not for brain cancer.

In another study, Floderus et al. [40] analyzed cancer incidence data for electrical railroad workers and found a nonsignificant increase in CLL, ALL, breast cancer, pituitary cancer, and lymphoma in the first decade of data, but not in later data. No increase in leukemia or in brain cancer was seen. No exposure estimates or measurements were made.

Sahl et al. [41] considered brain cancer in a study at Southern California. The analysis included 32 deaths from brain cancer. In this study, the OR by commutative exposure category was close to 1.

Theriault et al. [32] examined the risk of brain cancer among workers at three large electric utility companies. In all, 250 cases of brain cancer were included in the study. A nonsignificant increase in risk of brain cancers was observed for workers with cumulative exposure to magnetic fields greater than 3.15 μT. However, a significantly increased risk was seen among the workers, based on five exposed cases.

Considering a study conducted by Savitz et al. [33], brain cancer mortality was elevated in relation to duration of work in exposed jobs and much more strongly associated with magnetic field exposure indices. It was noticed that brain cancer risk increased by an estimated 1.94 per μT-year of magnetic field exposure in the previous 2-10 years, with a mortality rate ratio of 2.6 in the highest exposure category. This study did not support an association between occupational magnetic field exposure and leukemia but did suggest a connection to brain cancer.

Wilkins et al. [42] reported a possible association between occupational exposure of men to ELF fields and the risk of childhood brain tumors in offspring by re-analyzing case-referent interview data from a study of environmental factors and childhood brain tumors conducted by one of the authors and first reported in 1990. Analyses of the data were limited to the 94 cases and 166 individually matched referents for which data on the biological fathers were available. Paternal exposure to occupational ELF fields was inferred from a list of job titles compiled for that purpose. OR for individually matched cases and referents were estimated for various definitions of field exposure. The findings suggested very small increase in risk for jobs associated with the occupational field exposure of fathers during the one-year period prior to conception. OR values ranged from 1.12 to 1.31. The results of re-analysis indicate that paternal occupational exposure to ELF fields is at best only weakly associated with the risk of childhood brain tumors. On the other hand, the findings for paternal welding are somewhat intriguing since relatively strong fields have been measured in association with welding. Further studies of welding, as a potential risk factor is required since welders can be exposed to a wide range of toxic agents in addition to ELF fields.

Another case-control study was conducted by Harrington et al. [43], in the United Kingdom, to investigate the death from brain cancer nested in a cohort of 84,018 male and female electric utility workers who had been employed between 1972 and 1984. The cohort was defined from the employment record. Exposure from different jobs and locations was assessed from a survey of 258 staff in the British electricity supply industry. No association was observed between brain cancer and exposure to magnetic fields.

Asymmetry in the degree of effort in classifying cases and controls also continues to occur. For example, Guenel et al. [44] indicated an association between power-line fields and brain tumors in French electric utility workers. The cases were identified on the basis of cancer diagnoses reported to the health insurance system, but the controls were matched simply on the basis of year of birth. The presumption was made that unless a subject was seen by a physician, diagnosed as having cancer, and reported to the health insurance system, the subject could not be considered having cancer.

Rodvall et al. [45] conducted a case-control study of brain cancer and occupational exposure to 50-Hz magnetic fields. Exposure estimates were based on occupational industry. A statistically insignificant increase in brain cancer rates was found for some definitions of exposure.

In 1999, Kheifets et al. [46] published a combined re-analysis of previously published studies of electric utility workers that examined the relation between occupational exposure to power-frequency magnetic fields and risk of brain cancer and leukemia. The connected analysis shows a weak association between exposure to power-frequency fields and both brain cancer and leukemia. Even in the most highly exposed groups, the associations were not strong or statistically significant.

4.3.4 Breast Cancer

Breast cancer refers to the erratic growth and proliferation of cells that originate in the breast tissue. Usually, breast cancer refers to a malignant tumor that has developed from cells in the breast. It is a most ubiquitous cancer among adults and women, in particular. Because of earlier investigations [47] reporting ELF fields effect on melatonin levels, a hypothesis was developed that exposure to magnetic fields could be a risk factor for breast cancer. This hypothesis is based on the demonstrated capability of such exposures to decrease the production of the hormone melatonin, and on the observation that melatonin, in turn, protects against certain types of cancer.

Norwegian researchers reported breast cancer incidences [48, 49]. Breast cancer appeared to occur more frequently among men who worked in electrical occupations in Norway. Number of cases was small (12) but more than might be expected by chance alone.

A subsequent study by Demers et al. [50] of men who had breast cancer reported that men were more likely than a comparison group without breast cancer to have had jobs in electrical occupations.

Matanoski et al. [51] reported an excess of male cancer, based on two cases among central office technicians in a cohort of employees. The peak exposure to magnetic fields was a significant risk factor in the study of leukemia in 1993 by the same group.

Floderus et al. [52] analyzed the risk of breast cancer among all Swedish men (20-64 years old) who had been employed as railway workers. Cases of breast cancer were collected from the National Cancer Registry for the period 1960-1979. Exposures were assessed by the railroad job titles that were associated with high exposure according to earlier personal monitoring. Significantly increased relative risks were reported for men in the most exposed occupations: engine drivers, conductors, and railway workers in the first decade, based on two, three, and four cases, respectively. In the second decade, only four cases of breast cancer were seen, none of which were in men with the occupations listed above.

Another Swedish case-control study of residential exposure and breast cancer was reported by Feychting et al. [53]. The investigators estimated the exposure based on historic field reconstruction. As a result, no significant associations were found for either male or female breast cancer.

Dr. Patricia Coogan and coworkers [54] in the School of Public Health at Boston University found a 43% increase in breast cancer in a large case-control study among women with high potential for occupational exposures to magnetic fields, notably those working with mainframe computers. There were over 6800 cases of breast cancer diagnosed between 1988 and 1991 among women 74 years of age or younger from the cancer registries in Maine, Wisconsin, and Massachusetts. Usual occupations were grouped into three categories (low, medium, and high) of potential exposure to 60 Hz magnetic fields above background by an industrial hygienist. The remaining occupations were aggregated into a background category. Conditional logistic regression stratified on age and state was used to calculate OR, with adjustment for risk factors of breast cancer. ORs by category were 1.0 for low exposure, 1.1 for intermediate exposure, and 1.4 for high exposure.

In a Finnish cohort study by Verkasalo [55], the risk for breast cancer in relation to calculated residential exposure to magnetic fields was examined. 1229 cases of breast cancer were found among women in the cohort. However, no significant association was observed.

Johansen and Olsen [37] also considered breast cancer of women in their retrospective cohort mortality study of electric utility workers in Denmark. No association was seen between death from breast cancer (96 cases) and exposure to magnetic fields, based on very small numbers of exposed cases: two in the low-exposure category (0.1-0.29 µT), none in the intermediate category, and one in the highest category (>1.0 µT).

Gammon et al. [56] carried out a case-control study of electric blankets and the risk of female breast cancer. The 2,199 case patients were under age 55 years and had been newly diagnosed with breast cancer between 1990 and 1992. The 2,009 controls were frequency-matched to cases by 5-year age group and geographic area. It was observed, however, that there was little or no risk associated with ever having used electrical appliances such as blankets, mattress pads, or heated waterbeds (OR =1.01).

Petralia et al. [57] investigated occupational exposure to power-frequency fields and female breast cancer in Shanghai. Exposure was based on job history.

OR for always having been exposed to ELF fields was 1.0 (0.9-1.0). When stratified for probability or level of exposure, there were no elevated risks.

In a recent case-control study reported by Forssén et al. [58], the authors investigated the association of female breast cancer with residential and occupational exposure to power-frequency fields. The incidence of breast cancer was not raised for occupational exposure, for residential exposure, or for occupational and residential exposures together.

4.3.5 Lung Cancer

Lung cancer has been one of the more appealing findings in relation to EM field exposure because no obvious causal mechanism could be discovered. The association between EM field exposure and lung cancer has been considered in few studies. Erren [59] reviewed five major studies, three occupational and two residential, in which a statistically significant excess of lung cancer was found in relation to ELF field exposure.

Armstrong et al. [60] examined the association between exposure to EM fields and cancer between the Hydro Québec and cohorts included by Thériault et al. [31]. This analysis was based on about 1000 person-weeks of measurements of exposure to high frequency EM transients, 508 lung cancer cases, and 508 controls. A significant association was observed between the risk for lung cancer and cumulative exposure to ELF fields (OR = 3.1).

Miller et al. [37] also analyzed the risk for lung cancer in the Ontario Hydro cohort of Thériault et al. [31] (indicating that workers with exposure to power-frequency fields have less lung cancer than anticipated) in relation to exposure to both electric and magnetic fields. They reported an increase in lung cancer risk of 1.84, although this was statistically nonsignificant.

Researchers at the Medical Physics Research Centre of the Bristol University in the United Kingdom [61] have demonstrated the ability of electric field components of power frequency fields to attract and concentrate airborne radon progeny in their vicinity. Radioactive radon progeny atoms when formed rapidly attract water molecules in air growing into a so-called *ultrafine aerosol* around 10 nm in size. The possibility of increased lung cancer in relation to ELF field exposure constitutes one prediction from the Bristol observations.

Savitz et al. [62] reexamined the cohort from a study of five U.S. utilities of Savitz and Loomis [63]. As a result, no association was seen between the risk for lung cancer and exposure to 60 Hz magnetic fields.

4.3.6 Skin Cancer

Skin cancer is the most common type of cancer and accounts for half of all new cancers in Europe and the United States. Although anyone can get skin cancer, the risk is greatest for people who have fair skin that freckles easily—often those with red or blond hair and blue or light-colored eyes.

A number of studies of ELF fields and cancer have found indications for a skin cancer risk. Dr. Alan Preece and his group at Bristol University examined the incidence of cancer under power lines in Devon and Cornwall [64]. They have found a significant increase in skin cancer in persons living within a range of 20 meters of a power line. When Dr. Preece divided the population into areas with high and low indoor radon levels, the risk of skin cancer in persons living close to power lines in the high radon group was further increased.

4.3.7 Prostate Cancer

Prostate cancer is a common type of cancer in men. It is usually found in older men, and the risk of having prostate cancer increases with age. Prostate cancer is mainly found in men of 55 years and above. In this disease, cancer cells are first formed in the prostate and can then spread (metastasize) to other parts of the body, particularly bones and other selected structures.

Zhu et al. [65] conducted a prostate cancer study involving the use of electric blankets or heated waterbeds. They found that the incidence of prostate cancer was not significantly raised and there was no increase in risk with increased duration of exposure.

4.4 EPIDEMIOLOGICAL STUDIES—NONCANCER

Other than cancer, various studies have been carried out to investigate the health of people working or living near ELF sources. After screening available studies, the review concentrated on those concerning neurodegenerative diseases, CNS, cardiovascular functions, reproductive or pregnancy outcomes, etc.

4.4.1 Studies Relevant to Neurodegenerative Diseases

Alzheimer's Disease and Dementia

Alzheimer's disease (AD) is the most common age-related neurodegenerative disorder, which affects nearly 20 million people worldwide. German Physician

Alois Alzheimer described it in 1906 as a degenerative disorder that bears his name. It is a progressive, irreversible degenerative disease, which affects specific areas of brain usually in people over the age of 65. The diagnosis includes symptoms of *dementia* (loss of memory and mental function) and excludes other causes such as Parkinson's disease, head trauma, alcoholism, and stroke.

Regarding the causes of AD, several possibilities exist, including indirect genetic alterations initiated by exposure to EM fields. Significant increase in AD is supported by relevant epidemiological studies, which have been conducted in this regard. Sobel et al. [66-69] reported an association between occupations with EM field exposure and AD during the period 1994-1995 using three different clinical case-control series, two from Finland (University of Helsinki) and one from the United States (University of Southern California) involving 386 AD patients and 475 controls. The estimated ORs for men and women combined were 2.9, 3.1, and 3.0. Combining the data led to an OR estimate of 3.0. Also, the researchers studied the cases of 326 AD patients over the age of 65 who were hospitalized at the Alzheimer's Disease Treatment and Diagnostic Center, Rancho Los Amigos Medical Center in California, and compared them to 152 non-AD patients. They found males with AD were 4.9 times as likely to have had a high occupational exposure to fields, while females were 3.4 times as likely. Generally, these results indicate that people who were exposed to high exposure levels on the job (for example, sewing machine operators) have three to five times the normal risk of contracting the harmful disease of aging. The risk is also high for carpenters, electricians, electrical and electronic assemblers, and those who use electrically powered tools held close to their body.

Another case-control study of AD was conducted by Graves et al. [70]. Subjects were identified from a large health maintenance organization in Seattle, Washington, and matched by age, sex, and proxy type. A complete occupational history was obtained from proxies and controls. Exposures to EM fields were rated as probable intermittent exposure or probable exposure for extended periods to levels above threshold. The OR for having always been exposed to EM fields was 0.74. As a result, the researchers found no association between the disease and occupational exposure to EM fields.

Feychting et al. [71] examined exposure to magnetic fields in the population of a study of dementia among Swedish twins, in which twins in the Swedish Registry were screened for dementia by a complete clinical work-up, including neurological and neuropsychological assessments and neuroimaging. All 77 cases in this study were dementia, and 71% (55) were AD. Risk estimates were adjusted for age at onset, education, and birth date. The results indicate that occupational magnetic field exposure may possibly influence the development of dementia. The study provides weak support, primarily because of its small size.

It can be concluded that there could be moderate support for an association between occupations presumed to have resulted in elevated ELF fields and AD, with fairly less support for a direct association between the exposure and AD.

Amyotrophic Lateral Sclerosis

Amyotrophic lateral sclerosis (ALS) is a progressive and fatal neurological disease. It is an advancing degeneration of motor nerve cells in the brain (upper motor neurons) and spinal cord (lower motor neurons). When the motor neurons can no longer send impulses to the muscle, the muscle begins to waste away (atrophy) causing increased muscle weakness leading to paralysis. ALS does not damage a person's intellectual reasoning, vision, hearing, sense of taste and smell, and sexual, bowel, and bladder functions.

Deapen and Henderson [72] reported some findings that implicated electrical work in the development of ALS. Their orientation, however, was that a chemical exposure might be the causative agent.

In 1996, Davanipour et al. [73] reported increased risk of ALS associated with likely increased lifetime or average ELF occupational exposure. The authors used an expert classification based on job description and tasks for jobs occupied.

Depression and Suicide

Depression is a common illness that may affect anyone. It is more than feeling down or being sad. Depression is a medical disorder that affects thoughts, feelings, physical health, and daily behavior. Depression is a possible risk factor for suicide. The majority of studies that evaluate depression and suicide have, with a few exceptions, produced negative results.

Poole et al. [74] provided a moderate support for an association between depression and exposure to magnetic fields. Meanwhile, Verkasalo et al. [75] provided no support.

Baris et al. [76] reviewed the link between exposure to ELF fields and suicide. They used death certificate data for cases and controls. The researchers conducted a case-cohort study with individual specific data available, and therefore were able to control data for demographic variables, alcohol use, and mental disorders. Exposure was determined through occupational histories and estimated magnetic field levels. No association between the suicide and exposure to ELF fields was found.

A very large and detailed study conducted by Wijngaarden et al. [77] at the University of North Carolina has uncovered what appears to be a distinct association between exposure to ELF fields and suicide among electric utility workers. A group of 138,905 male U.S. electric utility workers from five companies were considered in the study. Electricians faced twice the expected risk of suicide. Linemen faced one-and-a-half times the expected risk. Meanwhile, suicides among power plant operators occurred at a rate slightly lower than expected.

4.4.2 Studies Relevant to Other Symptoms

Positive and negative associations between many symptoms and ELF exposure were reported in the literature. After screening available studies, the review concentrated on those concerning mainly the CNS, congenital malformations, and cardiovascular diseases.

An occupational study by Stopps and Janischewsky [78], in Canada examined a wide range of health problems and reported no significant effects on the CNS, cardiovascular function, or other physical functions.

In the United Kingdom, Broadbent et al. [79] observed no critical health risk from exposure of 287 power transmission workers.

Savitz et al. [80] reported the results of an analysis of mortality from specific types of cardiovascular disease in their study of five utilities [33] related to exposure to magnetic fields. The investigation motivated by clinical findings suggested a decrease in heart rate variability in people exposed to 20-μT, 60-Hz magnetic fields. Various categories of death causes from heart disease were combined into four groupings: arrhythmia-related (212 deaths), acute myocardial infarct (4238 deaths), atherosclerosis (142 deaths), and chronic coronary heart disease (2210 deaths). These causes accounted for 88% of all cardiovascular deaths identified in the cohort. The researchers found no link between exposure to magnetic fields and risk for atherosclerosis or chronic coronary heart disease.

4.4.3 Studies Relevant to VDTs

Over the years, research institutions as well as industries have conducted numerous studies to determine health hazards, which may exist from extended exposure to video display terminals (VDTs). The studies always assure that all kinds of VDTs, if manufactured according to existing guidelines and standards do not present a significant health hazard to the users. However, a wide array of opinions still exists on the subject of health hazards from VDTs.

Several physical and biophysical mechanisms are involved when humans are exposed to VDTs. Eyestrain, headaches, and blurred vision rank as the top three vision complaints associated with the use of VDTs. When a person stares at a computer screen for some time, his/her eye muscles become tired. Tired eye muscles leads to symptoms such as drying, burning, irritation, headache, blurred vision, dizziness, and even slight nausea. Although visual fatigue does not appear to have any serious consequences, a person with tired eyes is more likely to work at a slower pace and probably make more errors. It is also expected that VDT operators suffer from neck, back, wrist, and hand and shoulder pain, which doctors sometimes refer to as repetitive strain injuries. Psychological stress is also frequently expected.

There have been many epidemiological studies of individuals exposed to VDTs, but all studies have been limited by inadequate assessment of field exposure to the individual subjects. A few studies have dealt with effects on vision and the musculoskeletal system. Ocular studies of workers have not shown any relationship between VDT use and ophthalmologic disease or abnormalities, including cataracts [81-84].

Some studies were prompted when women who used VDTs during pregnancy reported several small clusters of miscarriages and birth defects. Higher miscarriage rates may have several explanations, which include field exposure, ergonomic factors, sitting for lengthy periods, and psychological stress related to job conditions. Interest was enhanced by reports that women who spent more time in front of VDTs had more miscarriages. In that regard, women receiving prenatal health care from a large health care group in California were interviewed to obtain data relating the amount of time spent in front of VDTs to the occurrence of miscarriages. The self-reported duration of daily VDT use was correlated with miscarriage frequency at OR of 1.8. Because miscarriage rates were not consistently affected within specific occupational categories, the validity of the association of VDTs and miscarriage is controversial [84].

A study by McDonald et al. [85] indicated a small risk, but the majority of studies that followed found that use of VDTs did not increase the risk of miscarriage, birth defects, or spontaneous abortion [86, 87].

A Finnish case-control study [88] by Lindbolm et al. examined the relationship between work with the VDT and spontaneous abortion, was conducted among women employed as bank clerks and clerical workers in three companies. They reported that women who miscarried at one of three companies were more likely to have used models of VDTs that could produce 50-Hz magnetic fields above 3 mG. As a result, the investigators did not find an overall link between miscarriage or birth defects and VDT use, nor was there a relationship between increased incidences of miscarriage and increasing fields.

A large study [89] at Yale focused on the effects of ELF exposure on the growth rate of the unborn child. The researchers obtained information about magnetic field exposure from power lines and home sources. It was found that VDT use over 20 hours a week did not affect the weight or growth rate of the baby, nor did the mother's exposure to higher magnetic fields or to high-field sources such as electrically heated beds.

4.4.4   Studies Relevant to Other Appliances

Electric appliances such as waterbeds, blankets, and other domestic equipment may have positive and negative impact on our life. Wertheimer and Leeper [90] investigated the relationship between utilization of electrically heated waterbeds and electric blankets and pregnancy outcome; especially, length of gestation, birth weight, congenital abnormalities, and fetal loss in Colorado. The study population consisted of 1806 (out of 4271) families in which a birth had occurred in two Denver-area hospitals in 1982, where birth announcement had been published. Seasonal patterns of occurrence of slow fetal development were observed among users of electric waterbeds and blankets, suggesting that use of such appliances at the time of conception might cause adverse health effects.

Dlugosz et al. [91] investigated a possible relationship between ELF fields from electric bed heaters and birth defects. They asked mothers of children born with cleft palate or neural tube defects if they had used an electric bed heater during the four months around the estimated date of conception of the child. A total of 663 case mothers were matched with a similar number of control women who had given birth to children without birth defects at approximately the same time. The comparison showed that mothers of children with birth defects were no more likely to have used an electric bed heater than other mothers.

Juutilainen et al. [92] conducted a case-control study on the association between loss in early pregnancy and domestic exposure to ELF fields in Finland. The study was nested within a cohort study of work and fertility in 443 healthy volunteer women who were trying to become pregnant over the period 1984-1986. For exposure classification, only average magnetic field strengths were associated with loss in early pregnancy.

No significant association was found between the incidence of spontaneous abortion and any measure of exposure to ELF fields from electric blankets. This finding was reported by Belanger et al. [93] on 135 spontaneous abortions that occurred in the same cohort between 7 and 25 weeks.

4.5   CONCLUDING REMARKS

Epidemiological studies have the advantage of providing information about human beings rather than cellular or animal studies. However, epidemiological studies have significant detailed limitations that arise, at least from the way the studies are carried out. Considering all the epidemiological evidence concerning ELF exposure, the conclusion is that there is no solid evidence linking electric and magnetic field exposure to cancer. Certainly the positive evidence for associated adverse effects have come from epidemiological studies, but the weaknesses, such as lack of reliable characteristics of the exposure source, lack of reliability of exposure data, and limited number of cases to look at effects, make it impossible to strongly prove this association. This level of evidence, although weak, is still enough to warrant limited concern. Therefore, epidemiological studies and statistical studies in general are quite important for hypothesis development, but they are not suitable for making conclusions.

Even if the epidemiological studies demonstrate a statistical association between ELF fields and health risks it does not mean those fields are the cause of disease. There may be additional factors that need to be considered in assessing any possible health effects. For example, populations as a whole are not genetically homogeneous and people may vary in their susceptibility to environmental hazards. In addition, epidemiology can only describe associations and may never prove the cause and effect. To establish links, it would be essential to have a systematic approach by which the fields implicated by the epidemiology interact with the living system. So far no such approach exists. The difficulty is that the encountered field levels and induced currents are very small; hence, it is difficult to say that any mechanism can depend entirely on the induced currents.

So far, a good number of studies have been conducted, but the results are not satisfying those who need a conclusive answer to the existence or absence of harmful effects. Considering the evidence now available, there are indications that the risk might exist. Although there is no theoretical or experimental basis to suggest this existence, the pervasive character of ELF fields in our environment makes it impossible to ignore even the most remote suggestion of such a hazard.

REFERENCES

[1]   Goldberg, R. B., The EMF Rapid Program Group Report Provides Comprehensive Assessment of Power-Frequency EMF Hazards, EMF Health Report 6, 1998.

[2]   Swanson, J., and D. C. Renew, Power-Frequency Fields and People, *Engineering Science and Education Journal*, pp. 71-79, 1994.

[3]   Becker, R. O., Microwave Radiation, *New York State Journal of Medicine* 77, p. 2172, 1977.

[4]   Zaret, M., Potential Hazards of Hertzian Radiation and Tumors, *New York State Journal of Medicine* 7, p. 146, 1977.

[5]   Hulbert, A. L., J. C. Metcalfe, and R. Hesketh, Biological Responses to Electromagnetic Fields, *The Federation of American Societies for Experimental Biology Journal* 12, pp. 395-420, 1998.

[6]   Moulder, J. E., and K. R. Foster, Is There a Link between Exposure to Power-Frequency Electric Fields and Cancer? *IEEE Engineering in Medicine and Biology* 18, pp. 109-116, 1999.

[7]   NIEHS Report on Health Effects from Exposure to Power-Line Frequency Electric and Magnetic Fields, National Institute of Environmental Health Sciences, National Institutes of Health, Research Triangle Park, NC, 1999.

[8] Cherry, N., Evidence that Electromagnetic Fields from High Voltage Powerlines and in Buildings, are Hazardous to Human Health, Especially to Young Children, Lincoln University, New Zealand, 2001.

[9] Poole, C., and D. Ozonoff, Magnetic Fields and Childhood Cancers, *IEEE Engineering in Medicine and Biology* 15, pp. 41-49, 1996.

[10] Cartwright, R., Childhood Leukaemia and Electromagnetic Fields-The Epidemiological Studies, *Electromagnetics Meeting*, Bristol, UK, 24-25 September 1998.

[11] Wertheimer, N., and E. Leeper, Electrical Wiring Configurations and Childhood Cancer, *American Journal of Epidemiology* 109, pp. 273-284, 1979.

[12] Fulton, J. T., S. Cobb, L. Prevle, L. Leone, and E. Forman, Electrical Wiring Configurations and Childhood Leukemia in Rhode Island, *American Journal of Epidemiology* 111, p. 292, 1980.

[13] Savitz, D. A., Case-Control Study of Childhood Cancer and Residential Exposure to Electric and Magnetic Fields, Contractor's Final Report, New York State Power Lines Project Contract 218217, March 30, 1987.

[14] Savitz, D. A., H. Wachtel, F. A. Barnes, E. M. John, and J. G. Tvrdik, Case-Control Study of Childhood Cancer and Exposure to 60 Hz Magnetic Fields, *American Journal of Epidemiology* 128, pp. 21-38, 1988.

[15] Savitz, D. A., and W. T. Kaune, Childhood Cancer in Relation to a Modified Residential Wire Code, *Environmental Health Prospect* 10, pp. 76-80, 1993.

[16] London, S. J., D. C. Thomas, J. D. Bowman, E. Sobel, T. S. Chen, and J. M. Peters, Exposure to Residential Electric and Magnetic Fields and Risk of Childhood Leukemia, *American Journal of Epidemiology* 134, pp. 923-937, 1991.

[17] Bowman, J., D. Thomas, S. London, and J. Peters, Hypothesis: The Risk of Childhood Leukemia is Related to Combinations of Power-Frequency and Static Magnetic Fields, *Bioelectromagnetics* 16, pp. 48-59, 1995.

[18] Feychting, M., and A. Ahlbom, Magnetic Fields and Cancer in Children Residing Near Swedish High-Voltage Power Lines, *American Journal of Epidemiology* 38, pp. 467-481, 1993.

[19] Olsen, J. H., A. Nielsen, and G. Schulgen, Residence Near High-Voltage Facilities and the Risk of Cancer in Children, *British Medical Journal* 307, pp. 891-895, 1993.

[20] Verkasalo, P. K., E. Pukkala, M. Y. Hongisto, J. E. Vajus, P. J. Jarvinen, K. V. Heikkila, and M. Koskenvuo, Risk of Cancer in Finnish Children Living Close to Power Lines, *British Medical Journal* 307, pp. 895-899, 1993.

[21] Kraut, A., R. Tate, and N. Tran, Residential Electric Consumption and Childhood Cancer in Canada (1971-1986), *Archives of Environmental Health* 49, Department of Community Health Sciences, pp. 156-159, University of Manitoba, Winnipeg, MB, 1994.

[22] Possible Health Effects of Exposure to Residential Electric and Magnetic Fields, National Academy of Sciences, Commission on Life Sciences, National Research Council, National Academy Press, Washington, DC, 1997.

[23] Linet, M. S., E. E. Hatch, R. A. Kleinerman, L. L. Robison, W. T. Kaune, D. R. Friedman, R. K. Severson, C. M. Haines, C. T. Hartsock, S. Niwa, S. Wacholder, and R. E. Tarone, Residential Exposure to Magnetic Fields and Acute Lymphoblastic Leukemia in Children, *The New England Journal of Medicine* 337,

pp. 1-7, 1997.

[24] Hatch, E. H., M. S. Linet, R. A. Kleinerman, R. E. Tarone, R. K. Severson, C. T. Hartsock, C. Haines, W. T. Kaune, D. Friedman, L. L. Robison, and S. Wacholder, Association Between Childhood Acute Lymphoblastic Leukemia and Use of Electrical Appliances During Pregnancy and Childhood, *Epidemiology* 19, pp. 234-245, 1998.

[25] Tynes, T., and T. Haldorsen, Electromagnetic Fields and Cancer in Children Residing Near Norwegian High-Voltage Power Lines, *American Journal of Epidemiology* 145, pp. 219-226, 1997.

[26] Michaelis, J., J. Schüz, R. Meinert, E. Zemann, J. –P. Grigat, P. Kaatsch, U. Kaletsch, A. Miesner, K. Brinkmann, W. Kalkner, and H. Kärner, Combined Risk Estimates for Two German Population-Based Case-Control Studies on Residential Magnetic Fields and Childhood Acute Leukemia, *Epidemiology* 9, pp. 92-94, 1998.

[27] Li, C. -Yi, W. Lee, and R. S. Lin, Risk of Leukemia in Children Living Near High-Voltage Transmission Lines, *Journal of Occupational and Environmental Medicine* 40, pp. 144-147, 1998.

[28] McBride, M. L., R. P. Gallagher, G. Thériault, B. G. Armstrong, S. Tamaro, J. J. Spinelli, J. E. Deadman, B. Fincham, D. Robson, and W. Chaoi, Power-Frequency Electric and Magnetic Fields and Risk of Childhood Leukemia in Canada, *American Journal of Epidemiology* 149, pp. 831-842, 1999.

[29] Green, L. M., A. B. Miller, D. A. Agnew, M. L. Greenberg, J. Li, P. J. Villeneuve, and R. Tibshirani, Childhood Leukemia and Personal Monitoring of Residential Exposures to Electric and Magnetic Fields in Ontario, Canada, *Cancer Causes and Control* 10, pp. 233-243, 1999.

[30] Sahl, J. D., M. A. Kelsh, and S. Greenland, Cohort and Nested Case-Control Studies of Hematopoietic Cancers and Brain Cancer Among Electric Utility Workers, *Epidemiology* 4, pp. 104-114, 1993.

[31] Matanoski, G. M., E. A. Elliott, P. N. Breysse, and M. C. Lynberg, Leukemia in Telephone Linemen, American *Journal of Epidemiology* 137, pp. 609-619, 1993.

[32] Theriault, G., M. Goldberg, A. B. Miller, B. Armstrong, P. Guenel, J. Deadman, E. Imbernon, T. To, A. Chevalier, D. Cyr, and C. Wall, Cancer Risks Associated with Occupational Exposure to Magnetic Fields Among Electric Utility Workers in Ontario and Quebec, Canada, and France: 1970-1989, *American Journal of Epidemiology* 139, pp. 550-572, 1994.

[33] Savitz, D. A., and D. P. Loomis, Magnetic Field Exposure in Relation to Leukemia and Brain Cancer Mortality Among Electric Utility Workers, *American Journal of Epidemiology* 141, pp. 123-134, 1995.

[34] Floderus, B., T. Persson, and C. Stenlund, Magnetic Field Exposure in the Workplace: Reference Distributions and Exposures in Occupational Groups, *International Journal of Occupational and Environmental Health* 2, pp. 226-238. 1996.

[35] Feychting, M., U. Forssen, and B. Floderus, Occupational and Residential Magnetic Field Exposure and Leukemia and Central Nervous System Tumors, *Epidemiology* 8, pp. 384-389, 1997.

[36] Johansen, C., and J. Olsen, Risk of Cancer Among Danish Utility Workers-A Nationwide Cohort Study, *American Journal of Epidemiology* 147, pp. 548-555,

1998.

[37] Miller, A. B., T. To, D. A. Agnew, C. Wall, and L. M. Green, Leukemia Following Occupational Exposure to 60 Hz Electric and Magnetic Fields Among Ontario Electricity Utility Workers, *American Journal of Epidemiology* 144, pp. 150-160, 1996.

[38] Villeneuve, P., D. A. Agnew, A. B. Miller, P. Coery, and J. Purdham, Leukemia in Electric Utility Workers: The Evaluation of Alternative Indices of Exposure to 60 Hz Electric and Magnetic Fields, *American Journal of Industrial Medicine* 37, pp. 607-617, 2000.

[39] Floderus, B., T. Persson, C. Stenlund, A. Wennberg, A. Ost, and B. Knave, Occupational Exposure to Electromagnetic Fields in Relation to Leukemia and Brain Tumors, A Case-Control Study in Sweden, *Cancer Causes and Control* 4, pp. 465-476, 1993.

[40] Floderus B., S. Tornqvist, and C. Stenlund, Incidence of Selected Cancers in Swedish Railway Workers, 1961-1979, *Cancer Causes and Control* 5, pp. 189-194, 1994.

[41] Sahl, J. D., M. A. Kelsh, and S. Greenland, Cohort and Nested Case-Control Studies of Hematopoietic Cancers and Brain Cancer Among Electric Utility Workers, *Epidemiology* 4, pp. 104-114, 1993.

[42] Wilkins, J. R., and L. C. Wellage, Brain Tumor Risk in Offspring of Men Occupationally Exposed to Electric and Magnetic Fields, *Scandinavian Journal of Work and Environmental Health* 22, pp. 339-345, 1996.

[43] Harrington, J. M., D. I. McBride, T. Sorahan, G. M. Paddle, and M. Van Tongeren, Occupational Exposure to Magnetic Fields in Relation to Mortality from Brain Cancer Among Electricity Generation and Transmissions Workers, *Occupational and Environmental Medicine* 54, pp. 7-13, 1997.

[44] Guenel, P., J. Nicolau, E. Inbernon, A. Chevalier, and M. Goldberg, Exposure to 50-Hz Electric Field and Incidence of Leukemia, Brain Tumors, and Other Cancers Among French Utility Workers, *American Journal of Epidemiology* 144, pp. 1107-1121, 1996.

[45] Rodvall, Y., C. Stenlund, A. Ahlbom, S. Preston-Martin, and T. Lindh, Occupational Exposure to Magnetic Fields and Brain Tumors in Central Sweden, *European Journal of Epidemiology* 14, pp. 563-569, 1998.

[46] Kheifets, L. I., E. S. Gilbert, S. S. Sussman, P. Guenel, J. D. Sahl, D. A. Savitz, and G. Theriault, Comparative Analyses of the Studies of Magnetic Fields and Cancer in Electric Utility Workers: Studies from France, Canada, and the United States, *Occup. Environ. Med.* 56, pp. 567-574, 1999.

[47] Stevens, R. G., Electric Power Use and Breast Cancer: A Hypothesis, *American Journal of Epidemiology* 125, pp. 556-561, 1987.

[48] Tynes T., and A. Andersen, Electromagnetic Fields and Male Breast Cancer, *The Lancet*, p. 1596, 1990.

[49] Tynes, T., A. Andersen, and B. Langmark, Incidence of Cancer in Norwegian Workers Potentially Exposed to Electromagnetic Fields, *American Journal of Epidemiology* 136, pp. 81-86, 1992.

[50] Demers, P. A., D. B. Thomas, K. A. Rosenblatt, L. M. Jiminez, A. McTiernan, H. Stalsberg, A. Stemhagen, W. D. Thompson, M. Curnen, A. Satariano, D. F. Austin,

P. Isacson, R. S. Greenberg, C. Key, L. Kolonel, and D. West, Occupational Exposure to Electromagnetic Radiation and Breast Cancer in Males, *American Journal of Epidemiology* 134, pp. 340-347, 1991.

[51] Matanoski, G. M., P. N. Breysse, and E. A. Elliott, Electromagnetic Field Exposure and Male Breast Cancer, *The Lancet*, p. 337, 1991.

[52] Floderus, B., T. Persson, C. Stenlund, A. Wennberg, A. Ost, and B. Knave, Occupational Exposure to Electromagnetic Fields in Relation to Leukemia and Brain Tumors: A Case-Control Study in Sweden, *Cancer Causes and Control* 4, pp. 465-476, 1993.

[53] Feychting, M., U. Forssen, L. E. Rutqvist, and A. Ahlbom, Magnetic Fields and Breast Cancer in Swedish Adults Residing Near High-Voltage Power Lines, *Epidemiology* 9, pp. 392-397, 1998.

[54] Coogan, P. F., R. W. Clapp, P. A. Newcomb, T. B. Wenzl, G. Bogdan, R. Mittendorf, J. A. Baron, and M. P. Longnecker, Occupational Exposure to 60-Hertz Magnetic Fields and Risk of Breast Cancer in Woman, *Epidemiology* 7, pp. 459-464, 1996.

[55] Verkasalo, P. K., Magnetic Fields and Leukemia Risk for Adults Living Close to Power Lines, *Scandinavian Journal of Work, Environment and Health* 22, pp. 1-56, 1996.

[56] Gammon, M. D., J. B. Schoenberg, J. A. Britton, J. L. Kelsey, J. L. Stanford, K. E. Malone, R. J. Coates, D. J. Brogan, N. Potischman, C. A. Swanson, and L. A. Brinton, Electric Blanket Use and Breast Cancer Risk Among Younger Women, *American Journal of Epidemiology* 148, pp. 556-563, 1998.

[57] Petralia, S. A., W. H. Chow, J. McLaughlin, F. Jin, Y. T. Gao, and M. Dosemeci, Occupational Risk Factors for Breast Cancer Among Women in Shanghai, *American Journal of Industrial Medicine* 34, pp. 477-483, 1998.

[58] Forssén, U. M., M. Feychting, L. E. Rutqvist, B. Floderus, and A. Ahlbom, Occupational and Residential Magnetic Field Exposure and Breast Cancer in Females, *Epidemiology* 11, pp. 24-29, 2000.

[59] Erren, T. C., Association between Exposure to Pulsed Electromagnetic Fields and Cancer in Electric Utility Workers in Quebec, Canada, and France, *American Journal of Epidemiology* 143, p. 841, 1996.

[60] Armstrong, B., G. Thériault, P. Guénel, J. Deadman, M. Goldberg, and P. Heroux, Association between Exposure to Pulsed Electromagnetic Fields and Cancer in Electric Utility Workers in Quebec, Canada, and France, *American Journal of Epidemiology* 140, pp. 805-820, 1994.

[61] Henshaw, D. L., A. N. Ross, A. P. Fews, and A. W. Preece, Enhanced Deposition of Radon Daughter Nuclei in the Vicinity of Power Frequency Electromagnetic Fields, *International Journal of Radiation Biology* 69, pp. 25-38, 1996.

[62] Savitz, D. A., V. Dufort, B. Armstrong, and G. Thériault, Lung Cancer in Relation to Employment in the Electrical Utility Industry and Exposure to Magnetic Fields, *Occupational and Environmental Medicine* 54, pp. 396-402, 1997.

[63] Savitz, D. A., and D. P. Loomis, Magnetic Field Exposure in Relation to Leukemia and Brain Cancer Mortality Among Electric Utility Workers, *American Journal of Epidemiology* 141, pp. 123-134, 1995.

[64] Preece, A. W., G. R. Iwi, and D. J. Etherington, Radon, Skin Cancer and Interaction

with Power Lines, *US Department of Energy Contractors Review Meeting*, San Antonio, Texas, 17-21 November, 1996.

[65] Zhu, K., N. S. Weiss, J. L. Stanford, J. R. Daling, A. Stergachis, B. McKnight, M. K. Brawer, and R. S. Levine, Prostate Cancer in Relation to the Use of Electric Blanket or Heated Water Bed, *Epidemiology* 10, pp. 83-85, 1998.

[66] Sobel, E., Z. Davanipour, R. Sulkava, T. Erkinjuntti, J. Wikstrom, V. W. Henderson, G. Buckwalter, J. D. Bowman, and P. –J. Lee, Occupations with Exposure to Electromagnetic Fields: A Possible Risk Factor for Alzheimer's Disease, *American Journal of Epidemiology* 142, pp. 515-524, 1995.

[67] Sobel, E. and Z. Davanipour, Electromagnetic Field Exposure may Cause Increased Production of Amyloid Beta and may Eventually Lead to Alzheimer's Disease, *Neurology* 47, pp. 1594-1600, 1996.

[68] Sobel, E., M. Dunn, Z. Davanipour, Z. Qian, and H. C. Chui, Elevated Risk of Alzheimer's Disease Among Workers with Likely Electromagnetic Field Exposure, *Neurology*, 1997.

[69] Sobel, E., Neurodegenerative Diseases and EMF Exposure, *Electromagnetics Meeting*, Bristol, 24-25 September 1998.

[70] Graves, A. B., D. Rosner, D. Echeverria D, M. Yost, and E. B. Larson, Occupational Exposure to Electromagnetic Fields and Alzheimer Disease, *Alzheimer Disorder Association* 13, pp. 165-170, 1999.

[71] Feychting, M., N. Pedersen, P. Svedberg, B. Floderus, and M. Gatz, Dementia and Occupational Exposure to Magnetic Fields, *Scandinavian Journal of Work, Environment and Health* 24, pp. 46-53, 1998.

[72] Deapen, D. M., and B. E. Hendersen, A Case-Control Study of Amyotrophic Lateral Sclerosis, *American Journal of Epidemiology* 123, pp. 790-799, 1986.

[73] Davanipour, Z., E. Sobel, J. D. Bowman, Z. Qian, and A. D. Will, Amyotrophic Lateral Sclerosis and Occupational Exposure to Electromagnetic Fields, *Bioelectromagnetics* 18, pp. 28-35, 1997.

[74] Poole, C., R. Kavet, D. P. Funch, K. Donelan, J. M. Charry, and N. Dreyer, Depressive Symptoms and Headaches in Relation to Proximity of Residence to Alternating Current Transmission Line Right of Way, *American Journal of Epidemiology* 137, pp. 318-330, 1993.

[75] Verkasalo, P. K., J. Kaprio J. Varjonen, K. Romanov, K. Heikkila, and M. Koskenvuo, Magnetic Fields of Transmission Lines and Depression, *American Journal of Epidemiology* 146, pp. 1037-1045, 1997.

[76] Baris, D., B. G. Armstrong, J. Deadman, and G. Thériault, A Case-Cohort Study of Suicide in Relation to Exposure to Electric and Magnetic Fields Among Electrical Utility Workers, *Occupational and Environmental Medicine* 53, pp. 17-24, 1996.

[77] Wijngaarden, E., D. A. Savitz, R. T. C. Kleckner, J. Cai, and D. Loomis, Exposure to Electromagnetic Fields and Suicide Among Electric Utility Workers: A Nest Case-Control Study, *Occupational and Environmental Medicine* 57, pp. 258-263, 2000.

[78] Stopps, G. J., and W. Janischewsky, Epidemiological Study of Workers Maintaining HV Equipment and Transmission Lines in Ontario, Research Report, Canadian Electrical Association, Montreal, Canada, 1997.

[79] Broadbent, D. E., M. H. P. Broadbent, J. C. Male, and M. R. L. Jones, Health of

Workers Exposed to Electric Fields, *British Journal of Industrial Medicine* 42, pp. 75-84, 1985.

[80] Savitz, D. A., D. Liao, A. Sastre, and R. C. Kleckner, Magnetic Field Exposure and Cardiovascular Disease Mortality Among Electric Utility Workers, *American Journal of Epidemiology* 149, pp. 135-142, 1999.

[81] Boos, S. R., B. M. Calissendorff, B. G. Knave, K. G. Nyman, and M. Voss, Work with Video Display Terminals Among Office Employees. III. Ophthalmologic Factors, *Scand. J. Work Environ. Health* 11, pp. 475-481, 1985.

[82] Ong, C. N., S. E. Chia, J. Jeyaratnam, and K. C. Tan, Musculoskeletal Disorders Among Operators of Visual Display Terminal, *Scandinavian Journal of Work, Environment and Health* 21, pp. 60-64, 1995.

[83] Bonomi, L., and R. Bellucci, Consideration of the Ocular Pathology in 30,000 Personnel of the Italian Telephone Company (SIP) Using VDTs, *Bollettion Di Oculistica* 68(S7), pp. 85-98, 1989.

[84] Goldhaber, M. K., and M. R. Polen, The Risk of Miscarriage and Birth Defects Among Women Who Use Visual Display Terminals During Pregnancy, *American Journal of Industrial Medicine* 13, pp. 695-706, 1988.

[85] McDonald, A. D., J. C. McDonald, B. Armstrong, N. Cherry, A. D. Nolin, and D. Robert, Work with Visual Display Units in Pregnancy, *British Journal of Industrial Medicine* 45, pp. 509-515, 1988.

[86] Ericson, A., and B. Kallen, An Epidemiological Study of Work with Video Screens and Pregnancy Outcome: II. A Case-Control Study, *American Journal of Industrial Medicine* 9, pp. 459-475, 1986.

[87] Schnorr, T. M., B. A. Grajewski, R. W. Hornung, M. J. Thun, G. M. Egeland, W. E. Murray, D. L. Conover, and W. E. Halperin, Video Display Terminals and the Risk of Spontaneous Abortion, *The New England Journal of Medicine* 324, pp. 727-733, 1991.

[88] Lindbolm, M. L., M. Hietanen, P. Kryonen, M. Sallmen, P. Von Nandelstadh, H. Taskinen, M. Pekkarinen, M. Ylikoski, and K. Hemminki, Magnetic Fields of Video Display Terminals and Spontaneous Abortion, *American Journal of Epidemiology* 136, pp. 1041-1051, 1992.

[89] Bracken, M. B., K. Belanger, K. Hellenbrand, L. Dlugosz, T. R. Holford, J. E. McSharry, K. Addesso, and B. Leaderer, Exposure to Electromagnetic Fields During Pregnancy with Emphasis on Electrically Heated Beds: Association with Birth Weight and Intrauterine Growth Retardation, *Epidemiology* 6, pp. 263-270, 1995.

[90] Wertheimer, N., and E. Leeper, Possible Effects of Electric Blankets and Heated Waterbeds on Fetal Development, *Bioelectromagnetics* 7, pp. 13-22, 1986.

[91] Dlugosz, L., J. Vena, T. Byers, L. Sever, M. Bracken, and E. Marshall, Congetial Defects and Electric Bed Heating in New York State: A Register-Based Case-Control Study, *American Journal of Epidemiology* 135, pp. 1000-1011, 1992.

[92] Juutilainen, J., P. Matilainen, S. Saarikoski, E. Laara, and S. Suonio, Early Pregnancy Loss and Exposure to 50 Hz Magnetic Fields, *Bioelectromagnetics* 14, pp. 229-236, 1993.

[93] Belanger, K., B. Leaderer, K. Kellenbrand, T. Holford, J. -E. McSharry, M. -E. Power, and M. Bracken, Spontaneous Abortion and Exposure to Electric Blankets and Heated Water Beds, *Epidemiology* 9, pp. 36-42, 1998.

5

Regulatory Activities and Safety Trends

5.1 INTRODUCTION

Can electric and magnetic fields that are created by devices that use, carry, or produce electricity cause health hazards? This is one of the more controversial questions looming in the mind of the scientific community today. It has caused much public concern, which largely dates to 1979, when epidemiologists Wertheimer and Leeper [1] reported a link between childhood leukemia and the proximity of residences to certain types of power lines in Denver, Colorado [see Section 4.3 for more details]. In the years following, numerous studies have produced contradictory results, but yet a few experts believe that the threat is still there.

It is perhaps understandable why many national and international regulatory agencies have found it difficult to set accurate protection guidelines for maximum human exposure levels to ELF fields. Accordingly, the authorities are still unable to tell the public for sure whether or not ELF exposure is safe. Although the possibility of risk exists, it may not be considered established since it is not biologically creditable.

Today, most scientists agree that more research and investigation is needed. There is insufficient data to determine whether specific types of exposure are riskier than other types, or whether they may be risky for certain groups of people whose normal compensating processes do not function properly.

An increasing number of scientists have accepted ELF fields as a proven health risk within certain levels higher than those available in the environment— A fact that urges keeping exposure levels under recommended limits.

131

5.2   SAFETY STANDARDS

The concept of *safety* or *safety standard* needs closer examination. The expression "safety standard" means an accepted level that is free from hazard. The development of safety standards presuppose the following [2]:

1.   Identification of the hazard.
2.   Selection of the level that produces an environment free from the hazard.

Practically, the better the hazard is understood, the sooner the safety standard is identified. A safety limit indicates that below a threshold, an EM field level is safe according to the available scientific knowledge. The safety limit is not an exact line between safety and hazard, but a possible risk to human health constantly increases with higher exposure level. The stumbling block for the regulatory agencies setting standards for both residential and occupational environments has been a lack of recognized interaction mechanisms showing how such low-level EM fields could possibly affect biological processes.

5.2.1   Early Worldwide Standards

Emphasis on the ELF portion of the electromagnetic spectrum as well as the RFR portion over the past thirty years resulted in introducing many safety standards. The USSR established the earliest exposure guideline for the ELF portion of the spectrum in 1975. However, the standard that is most relevant to use is the consensus standard, which was composed by the Institute of Electrical and Electronic Engineers (IEEE) in 1991 [2]. The American National Standards Institute (ANSI) approved this standard in 1992 as ANSI C95.1-1992. The ANSI/IEEE standard recommends that exposure averaged over any six-minute period and over a cross section of the human body should not exceed 0.614 kV/m for the electric field and 163 A/m (205 µT) for the magnetic field. The ANSI/IEEE standard is designed to keep the induced current in human body at least of ten below the lowest reported stimulation thresholds for electrically excitable cells. The current standard is less stringent than the 1982 version of the standard (ANSI C95.1-1982). More details are discussed in Chapter 10.

Besides the ANSI/IEEE standard, there are other worldwide institutions and organizations that have recommended ELF exposure limits, even stricter than the limits suggested in the ANSI/IEEE standard. Among these are the Australian Radiation Laboratory (ARL) and the National Health and Medical Research Council (NH & MRC), the Canadian health regulations [3], the Commonwealth of Massachusetts labor regulations [4], the Federal Republic of Germany (FRG) [5], the North Atlantic Treaty Organization (NATO) [6], the United States Air

Table 5-1   Standards and Guidelines Limits for Magnetic Field Exposure

Institution/Country	Level (μT)*	
	Occupational	General Public
ANSI/IEEEE (1991)	205	205
Australia: NH & MRC (1989)	500	100
Canada (1989)	5.01	2.26
Comm. of Massachusetts (1986)	1.99	-
FRG (1986)	314	314
NATO (1979)	3.27	-
USAF (1987)	1.99	1.99
USSR (1985)	1760	-

* 0.1 μT = 1 mG.

Force (USAF) [7], and the USSR. These exposure limits are given in Table 5-1.

5.2.2 ELF Standards in Europe

The Swedish Standards

Sweden has been a leader in developing recommended visual ergonomic and electromagnetic emission standards for computer displays. The Swedish standards are basically different from the standards developed by the agencies discussed in 5.2.1. Two prominent measurement and emission guidelines for monitors have emerged during the past few years. One, known as MPR II, prescribes limits on electric and magnetic field emissions in the ELF and VLF ranges, as well as electrostatic fields. A recent and more restrictive standard, promoted by a major Swedish union, limits monitor emissions also, and was expanded in 1995 to address the entire computer.

MPR-I

The National Board on Occupational Safety and Health and the Swedish Radiation Protection Institute, MPR (Mät-och Provningsrådet), were given the task to investigate the need for requirements and consequences of the introduction of compulsory or obligatory testing of video display terminals (VDTs). In 1987, a nonmandatory testing procedure for VDTs was introduced.

The method, called MPR-I, specified a maximum of 50 nT (0.5 mG) of peak VLF magnetic field strength in the 1-400 kHz range at 50 cm from the front of the screen. The full test procedure called for 16 measurements taken on 5 horizontal planes at 22.5-degree intervals all around the display units for a total of 80 measurements in all [8].

MPR-II

MPR-I was recognized as too cumbersome and difficult to evaluate. Therefore, another committee was formed to set up new recommendations. On July 1991, the new test methods, called MPR-II, specified less than 2.5 mG RMS of ELF magnetic emissions in the 5 Hz to 2 kHz range (band 1) and less than 0.25 mG RMS of VLF magnetic emissions in the 2 kHz to 400 kHz range (band 2). The number of measurements was fixed to 48 for each band taken at 50 cm starting from the front of the screen and every 22.5-degree all around the display (16 points) on each of three horizontals planes 25-cm apart.

MPR-II provides guidelines for visual ergonomics (such as focus, jitter, and character distortion), X-ray, electrostatic potential, electrostatic discharge, and AC electric fields [9, 10].

TCO

Many major manufacturers of computer displays have embraced the Swedish guidelines. However, the Swedish Confederation of Professional Employees, or TCO, which represents over a million workers, requested more restrictive limits and test protocols as low as 2 mG for ELF magnetic fields at 30 cm from the front of the screen and 50 cm around the monitor. Their justification is that levels above 2 mG have been linked to increased risks of cancer, and that VDT users' heads, hands and/or breasts are often closer than 50 cm from the screen. TCO published its own series of guidelines: TCO'90, TCO'92, TCO'95, and TCO'99, which in reality are a copy of MPR-II with some adjustment [11, 12]. In addition, recent TCO guidelines include guidelines for energy consumption, screen flicker, luminance, and keyboard use. Table 5-2 shows the emission limits recommended by both MPR-II and TCO.

A number of experts have questioned the validity of 0.25 mG for VLF fields, pointing out that VLF fields contain more energy than ELF fields. These experts say if induction levels are used to measure the amount of energy in the radiation, then 2.5 mG of ELF fields is equal to 0.01 mG of VLF fields. The answer is the nonexistence of proven biological reason for limiting ELF fields.

Table 5-2 Swedish Limits by MPR-II and TCO

Frequency Range	MPR II	TCO
Electric Fields		
Static fields	+/-500 V	+/-500 V
ELF (5 Hz-2 kHz)	</=25 V/m	</=10 V/m
VLF (2 kHz-400 kHz)	</=2.5 V/m	</=1 V/m
Above 400 kHz	none	none
Magnetic Fields		
ELF (5 Hz-2 kHz)	</=2.5 mG	</=2.0 mG
VLF (2 kHz-400 kHz)	</=0.25 mG	</=0.25 mG
Above 400 kHz	none	none

United Kingdom

In the United Kingdom, the National Radiological Protection Board (NRPB) started providing guidance on restrictions to the exposure of people to EM fields. The NRPB was created by the Radiological Protection Act 1970. The NRPB aims to advance the acquisition of knowledge about the protection of mankind from ionizing and nonionizing radiation hazards. It provides information and advice to persons (including government departments) with responsibilities in the U.K. in relation to the protection from radiation hazards either of the community as a whole or of particular sections of the community.

The NRPB fixed its exposure guidelines for 50/60 Hz fields on the same basis as the IRPA committee in fixing its interim guidelines. The recommended NRPB guidelines are same for occupational and public environments. The field levels are 1600 μT and 1330 μT for 50 Hz and 60 Hz, respectively. They are associated with large-scale induced currents in the body and are not relevant to the public concern about cancer and other possible health effects. Table 5-3 gives the NRPB exposure guidelines.

Germany

A basic precautionary limit has been used in German legislation to derive maximum limits for electric and magnetic field strengths at a frequency of 50 Hz. These values are legally binding under the provisions of the 26th Ordinance [13], in force since 1st January 1997, regulating the Federal Pollution Control Law.

Table 5-3 NRPB ELF Exposure Guidelines

Frequency	Electric Field kV/m	Magnetic Field μT
50 Hz	12	1600
60 Hz	10	1330

The limits for electric and magnetic fields for transformation and transmission of electricity at a voltage of 1000 V or more are 5 kV/m and 100 μT (50 Hz); and 10 kV/m and 300 μT (16 2/3 Hz), respectively. Under certain circumstances, the limits for magnetic flux density may by exceeded by 100% for a short duration, and electric field strength may be exceeded by 100% within a small area.

5.2.3   Guidelines in the United States

Currently, there are no federal governmental standards for exposure to 60 Hz electric and magnetic fields in the United States. However, a few states have set protection guidelines for electric fields near rights-of-way (ROW) (land around power lines). Only two states (New York and Florida) have fixed magnetic field guidelines, which range from 150 to 250 mG at the edge of utilities' ROW. The guidelines were set up to ensure that future power lines do not exceed current ELF field levels. They are not pledged to be health-based standards. Other states have resisted the temptation to set limits, because of the risk uncertainty. Table 5-4 summarizes the state power-line ELF electric field guidelines. Further, Table 5-5 gives the power-line magnetic field guidelines in New York and Florida.

ACGIH Standard

The independent National Conference of Governmental Industrial Hygienists (NCGIH) convened on June 27, 1938, in Washington, D.C., with 76 members, representing 24 states, 3 cities, 1 university, the U.S. Public Health Service, the U.S. Bureau of Mines, and the Tennessee Valley Authority. In 1946, the organization changed its name to the American Conference of Governmental Industrial Hygienists (ACGIH) and offered full membership to all industrial hygiene personnel within the agencies as well as to governmental industrial hygiene professionals in other countries. The ACGIH develops the threshold limit

Table 5-4   ELF Electric Field Guidelines for Some States in the United States

State	Electric Field	
	ROW	Edge of ROW
Florida	8 kV/m[1]	2 kV/m
	10 kV/m[2]	
Minnesota	8 kV/m	
Montana	7 kV/m[3]	1 kV/m
New Jersey		3 kV/m
New York	11.8 kV/m	1.6 kV/m
	11 kV/m[4]	
	7 kV/m[3]	
Oregon	9 kV/m	

[1] For double-circuit lines (69-230 kV).
[2] For single-circuit 500-kV lines.
[3] Maximum for highway crossings.
[4] For 500-kV lines on certain existing ROW.

Table 5-5   ELF Magnetic Field Guidelines for New York and Florida

State	Magnetic Field at the Edge of ROW
Florida	150 mG[1]
	200 mG[2]
	250 mG[3]
New York	200 mG[4]

[1] For double-circuit lines (69-230 kV).
[2] For single-circuit 500-kV lines.
[3] For 500-kV lines on certain existing ROW.
[4] For lines greater than 230 kV.

values (TLVs) and biological exposure indices (BEIs) on chemical substances and physical agents to which humans might be exposed in the workplace. The TLV is 614 V/m for electric field strength over the frequency range 30-3000 kHz and 205 μT for magnetic flux density over the frequency range 30-100 kHz. With

Table 5-6 ACGIH 60 Hz Occupational Exposure Guidelines

Frequency 60 Hz	Electric Field kV/m	Magnetic Field G
Limits	25	10
Workers with cardiac pacemakers	1 or below	1

respect to ELF exposure at 60 Hz only, the ACGIH guidelines are illustrated in Table 5-6 [14, 15].

5.2.4   ICNIRP Standard

In 1989, the International Radiation Protection Association (IRPA) approved interim ELF fields exposure guidelines prepared by its International Commission on Non-Ionizing Radiation Protection (ICNIRP) [see Table 5-7] [16-18]. These guidelines were a result of cooperation with the World Health Organization (WHO) and the United Nations Environment Program (UNEP). The guidelines are intended to prevent effects, such as induced currents in cells or nerve stimulations, which are known to occur at high magnitudes, much higher than levels found typically in occupational and residential environments.

It is significant to note that these guidelines were only designed to avoid immediate high-level hazards and do not consider prolonged low-level exposures. In April 1998, the ICNIRP published revised guidelines for limiting exposure to EM fields [19]. For the general public, the exposure standard is 100 µT at 50 Hz and 84 µT at 60 Hz. However, for occupational exposures the standard is 500 µT at 50 Hz and 420 µT at 60 Hz.

Several institutions have criticized the guidelines as lacking clear interpretation on exposure safety or direct application to equipment in use. Concerns have been expressed about the use of safety factors, precautionary aspects, and long-term exposure. Accordingly, a statement clarifies the way in which the protection guidelines should be applied in a regulatory and legislative context was issued [20].

The Australian regulatory authorities such as the NH & MRC have recommended the ICNIRP guidelines as the standard for Australia [21]. The occupational limit accepted in Australia is 5 G for AC-induced fields on a continuous 8-hour basis, and up to 50 G for 2-hour exposure basis. The nonoccupational limit is 1 G.

Table 5-7   IRPA/ICNIRP 50 Hz Exposure Guidelines

	Electric Field kV/m (RMS)	Magnetic Field G (RMS)
Occupational		
Whole day	10	5
Short period (2 hours/day)	30	50
For limbs	-	250
General Public		
Whole day	5	1
Few hours per day	10	10

5.3   MEASUREMENT TECHNIQUES

To realize electric and magnetic fields, a common lamp is good example for consideration. Electric fields are present when the lamp is plugged in, while magnetic fields are created when the lamp is plugged in and turned on, as illustrated in Figure 5-1.

5.3.1   Frequency and Object Size

Electric and magnetic fields near a source are characterized by frequency. Therefore, any measurement of ELF fields should likely be frequency weighted. This means it should read the product of electric or magnetic field strength times the frequency. This frequency weighting should extend up to about 1000 Hz and then sensitivity should decrease at higher frequencies. To understand that; consider an external electric field of 20 kV/m at 50/60 Hz. This will produce high current inside the body. This current is proportional to field strength times the frequency. At 100/120 Hz (twice the frequency), only half as much field strength (10 kV/m) is necessary to produce the same current inside the body.

Another matter to be considered has to do with how magnetic fields (and not electric fields) induce current in the body. The current per area induced is proportional to field strength, frequency, conductivity, and length of the body. That is why children exposed to magnetic fields experience less current per area than do adults, and lab rats experience about 1/10 as much. The multiplication by body length does not apply to electric fields; as a result, both children and adults

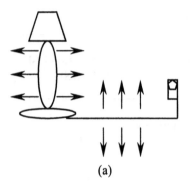   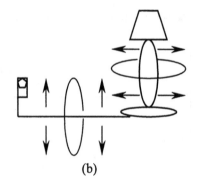

                    (a)   (b)

Figure 5-1   (a) Lamp off. (b) Lamp on.

would experience the same current when exposed to them. A reasonably strong
magnetic field (about 500 mG) and electric field (about 2 kV/m) exist in nature,
but these fields are static ($f = 0$), hence they produce no current inside the body.

   As discussed in previous chapters, the nature of electric fields is different
from that of magnetic fields; therefore, different measuring procedures are
necessary in order to assess emission levels for each type of field. In fact, there
are standard procedures that have been already fixed for the measurement of both
electric and magnetic fields.

5.3.2   Electric Field Measurements

Electric fields exist between objects, which are at different electric potentials, or
voltages. For example, if a 9-volt battery is connected to two metal plates at a
given distance apart, an electric field will exist between them given by voltage
divided by the distance, or 9 V/m. The measurement and calculation of such
fields are quite complex. Although several techniques of measurement are
available, the common one is the RMS (root-mean-square) average, taking the
maximum field strength reading in three planes and extracting the square root of
the sum of the squares of the individual readings. If the field is oscillating at a
constant frequency, an electric field meter can be set such that it has the
maximum sensitivity at that frequency. However, if the field is composed of
different frequencies, as is the case of VDT and other appliances, there will be a
need for a limited number of frequencies to be measured. The range of
frequencies, which is allowed in the RMS average, is called the *bandwidth* of the
instrument.

   Electric field measurements are performed with displacement current sensors
that operate on the basis of measuring displacement current that flows between
two closely spaced electrodes immersed inside the electric field. The sensors are

placed on a nonmetallic tripod to prevent the influence of the operator's body on the measured field value. Commercially available meters are sufficient for measurement near power lines and other sources. They are not suitable for measurements in laboratories because of their size. Yet, smaller meters are also available [22]. In order to avoid the error of field perturbation caused by the body of the person holding the meter during measurement, a horizontal distance of at least 2.5 meters should be maintained between the person and the meter.

5.3.3 Magnetic Field Measurements

Magnetic fields in the environment come from a number of sources. The level of these fields is called *background level*. The background level of schools, hospitals, homes, and workplaces is always increasing due to the rapid increase in the use of electricity. The background field must be considered while measuring the magnetic field from a particular source. Before any assessment of emissions from the source is possible, it is important to define the background field in the place. To do that, the source under measurement must be turned off and readings in the surrounding area must be taken. If the background field is relatively high (i.e., above 5 mG), the contribution of the assigned appliance to the environment may be unmeasurable. According to this fact, the Swedish specification MPR-II requires the background levels to be no greater than 0.4 mG in order for the measurement to be valid.

Differences among magnetic field meters are considerable. A good meter shows the strength of the field, its direction, and polarization of the magnetic field. The meter should measure fields in one direction at a time and display the maximum field strength at that location. However, a person under the exposure of the field is receiving the field from all directions.

To determine the maximum magnetic flux density at a particular location, the meter should be rotated through all possible angles so that the field can intersect with the sensor in such a way to display the maximum reading. This means, the maximum flux density in three orthogonal planes (B_x, B_y, and B_z) is measured and the resultant B_r, which is equal to the square root of the sum of the squares of the individual reading, is extracted [23].

To measure the polarization of the magnetic field, the user must adjust the orientation of the meter until the reading reaches a maximum (B_{max}). The field is linearly polarized when $B_r = B_{max}$, and is circularly polarized when $B_r = 1.41\ B_{max}$. The degree of polarization B_d is expressed by the axial ratio between the major and minor axes of the field ellipse. It is given by [24]

$$B_d = \sqrt{\left(B_r / B_{max}\right)^2 - 1}$$

(5.1)

Meters must be calibrated before use. The calibration of these instruments must be traceable to particular standard. Portable calibrators are usually available. Users must follow the recommendations of both the calibrator and the meter manufacturer.

5.3.4 The Gauss Meter

Gauss is a common unit of measurement of AC magnetic field strength. Still, some engineers prefer Tesla as a unit of measurement (for example, one µT equals 10 mG). A Gauss meter is the instrument to measure the strength of AC magnetic field. Inside the Gauss meter there is a coil of thin wire, typically with thousands of turns. As the magnetic field emanates through the coil, it induces a current, which is amplified by the electronic circuitry inside the Gauss meter. If the Gauss meter has an induction coil with approximately 40,000 turns, a relatively low magnetic field strength of 1 mG would induce enough current to be read directly with a voltmeter. It is more practical, however, to build a Gauss meter with fewer turns and, through operational amplification circuitry, to increase the voltage or current and then calibrate the meter to read either in Gauss (G) or milligauss (mG).

It is necessary to take three perpendicular readings, one for each axis. It is better to always take the readings in the same order. For example, take the first reading in the x-axis direction. For the second reading, rotate the meter 90 degrees and take the y-axis reading. For the third reading, rotate the meter 90 degrees and take the x-axis reading. Once the readings are completed, it is possible to calculate a single combined reading by squaring the reading for each axis, adding the three squared numbers, and then taking the square root of the sum. For example, suppose the observed x, y, and z readings from the Gauss meter are 5, 6 and 7 mG, respectively. To find the combined field strength, carry out the following calculation:

$$\text{Square root of total} = \sqrt{25 + 36 + 49} = 10.488 \text{ mG}$$

It is not necessary to be so precise as to actually use the formula, especially if the highest reading on one axis is much stronger than the rest. For example, readings of 3, 0.4, and 0.5 mG would result in combined field strength of about 3.067 mG. Thus, just by using the dominant axis reading, the result is nearly the same as carrying out the calculation. In case the readings for each axis are close to each other, the combined reading can be as much as 73% more than any one axis.

5.4 STANDARDS FOR MEASUREMENT

In order to measure adequately, one must have some standards to refer to. Key standards are listed below.

5.4.1 IEEE 644-1994 [22]

The purpose of this standard is to establish uniform procedures for the measurement of 50/60-Hz power-frequency electric and magnetic fields from AC overhead power lines. The procedures apply to the measurement of fields close to ground level. They can also be tentatively applied (with limitations, as specified in the standard) to electric fields near an energized conductor or structure. The standard sets 1 meter above the ground as the point for taking electric and magnetic field reading. Any deviation from this height should be reported.

According to the standard, the distance between the support holding the electric field strength meter and the operator should be 2.5 meters. This is to reduce the effect of the operator on the reading. Five percent proximity effect exists when the operator is between 1.8 and 2.1 meters away from the field strength meter. Usually, the meter comes with a 1.1-meter rod device that allows the meter to be held away from the body.

The operator can hold the magnetic field meter because the human body does not influence the magnetic field. But, metal objects may develop induced currents, which produce magnetic fields that can distort the measurements.

5.4.2 IEEE 1140-1994 [25]

The IEEE Electromagnetic Compatibility Society develops this standard. The standard sets procedures for the measurement of electric and magnetic fields in close proximity to VDTs in the frequency range of 5 Hz to 400 kHz. Existing international measurement technologies and practices are adapted to achieve a consistent and harmonious VDT measurement standard for testing in a laboratory-controlled environment. This standard largely follows the Swedish standard. The aim is to set distances and locations for measuring electric and magnetic fields emanating from VDTs.

5.4.3 IEEE P1140.1-1999 [26]

This standard is developed by the IEEE Computer Society. The aim is to define locations for recording measurements for VDTs. This may assure that the values would be comparable from one manufacturer's set to another. The protocol of measurement is in the form of a cylinder. A circle may be in the form used for appliances. Number of locations for taking the measurements needs concurrence.

5.5   FIELD MEASUREMENT SURVEYS

Safety regulations stipulate field limits in occupational and public environments, because of which a need for field measurement surveys arises. Such surveys are usually performed for one or more of the following reasons:

1.   To evaluate a commercial space where VDTs or other devices are being greatly affected by electrical installation systems or other EMI sources.
2.   To evaluate the impact of power lines or other electrical facilities, and to provide guidance in the installation of further structures.
3.   To assess the exposure conditions at homes or offices in order to assure compliance with relevant safety standards.
4.   To prevent overexposure conditions that may pose short- and long-term health problems.

5.5.1   Methods of Survey

The easiest method for performing ELF measurement surveys is through the use of handheld field meters and probes. More complicated devices are also used such as a mapping wheel attached to a programmable tri-axial Gauss meter that collects three-axis calculated resultant data at selected intervals along a path. As yet, there has been little progress in reducing the complexity of data collection and analysis methods posed to the user.

Measured magnetic field exposures to individuals in homes and in the workplace tend be *quasi-log-normally distributed* [27]. Log normal distributions are not symmetrical about the mean. The bulk of their values lie in the low range with fewer values in the range of higher exposures. The central inclination of values is preferred as a *geometric mean* (GM) and the variation around that mean given as a *geometric standard deviation* (GSD). Their *arithmetic mean* (AM) and *standard deviation* (SD) give some values. To change values from AM and SD to GM and GSD, the following equations may be used [28]:

$$GM = \frac{AM^2}{\sqrt{AM^2 + SD^2}} \qquad (5.2)$$

$$GSD = \exp\left(\sqrt{\ln\left[1+\left(\frac{SD}{AM}\right)^2\right]}\right) \qquad (5.3)$$

Another common measure is the median. Statistically it is easy to determine the median since it is the value in the middle. Regarding ELF exposure, it denotes the estimate of exposure for which 50% of the population has smaller exposure and 50% have larger exposure. Also, the estimate is presented for the portion of the population in the upper range of exposure [29].

5.5.2 Types of Survey

There are three common types of field survey: *spot*, *contour*, and *dosimetric*. A spot survey, suitable for residential and small commercial sites, collects data in spots such as the center of an area or other selected points, and arranges these data in a table format and referenced to a layout of the surveyed area.

A contour survey is suitable for most commercial applications and assessment of outdoor areas especially near power lines. In that sense, the mapping wheel is a suitable tool to conduct this survey.

A dosimetric survey collects field data at a fixed point in an area (residential or workplace) in timed increments over a defined period (hours or days). Field surveys should include measurements of the following:

1. Perimeter of the working areas and buildings.
2. Transmission/distribution lines and transformers to the nearest exterior walls.
3. Hallways, offices, all common areas, transformer vaults, electrical rooms, and feeders near offices.

In addition, all monitors should comply with the adopted standards. The grounding systems and water services should not carry any excessive and potentially dangerous ground or plumbing currents.

In general, only magnetic fields are recorded during a field survey, however, if there is a high-voltage power line near or over the area under evaluation, then electric fields should also be recorded. The final survey report, which should be prepared by an authorized survey engineer, includes:

1. Address of test site.
2. Detailed drawing of the property, building(s), etc.
3. Full identification and categorization of the potential sources of ELF fields.
4. Recorded spot or contour (with graphical 2-dimensional and 3-dimensional presentations of field intensity) measurements of the surveyed areas

including equipment, grounding, and plumbing problems.
5. Instrument data such as manufacturer, meter type and model number, probe type and model number, frequency response, and calibration date.

Technical protocols and standards, which are used as guidelines for field measurement surveys, should be followed [22, 30, 31].

5.5.3 Data Analysis

Measurement of fields at sufficient number of points in a site to obtain a fair picture of the field level and at a sufficient number of points in time is useful in order for the result to be reproducible. Documentation of the measuring methods is very important. The next step is to analyze the data collected and answer the main question of whether or not the site is, as far as health safety is concerned, agreeable for use. It is necessary to note that any source that generates a time-varying magnetic field at a magnitude exceeding 1 mG is considered a potential source. Data analysis results will present the site either acceptable for use or a candidate site for shielding in order to attain lower site fields. Next, we need to consider the shielding options available and their relative costs.

5.5.4 Survey Parameters

Any residential or commercial site is subject to coincident exposure from many ELF sources external and internal to the site itself [Figure 5-2] [32]. While evaluating fields at the surveyed site, it is helpful to note that relatively high local fields from magnetic-core devices such as transformers and motor-driven appliances decrease sharply with distance ($1/r^3$). Fields from high-current distribution busses decrease less quickly ($1/r^2$), and fields from ground currents through conductive paths in building structure decrease the least quickly ($1/r$).

It is useful to note the difference between types of measurements. According to Swanson and Kaune [28], certain parameters should be considered during the measurement: duration, location, and conditions at time of measurements.

Duration

Three categories of measurements are distinguished under the duration type. They are:

1. Spot measurements, which refer to measurements made in one or more places over a short period of time with a single answer at each location.

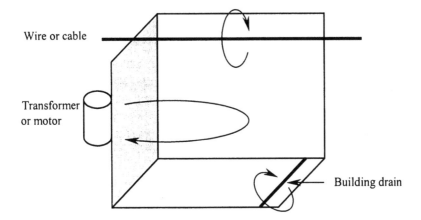

Figure 5-2 A typical site for an ELF measurement survey.

2. Long-term measurements, which are made by a logger placed in one position for, usually, a full day or even longer.
3. Personal-exposure measurements, which are made by asking the person under test to wear a small, portable data logger for, usually, a full day. These measurements pertain to exposures incurred outside homes as well as movement of individuals near field sources within homes.

Location

Measurements are conducted at various locations away from appliances. Sometimes a wall or door may separate instruments from sources of fields.

Conditions at Time of Measurements

Measurements are conducted when sources of field are either turned on or turned off. Conditions of measurements differ also according to the day, season, and even the year following largely the daily and pattern of loads, which in turn, depend on the balance of air conditioning.

5.6 REVIEW OF SURVEY STUDIES

Measurements of ELF away from ELF potential sources such as power lines, substations, and electrical appliances have been conducted in North America, Europe, and many other countries.

5.6.1 North America

Zaffanella [33] performed the largest spot and long-term measurement survey in the United States. He measured the magnetic fields within more than 900 homes using fixed meters. The survey provides a snapshot of residential fields, and the results are probably representative of residential conditions. A large measurement protocol was used including spot measurements inside rooms, field recordings in the home, measurements of field profiles from wiring outside the home, measurements of household appliances, and measurement of fields from currents in the grounding system. The survey showed that the median measured fields using monitors located for 24 hours in several places in the homes was 0.06 µT with about 28% of the homes exceeding 0.1 µT. He found also that about 11% of the homes exceeded 0.2 µT and about 2% exceeded 0.5 µT.

In 1998, Zaffanella and Kalton [27, 34] conducted a survey of two phases for personal magnetic field exposures under the EMF RAPID program. Phase I [26], was part of an effort to assess personal ELF exposures of the U.S. population by conducting personal exposure measurements for a statistical sample of the population. During Phase I, survey methodologies were developed and a small-scale survey was conducted to verify them. However, Phase II [33] included a large-scale survey using the methodologies developed in Phase I. As a result, they found that the average 24-hour personal magnetic field exposure for individuals in the U.S. population is about 0.09 µT. It was observed also that about 44% of the population have 24-hour exposures above 0.1 µT, about 14% above 0.2 µT, about 2.5% above 0.5 µT, and less than 1% above 0.75 µT.

Kaune et al. [35] reported the results of a study in which the rate of occurrence of magnetic field events with 2-200 kHz frequency content were measured over 24-hour or longer periods in 156 U.S. residences. A dual-channel meter was developed for the study that, during 20 seconds continuous intervals of time, counted the number of events with peak 2-200 kHz magnetic fields exceeding thresholds of 3.3 nT and 33 nT. Homes that were electrically grounded to a conductive water system and extended into the street and beyond had higher levels of 33 nT channel transient activity. Homes located in rural surroundings had less 33 nT transient activity than homes in suburban/urban areas.

In Canada, Donnelly and Agnew [36] conducted a spot (24 homes) and long-term (31 home) single-axis measurement survey in Toronto. They found reasonably high magnetic fields with 24-hour GM of 0.107 µT. Proximity to power lines could be a reason for such elevated fields.

Surveys were also conducted to measure ELF fields from common appliances. Kaune et al. [37] evaluated magnetic field exposures produced from 72 television (TV) sets used by children to watch TV programs and 34 TV sets used to play video games in Washington, D.C. and its Maryland suburbs. The resulting TV-specific magnetic field data were combined with information collected through questionnaires to estimate the magnetic field exposure levels associated with TV watching and video game playing. The GM of the ELF and VLF exposure levels so calculated were 0.0091 and 0.0016 μT, respectively, for children watching TV programs and 0.023 and 0.0038 μT, respectively, for children playing video games. GMs of ambient ELF and VLF levels with TV sets turned off were 0.10 and 0.0027 μT, respectively. Summed over the ELF frequency range (6-3066 Hz), the exposure levels were small compared to ambient levels. In restricted ELF frequency ranges (120 Hz and 606-3066 Hz) and in the VLF band, TV exposure levels were comparable to or larger than normal ambient levels. Even so, the strengths of the 120 Hz or 606-3066 Hz components of TV fields were small relative to the overall ambient levels. The results do suggest that any future research on possible health effects of magnetic fields from television sets might focus on the VLF electric and magnetic fields produced by TV sets because of their enhanced ability relative to ELF fields to induce electric currents.

5.6.2 Europe

Various residential survey studies have been conducted in the U.K. [38-40], Germany [41], France [42], and Scandinavian countries [43, 44].

Merchant et al. [38, 39] conducted long-term and a personal-exposure measurement over a year at around 200 homes in England and Wales with GMs of 37 and 54 nT, respectively. Meanwhile, Preece et al. [40] carried out spot, long-term and personal-exposure measurement surveys at homes in Avon, U.K., with GMs of 19, 29, and 42 nT, respectively.

In Germany, Michaelis et al. [41] investigated an association between increased exposure to residential ELF fields and childhood leukemia as part of a population-based case-control study carried out between 1992 and 1995 in the northwestern part of Germany. They conducted a spot measurement survey over a period of more than 3 years at more than 350 homes with GM of 32 nT.

Residential magnetic field measurements were conducted for the first time in a representative sample of French dwellings by Clinard et al. [42]. Exposure levels were assessed by two methods: indoor and outdoor measurements. Linear and logistic regression models were used to determine factors associated with the time-weighted average (TWA) home magnetic fields. TWA magnetic field magnitudes were approximately log-normally distributed with GMs under 0.010 μT for both indoor and outdoor measurements. Only 5% of the dwellings presented indoor levels greater than 0.120 μT. Both indoor and outdoor variations were explained by three factors: wiring configuration, the dwelling's location (i.e., urban or rural), and housing characteristics (houses or apartment building).

Juutilainen et al. [43] measured magnetic fields at 37 homes in Kuopio, Finland. In general, they found a 24-hour GM of 60 nT.

Vistnes et al. [44] carried out personal exposure measurements for 24 hours by 65 schoolchildren living 28-325 meters away from a 300 kV transmission line (current load was 200-700 A) in suburb of Oslo, Norway. The 24-hour personal exposure GM was 15 nT.

5.6.3 Summary of Survey Studies

A complete summary of measurement surveys is available at a review paper by Swanson and Kaune [28] published in 1999. They reviewed measurements of residential power-frequency magnetic fields made in different countries, considering 27 studies (14 from North America, 5 from the United Kingdom and 8 from other European countries). They summarized the papers by their GMs. The authors indicated that the GMs of long term background fields at homes in the United States is in the range of 0.06-0.07 μT, with lower levels in the United Kingdom (0.036-0.039 μT). This shows that the ratio of GM fields between the two countries is approximately between 1.5 to 1.9. This difference may be related to the type of appliances, wiring practices, and electricity used in both countries.

They have also recognized that measurements of personal exposure are higher than measurements of background fields. This is perhaps due to exposures from appliances and other sources in the home. They concluded that the ratio of personal exposure to background field seems, on average, to be 1.4.

5.7 FIELD MANAGEMENT

The ultimate demand of the user is always to achieve field management, which includes engineering changes to reduce, avoid, or eliminate certain fields or field characteristics. The process of field management requires techniques with tremendous energetic extent. It involves the level of field, which depends on the field strength, frequency, direction, and type of field source.

5.7.1 Mitigation Techniques for Power Lines

It is basically known, for example, that reduction of magnetic fields generated from power lines relies on many options including allocating larger ROW, using cancellation techniques, and replacing overhead power lines with underground cables.

Underground Cables

As discussed in Chapter 2, burying overhead power transmission lines can substantially reduce their ELF fields, especially electric fields. The reduction of magnetic field is not due to the burying itself, but occurs because underground power lines use plastic or oil for insulation rather than air. This lets the conductors to be placed closer together and therefore allows better phase cancellation. However, when high voltage cables are buried in the ground they must be kept at least 15-30 cm apart to limit mutual heating and they must be placed deep enough to provide clearance for activities on the ground surface (the depth increases with voltage). For cables operating at 33 kV and above, trenches wider than 1 meter have to be excavated and the swathe of land required for a number of cables, necessarily spaced, can be as much as 30 meters wide. Consequently, high voltage underground cables over long distances are expensive and involve extensive work during installation and maintenance. For example, the capital cost of installing an underground cable is greater than that for an equally rated overhead power line. The ratio ranges from about 2:1 at 11 kV to 20:1 or more at 400 kV and above.

It should also be noted that magnetic fields at the center of underground cable corridor might be much higher than those from overhead lines. This is due to the fact that ground-level magnetic fields from cables fall much more rapidly with distance than those from a corresponding overhead power lines, but can actually be higher at small distances from the cable. According to Swanson and Renew [45], the magnetic fields under overhead lines on the RoW were about 24 μT and more than 100 μT for the buried line. While, at 30 meters away, fields were about 4 μT for the overhead line and less than 1 μT for the buried line.

Accordingly, using underground cables remains unreal choice for power utilities and the liked choice by users. To realistically proceed with the advantages of this option, planned development to avoid hazards and pitfalls of existing power systems is required from the utilities. Offering guidance in new network construction may avoid much of the massive economic impact inevitable in mitigating suspected hazards associated with past and present technologies.

Rights-of-Way

The term rights-of-way (ROW) as used in this book covers use that will encumber real property by granting a right to use and alter the landscape through construction of overhead power and communication lines, or buildings (power plant, substation, radio tower, etc.). Generally, such uses are for a relatively long period of time; i.e., 10 years or longer.

It is important to know that the highest magnetic field strength from high-voltage power lines on the ROW during peak usage could be lower than the median measurement of magnetic field from many appliances. However, the duration of exposure from power lines is typically much longer than the duration of exposure to magnetic field from the appliances. Here indeed lies the reason for public concerns. Because of this lasting exposure, there is a demand to enlarge the ROW, although such action involves financial and land rights acquiring difficulties. Authorities in many countries now require from power utilities to have more land around overhead power lines.

Another solution could be achieved by increasing the height of towers, and therefore the height of conductors above the ground will reduce the field intensity at the edge of the ROW.

Cancellation Techniques

It is well known that currents oscillating together at the same amplitude, frequency, and direction can add to each other. This fact is called *in phase*, and it creates the highest magnetic fields. Likewise, fields that are precisely opposing each other achieve a significant cancellation. This means the phase current in a given conductor is opposed by current flowing in the opposite conductor. Such case is called *out of phase*. This fact is workable for both single-phase systems and three-phase systems. Cancellation techniques could be successful to a great extent if the phase currents are balanced, a state that is practically difficult, if not impossible, to achieve. In that sense, other procedures may be considered.

5.7.2 Reducing the Level of ELF Exposure

Importantly for the user, there appear to be general procedures and suggestions to reduce the levels of electric and magnetic fields in homes and in workplaces. Following are a few suggestions to minimize the level of ELF fields, as a procedure before resorting to various shielding techniques, especially when shielding is the most effective and least expensive alternative [46, 47]:

1. Determine sources of ELF fields. For example, a tri-axis Gauss meter could be used to determine the levels and locations of magnetic fields.
2. Use bundled and twisted power cable drops to reduce field generation.
3. Keep the drop, meter, service panels, and subpanels away from normally occupied rooms.
4. Fix up a thorough ground rod. Never provide a separate ground for subpanels. Affix an insulated bushing at the water meter to keep current imbalances from returning on the metal water pipes. Prevent metal-sheathed cabling from contacting water pipes, electrical conduit, or appliances by

providing a separate ground path.

5. Keep high load wiring from the main panel to a subpanel or to high current appliances away from frequently used spaces.

6. Avoid separating hot and neutral wires and ensure there is always a supply and return current in all wiring runs.

7. Place high load appliances such as electric dryers and electric hot water heaters away from bedrooms, kitchens, etc.

8. Avoid using devices such as alarm clocks or electric blankets near the bed.

9. As a last solution, use shielding techniques to reduce the level of fields. Shielding ELF fields requires either to divert the fields around the area considered sensitive to the magnetic fields or to contain fields within the source producing them.

5.7.3 Mitigation of Electric Fields

As discussed in Chapter 1, if the charges exist in a medium that permits the charges to move, the medium is considered conductive and the field can be adjusted in magnitude and direction with the movement of the charges. At ELF fields, air has a conductivity of less than 10^{-9} siemens, while metals have conductivity of greater than 10^7 siemens. The human body has a conductivity that ranges from 0.01 to 1.5 siemens [25]. Due to the huge difference in conductivity, placing any grounded metallic surface between the electric field source and user will eliminate the electric field. The metal surface can be any inexpensive mesh chicken wire screen.

Cancellation techniques are applicable for electric fields. This can be achieved by placing together two conductors carrying charges to and from an electrical appliance. For plug-in appliances, a switched-off appliance has a larger electric field than a switched-on appliance. This is because most of the switches break only one of the conductor circuits.

Although cancellation techniques are the only practical electric field management technique for specific cases, shielding is the usual and easier technique to apply. In this case, both the user and equipment can be shielded, simply by placing a metal shroud around the object. Therefore, management of electric fields is not that difficult a task compared to the management of magnetic fields. While both cancellation and shielding techniques are applicable to electric and magnetic fields, shielding could be the best solution.

5.7.4   Mitigation of Magnetic Fields

In general, there are two basic magnetic field mitigation methods: passive and active. They may be used either separately or together as is necessary.

Passive Shielding Techniques

Passive magnetic shielding is divided into two basic types based upon the selection of the shielding material: ferromagnetic and conductive. A ferromagnetic material shield is constructed with highly permeability (μ) material, especially annealed ferromagnetic Mumetal alloy (composed of 80% nickel and 15% iron, with the balance being copper, molybdenum or chromium, depending on the recipe being used), which exhibits high magnetic conductivity. The relative permeability μ_r of Mumetal ranges between 350,000-500,000 depending on the composition and annealing process.

Mumetal either surrounds or separates the victims from the magnetic sources. All shielding materials work by diverting the magnetic flux to them, so although the field from a magnet will be highly reduced by a shield plate, the shield plate will itself be attracted to the magnet. Closed shapes are the most effective for magnetic shielding such as cylinders with caps, and boxes with covers.

The electrical properties of ferromagnetic materials are complex functions of magnetic fields and frequencies. They have high saturation characteristics, which can be adjusted to achieve source shielding. Conducting material shields depend on the eddy-current losses that occur within highly conductive materials (copper and aluminum). When a conductive material is subjected to an ELF field, eddy currents are induced within the material, which flow in closed circular paths perpendicular to the inducing field. According to Lenz's law, these eddy currents oppose changes in the inducing fields, hence the magnetic fields produced by the circulating eddy currents attempt to cancel the larger external fields near the conductive surface, thereby generating a shielding effect. It is often effective but expensive to shield with multiple layers composed of highly conductive aluminum/copper plates, and highly permeable Mumetal sheets.

Practically, shielding design depends on the following factors:

1.   Maximum predicted worst-case magnetic field intensity and the earth's geomagnetic (DC static) field at that location.
2.   Type of material and properties such as conductivity, permeability, induction, and saturation, which are functions of material thickness.
3.   Number of shield layers and spacing between sheet materials and layers.

Small, fully enclosed shields for VDTs, electronic equipment, and electrical feeders follow simple formulas that guide the design engineer through the process to a functional, but not necessarily optimal, design. After assembling a prototype, the design engineer measures the *shielding factor* (SF) and modifies the design by adding materials and layers to achieve the maximum shielding requirements. This is a very iterative design process, from the concept to final product.

Shielding factor is the ratio between the unperturbed magnetic field B_o and the shielded magnetic field B_i. It is defined as

$$SF = \frac{B_o}{B_i}$$

or

$$SF = 20 \log 10 \left(\frac{B_o}{B_i} \right) (dB) \tag{5.4}$$

For example, if the field before shielding is 500 mG, and the field measured inside the shield is 10 mG, the SF is then 500/10 or 50 times. SF is usually expressed in dB (decibels). The ratio in dB for the above example is 34 dB.

Unfortunately, magnetic shielding is more of an art than a science, especially when shielding very large areas and rooms from multiple, high-level magnetic field sources. Currently, there are no reliable design formulas or field simulation programs that offer design engineers practical guidelines for shielding large exposed areas from multiple, high-level magnetic field sources.

Active Shielding Techniques

The use of active cancellation loops involves a system that senses the magnetic field in the region to be shielded and, via a feedback system, imposes a current on additional conductors such that it reduces the magnetic field in the region. Active shielding is therefore a technique that works best for full-room shielding of affected instrumentation once strong local sources have been moved or passively shielded. Design changes for power line mitigation include opposite phasing (or revising conductor arrangements to reduce fields), creating balanced currents, or other engineering design changes. For electrical equipment rooms, rearranging and moving electrical components is often the first step to consider since it is more cost effective than installing magnetic field shields.

5.7.5   Protection from VDTs

The source of electric fields in the VDT is the power supply and deflection coils. These components can create a surface potential of several kilovolts, depending upon humidity, temperature, air velocity, and ion concentration in the air. Reduction of the electrostatic potential and the electric fields is usually achieved by placing a conductive surface coating on the screen, which is connected to the power ground, together with metallic shielding of the power supply. Sometimes, the CRT-type VDT may include a metal cage around all the internal components, or a metal foil on the inside of the cabinet to shield electric fields.

There has been a public debate about whether exposure from VDTs poses health problems. As yet, there is no conclusive evidence to settle the matter once and for all. Some simple precautions could be followed to reduce the exposure:

1.   Use a low emission VDT.
2.   Reduce use of computers as the best step. It is also recommended that VDT operators reduce eyestrain by taking rest breaks, for example, after each hour or so of operating a VDT.
3.   Most of fields do not extend from the front of the screen of the VDT but from the inductive components located near the inside rear or sides of the equipment. Accordingly, avoid sitting or working at places where you expose yourself to the emission from the backs and sides of other computers. If you find you are close to any VDT (less than 120 cm), you should change your work environment to enhance your safety [Figure 5-3].
4.   Keep the computer screen as far away from you as you can manage (at least 70 cm) since magnetic field strength diminishes rapidly the farther you move from the VDT.
5.   VDT users should be aware of ergonomic problems, which can be improved by the use of antiglare screens and proper eyeglasses (avoid wearing metal objects, which concentrate fields while using a computer).
6.   Do not place a bed on the other side of the wall from a computer, as building materials cannot shield magnetic fields.
7.   Before you use a new computer, leave it turned on for a few days in an empty ventilated room to allow for chemical outgassing.
8.   Turn off the computer when it is not in use.
9.   A notebook with liquid crystal display (LCD), which requires much less power and narrow range of frequencies, could be a substitute to the desktop computer. The notebook emits virtually no fields. But it has been found that high fields emanate from the keyboards.

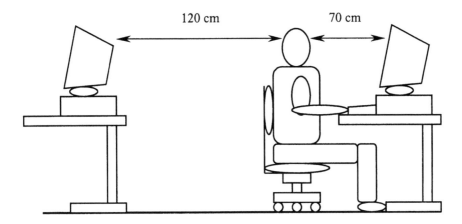

Figure 5-3 Minimum recommended distances between users and computers.

REFERENCES

[1] Wertheimer, N., and E. Leeper, Electrical Wiring Configurations and Childhood Cancer, *American Journal of Epidemiology* 109, pp. 273-284, 1979.

[2] IEEE Standard for Safety Levels with Respect to Human Exposure to Radio Frequency Electromagnetic Fields, 3 kHz to 300 GHz, Incorporation of Std C95.1-1991 and Std C95.1a-1998, IEEE Std C95.1, 1999, IEEE, New York, NY, 1999.

[3] Stuchly, M. A., Canadian and Other National RF Protection Guides, *The Joint Symposium on Interaction of Electromagnetic Waves with Biological Systems, 22nd General Assembly of the International Union of Radio Science*, Plenum Press, New York, NY, 1989.

[4] Fixed Facilities Which Generate Electromagnetic Fields in the Frequency Range of 300 kilohertz to 100 Gigahertz and Microwave Ovens, Code of Massachusetts Regulations 105 CMR 122.000, Commonwealth of Massachusetts Department of Labor and Industries, Boston, MA, 1986.

[5] Hazards by Electromagnetic Fields Protection of Persons in the Frequency Range from 10 kHz to 3000 GHz, VDT 0848 Teil 2 (Deutsche Elektrotechnische Kommission im DIN und VDE), Federal Republic of Germany, 1986.

[6] Control and Recording of Personnel Exposure to Radio Frequency Radiation, Standardization Agreement STANAG No. 2345, Military Agency for Standardization, NATO, Brussels, Belgium, 1979.

[7] Occupational Health Exposure to Radio Frequency Radiation, AFOSH Standard 161-9, USAF, Washington, D.C., 1987.

[8] Provning av Bildskärms-Terminaler, Technical Report, MPR-P, 1987.

[9] User's Handbook for Evaluating Visual Display Units, Technical Report MPR, 1990.

[10] Test Methods for Visual Display Units, Technical Report MPR, 1990.

[11] Measuring Methods for Environmental Labelling of Computers, Emission and

Energy Efficiency Characteristics, TCO'95 Certification, 1995.

[12] TCO'99 Certification, Display (CRT), TCO Report No. 1, Stockholm, Sweden, 20th July 1998.

[13] Verordnung zur Durchführung des Bundes-Imissionsschutzgesetzes 1996 (Verordnung über elektromagnetische Felder 26. BImSchV), 26. BImSchV 1996: Bundesgesetzblatt Jahrgang Teil 1 Nr. 66, Bonn, Germany, 1996.

[14] Editorial Comments: International & Australian EMF Guidelines and Cancer: Are We Protected? *Electromagnetic Forum* 1(3), 1997.

[15] Documentation of the Threshold Limit Values and Biological Exposure Indices, ACGIH, Cincinnati, Ohio, 1991.

[16] IRPA Guidelines on Limits of Exposure to Radio Frequency Electromagnetic Fields in the Frequency Range from 100 kHz to 300 GHz, *Health Physics* 54, pp. 115-123, 1988.

[17] IRPA Interim Guidelines on Limits of Exposure to 50/60 Hz Electric and Magnetic Fields, *Health Physics* 58, pp. 113-122, 1990.

[18] ICNIRP Guidelines on Limits of Exposure to Static Magnetic Fields, *Health Physics* 66, pp. 100-106, 1994.

[19] ICNIRP Guidelines for Limiting Exposure to-Time-Varying Electric, Magnetic, and Electromagnetic Fields (up to 300 GHz), *Health Physics* 74, pp. 494-522, 1998.

[20] Response to questions and Comments on ICNIRP Guidelines, *Health Physics* 75, pp. 438-439, 1998.

[21] Threshold Limit Values for Chemical Substances and Physical Agents and Biological Exposure Indices, ACGIH, Cincinnati, Ohio, 1996.

[22] IEEE Standard Procedures for Measurement of Power Frequency Electric and Magnetic Fields From AC Power Lines, IEEE Std 644-1994-Revision of IEEE Std 644-1987 IEEE, New York, NY, 1999.

[23] Silva, M., H. Hummon, D. Rutter, and C. Hooper, Power Frequency Magnetic Fields in the Home, *IEEE Transactions on Power Delivery* 4, pp. 465-478, 1989.

[24] Letters to the Editor: More on Measuring Polarization, *Microwave News* XX No. 3, p. 13, May/June 2000.

[25] IEEE Standard Procedures for the Measurement of Electric and Magnetic Fields From Video Display Terminals (VDTs) From 5 Hz to 400 kHz, IEEE Std 1140-1994, IEEE, New York, NY, 1999.

[26] IEEE Standard Measurement Techniques for ELF and VLF Magnetic Fields and Electrical Fields from Desktop Computer Displays and Associated Desktop Devices, IEEE P1140.1, IEEE, New York, NY, 1999.

[27] Zaffanella, L. E., and G. W. Kalton, Survey of Personal Magnetic Field Exposure, Phase I: Pilot Study and Design of Phase II, EMF RAPID Engineering Project #6, Enertech for Oak Ridge National Laboratory EMF Research Program, U.S. Department of Energy, 1998.

[28] Swanson, J., and W. T. Kaune, Comparison of Residential Power-Frequency Magnetic Fields Away from Appliances in Different Countries, *Bioelectromagnetics* 20, pp. 244-254, 1999.

[29] Health Effects from Exposure to Power-Line Frequency Electric and Magnetic Fields, National Institute of Environmental Health Sciences (NIEHS) and National Institutes of Health, 1999.

[30] IEEE Standard Procedures for Measurement of Power Frequency Electric and Magnetic Fields from AC Power Lines, ANSI/IEEE Standard 644, 1994.

[31] Yost, M. G., G. M. Lee, B. D. Duane, J. Fisch, and R. R. Neutra, California Protocol for Measuring 60 Hz Magnetic Fields in Residences, *Applied Occupational and Environmental Hygiene* 7, pp. 772-777, 1992.

[32] Dunnam, C. R., E. M. Site: Magnetic Fields: Sources, Surveys, and Solutions, Linear Research Associates, Trumansburg, NY, 1999.

[33] Zaffanella, L., Survey of Residential Magnetic Field Sources. Volume 1: Goals, Results and Conclusions, Volume 2: Protocol, Data Analysis, and Management, TR-102759-V1, TR-102759-V2, EPRI, Palo Alto, CA, 1993.

[34] Zaffanella, L. E., and G. W. Kalton, Survey of Personal Magnetic Field Exposure Phase II: 1000-Person Survey, EMFRAPID Program Engineering Project #6, Oak Ridge, TN: Lockheed Martin Energy Systems, Inc., 1998.

[35] Kaune, W. T., T. D. Bracken, R. S. Senior, R. F. Rankin, J. C. Niple, and R. Kavet, Rate of Occurrence of Transient Magnetic Field Events in U.S. Residences, *Bioelectromagnetics* 21, pp. 197-213, 2000.

[36] Donnelly, K. E., and D. A. Agnew, Exposure Assessment Methods for a Childhood Epidmiological Study, Ontario Hydro Report HSD-ST-91-39, Pickering, Canada, 1991.

[37] Kaune, W. T., M. C. Miller, M. S. Linet, E. E. Hatch, R. A. Kleinerman, S. Wacholder, A. H. Mohr, R. E. Tarone, and C. Haines, Children's Exposure to Magnetic Fields Produced by U.S. Television Sets Used for Viewing Programs and Playing Video Games, *Bioelectromagnetics* 21, pp. 214-227, 2000.

[38] Merchant, C. J., D. C. Renew, and J. Swanson, Origins and Magnitudes of Exposure to Power-Frequency Magnetic Fields in the UK, *CIGRE*, pp. 36-105, 1994.

[39] Merchant, C. J., D. C. Renew, and J. Swanson, Exposures to Power-Frequency Magnetic Fields in the Home, *Journal of Radiological Protection* 14, pp. 77-87, 1994.

[40] Preece, A. W., P. Grainger, J. Golding, and W. Kaune, Domestic Magnetic Field Exposure in Avon, *Physics in Medicine and Biology* 41, pp. 71-81, 1996.

[41] Michaelis, J., J. Schuz, J. Meinart, M. Menger, J. –P. Grigat, P. Kaatch, U. Kaletsch, A. Miesner, A. Stamm, K. Brinkmann, and H. Karner, Childhood Leukemia and Electromagnetic Fields: Results of a Population-Based Case-Control Study in Germany, *Cancer Causes Control* 8, pp. 167-174, 1977.

[42] Clinard, F., C. Milan, M. Harb, P. –M., Carli, C. Bonithon-Kopp, J. –P. Moutet, J. Faivre, and P. Hillon, Residential Magnetic Field Measurements in France: Comparison of Indoor and Outdoor Measurements, *Bioelectromagnetics* 20, pp. 319-326, 1999.

[43] Juutilainen, J., K. Saali, J. Eskelinen, P. Matilainen, and A. –L. Leinonen, Measurements of 50 Hz Magnetic Fields in Finnish Homes, Research Report IVO-A-02/89 Helsinki: Imatran Voima Oy, Finland, 1989.

[44] Vistnes, A. I., G. B. Ramberg, L. R. Bjornevik, T. Tynes, and T. Haldorsen, Exposure of Children to Residential Magnetic Fields in Norway: Is Proximity to Power Lines an Adequate Predictor of Exposure? *Bioelectromagnetics* 18, pp. 47-57, 1997.

[45] Swanson, J., and D. C. Renew, Power-Frequency Fields and People, *Engineering*

Science and Education Journal, pp. 71-79, 1994.

[46] *Handbook of Shielding Principles for Power System Magnetic Fields Volume* 1: *Introduction and Application*, EPRI (TR-103630-V1), Palo Alto, CA, 1994.

[47] MacMillen, A., Minimizing Home EMF Exposure, Internet Document at http://www.efn.org/~andrewm/hhd/emf.html, 1995.

Part II
Radio Frequency Radiation

6

Sources of Radio Frequency Radiation

6.1 INTRODUCTION

Radio was developed in 1909, when Italian-born British entrepreneur Guglielmo Marconi (1874-1937) put to use the innovations of his predecessors and sent the first wireless signal across the Atlantic Ocean. He bridged the 3000-km distance between St. John's (Newfoundland) and Poldhu (Cornwall), on the Southwest tip of England [1].

Later, wireless transmission came to be *radio,* as we know it. Since then, radio has become an essential part of our everyday life. Today, radio technology leads one of the biggest businesses in the global market, and the use of wireless devices, such as cellular phones, is increasing dramatically.

The term radio frequency (abbreviated RF) refers to alternating current (AC), which if fed to an antenna, generates electromagnetic fields. These fields are suitable for wireless communications, broadcasting, and other industrial, scientific, and medical applications. RF covers an important portion of the electromagnetic radiation spectrum, extending from a few kilohertz (within the range of human hearing) to thousands of gigahertz.

As defined by the Institute of Electrical and Electronics Engineers (IEEE), radio frequency radiation (RFR) is a band in the electromagnetic spectrum that lies in the frequency range of 3 kHz to 300 GHz. Microwave (MW) radiation is usually considered a subset of RFR, although an alternative convention treats RF and MW as two separate spectral regions. Microwaves occupy the spectral region between 300 GHz to 300 MHz, while RF includes 300 MHz to 3 kHz. Since they have similar characteristics, RF and MW are recognized together, and referred to as RFR throughout this book. Specific ranges and applications of RFR are given in Table 6-1 [1, 2].

Table 6-1 Range of RFR Applications [2, 3]

Application	Frequency Range
RFR range	3 kHz to 300 GHz
General	
AM radio	535-1705 kHz
FM radio	88-108 MHz
TV channels	54-88/174-220 MHz
UHF television	470-806 MHz
Commercial paging	35, 43, 152, 158, 454, 931 MHz
Amateur radio	1.81-2.0/3.5-4.0/7.0-7.3/
	10.1-10.15/14-14.35/
	18.068-18.168/21.0-21.45/
	24.89-24.99/28.0-29.7 MHz
Cellular Systems	
NMT 450	453-457.5/463-467.5 MHz
NMT 900	890-915/935-960 MHz
AMPS	825-845/870-890 MHz
TACS	890-915/935-960 MHz
E-TACS	872-905/917-950 MHz
GSM 900	890-915/935-960 MHz
DCS 1800	1710-1785/1805-1880 MHz
Cordless Systems	
CT-2	864-868 MHz
DECT	1880-1900 MHz
PHS	1895-1918 MHz
PACS	1910-1930 MHz
PCS	1850-1990 MHz
Industrial, Scientific, and Medical	
ISM	433, 915, and 2450 MHz
RF heaters/sealers	13.56, 27.12, 40.68, and 100 MHz
Microwave ovens	2450 MHz

RFR is described as a series of waves of electromagnetic energy composed of oscillating electric and magnetic fields that travel through space at the speed of light (3×10^8 m/s) in a vacuum and does not require a medium for transmission. RFR waves are slowed as they pass through media such as air, water, glass, biological tissues, etc. They radiate outward from their transmission source in energy packets that combine the characteristics of waves and particles. When generated, these waves of energy travel from their transmitter through space. They are reflected from, refracted around, or absorbed by their receivers or any object in their path.

Recognized applications of RF energy may include:

1. Radio and television broadcast stations.
2. Point-to-point microwave radio; mobile radio including cellular communications, paging, and ship-to-shore radio.
3. Amateur radio and citizen's band radio.
4. Navigation (ship and aircraft) and radar (military and civilian use for detection and guidance, flight surveillance around airports, weather surveillance and prediction, and traffic speed control).
5. Processing and cooking of food, RF sealers and heaters, high frequency welders, microwave drying equipment, and microwave ovens.
6. Power amplifiers used in electromagnetic compatibility (EMC) and metrology.

Consumers utilize the above applications according to their personal, social, and economic well being; however, the absorbed energy by the consumer's body is a matter of concern.

6.2   ELEMENTS OF A RFR SYSTEM

RFR is emitted from three basic elements of any wireless system. These elements are generator, transmission path, and antenna as shown in Figure 6-1.

6.2.1   Generators

RF sources, or generators, convert electrical power into radiation using certain technologies such as oscillators or magnetrons. The radiation requirements of the system determine the type of generator or RF source used. Important parameters are power output requirement, efficiency, size, bandwidth, frequency, and modulation technique.

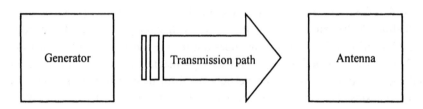

Figure 6-1 The basic elements of exposure from a wireless communication system.

An oscillator is the most basic RF source. It consists of a tuned resonant circuit that is usually equipped with amplification stages and positive feedback circuits. This source is often used as the input to other high power amplifiers. These amplifiers, such as *klystron* and *traveling wave tubes*, increase the output power of the oscillator. Both types of amplifiers are operated by the principles of velocity and current modulation. This is carried out by injecting a beam of electrons into a vacuum tube, which uses the input from the oscillator to alternately accelerate and decelerate the beam at the desired frequency. Figure 6-2(a) shows a high-power microwave generator (klystron).

A smaller generator is the *magnetron*, which is another microwave source with a vacuum tube and resonant cavities. Its static magnetic field bends the electron beam from the cathode to the anode. The bent electron beam passes the resonant cavities and induces current at the desired frequency for radiation. This generator does not require an oscillating source or amplifier. Figure 6-2(b) shows a magnetron from a typical microwave oven.

6.2.2 Transmission Lines

Transmission lines are commonly used for high bandwidth communication and power transfer. They come in a wide variety of geometries and sizes and operate over broad frequency ranges. When RF energy is generated and information is imparted to the signal through electronic stages, the next task is to guide the energy from the generator to the antenna. Using a two-conductor transmission line, coaxial cable, or waveguide may accomplish this.

Two-conductor Lines

The two-conductor (predominantly copper) line is one of the oldest types of communication channels. It was designed mainly for telephone systems. It represents the simplest type of geometry in that the two conductors are of equal size and are spaced apart by a constant separation.

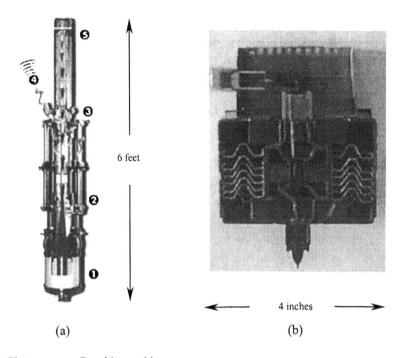

6 feet

4 inches

(a)   (b)

Electron gun   Bunching cavities
Output cavity   Waveguide   Beam stop

Figure 6-2 Microwave generators. (a) Klystron. (b) Magnetron. [Courtesy of Stanford Linear Accelerator Center.]

The two-conductor line is usually twisted. The twist reduces the EM radiation from signal propagating over the wires as well as the pickup of unwanted signals when EM fields surround the wire. In the past, paper was used as insulator between the wires, but today the polyethylene is common. Two-conductor lines are usually used in telephone networks and their use is generally restricted to operation up to about 100 MHz.

Two-conductor lines are combined in cables of various sizes ranging from a couple in the user's premises and distribution section to few hundred pairs in the feeder section. A capacitive or inductive coupling takes place between various wires in the same cable. The coupling increases, as the wires are placed closer, causing unwanted crosstalk.

The two-conductor transmission line is described in terms of its line parameters, which are its resistance per unit length R, inductance per unit length L, conductance per unit length G, and capacitance per unit length C as shown in Figure 6-3.

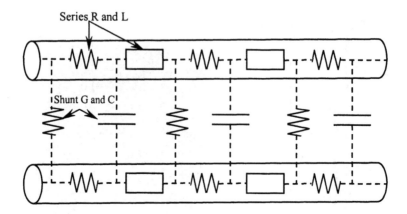

Figure 6-3 Distributed parameters for a two-conductor transmission line.

Coaxial Cables

Coaxial cables are the most widely used transmission lines for high-frequency applications. The two conductors required for transmission of energy are the center conductor and an enclosing conducting shield as shown in Figure 6-4. An insulating material separates the center conductor and the shield. Coaxial cables are used wherever there is a need for long distance, low attenuation, and ability to support high data transmission rates with high immunity to electrical interference. Coaxial cables are widely used in telephone networks and cable TV.

Waveguides

Waveguides are found in several forms. They can have a circular or a rectangular cross section. They may have other shapes as well, if utilized and manufactured for specific applications. Waveguides normally consist of metallic hollow structures used to guide EM waves as shown in Figure 6-5. They are used for transferring signals, where the wavelengths involved are so short that they are of the same size range (2 GHz and higher). Large waveguides would be required to transmit RF power at longer wavelengths. Waveguides are low loss, which means the wave travels along the waveguide without greatly attenuating as it goes. Waveguides can be gently twisted without losing contact with the wave, without generating reflections, and without incurring much additional loss.

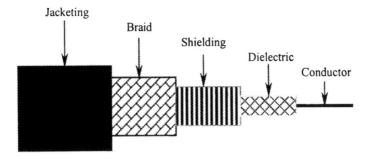

Figure 6-4 The geometry of a coaxial cable.

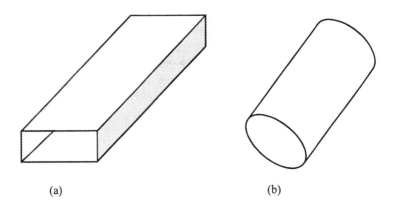

(a)   (b)

Figure 6-5 (a) A rectangular waveguide. (b) A circular waveguide.

6.2.3 Antennas

The antenna is the last component in the wireless transmitting system. The antenna is a device that provides the transition from a guided EM wave on a transmission line to an EM wave propagating in free space. Also the antenna may also be considered as a transducer used in matching the transmission line or waveguide to the surrounding medium.

Most antennas are *reciprocal* devices, which means the antenna performs equally well as either transmitting antenna or receiving antenna. The purpose of the transmitting antenna is to radiate electromagnetic waves into free space (usually, but not necessarily, air). Antennas are also used for reception to collect radiation from free space and deliver the energy contained in the propagating wave to a feeder and receiver.

Antenna Properties

The design of antenna is influenced by requirements such as size, frequency range, power output, directivity, gain, propagation technique, polarization, and electrical impedance. These requirements justify the wide range of antenna designs available for different applications. In general, the properties of antennas are the most important aspect of radiation hazard evaluation:

Bel: This term was originally developed from measurement of sound. It reflects the fact that the human ear has a logarithmic response. The bel is a ratio of two powers, the output power P_o and the input power P_i.

Decibel: In order to deal with the wide range of numbers in a telecommunication system, it is convenient to use a logarithmic scale for comparing power levels. It is common to use a base-10 logarithm in such case. We also multiply the result by 10. The unit is decibel, but people usually say dB. In case of work in voltages or currents, multiply the result by 20. For an amplifier, the gain can be written in dB as

$$G = 10 \log\left(\frac{P_o}{P_i}\right) \text{dB}$$ (6.1)

Directivity: This is the ability of an antenna to concentrate the radiation in the desired direction. The directivity is also the ratio of the radiation intensity in a given direction from the antenna to the radiation intensity averaged over all directions. This average radiation intensity is equal to the total power of the antenna divided by 4π. If the direction is not specified, the directivity refers to the direction of maximum radiation intensity.

Gain: The gain of any antenna is the most important parameter in the design and performance of the antenna system. It is defined as the product of the antenna efficiency and its directivity. The gain is obtained by concentrating the radiated power into a narrow beam. The gain in any direction (θ, ϕ) is the power density radiated in the direction (θ, ϕ) divided by the power density, which would have been radiated at (θ, ϕ) by an isotropic radiator having the same input power. A high gain is achieved by increasing the effective aperture area A_e of the antenna square meters (m^2). We write the gain G as

$$G = \frac{4\pi A_e}{\lambda^2}$$ (6.2)

The gain is normally expressed in dBs by taking 10 log (G). The term dB_i refers to antenna gain with respect to an isotropic antenna, while the term dB_d is used to refer to the antenna gain with respect to a half-wave dipole antenna (0 dB_d = 2.1 dB_i).

Polarization: The polarization of an EM wave is the orientation of the electric field intensity vector **E** relative to the surface of the Earth. The propagating wave has a transverse direction for the electric field called the *polarization direction*. This normally lies along the direction of the electric field. There are two basic types of polarization: linear and elliptical. Linear polarization is divided into two classes, vertical and horizontal. Circular polarization is the more common form of elliptical polarization. Two classes of circular polarization exist: right-hand circular and left-hand circular.

Effective area: The effective aperture area A_e of an antenna is related to the gain G and free space wavelength λ [see Equation 6.2].

Near-field zone: It is a region generally in close proximity to the antenna or other radiating structure in which the electric and magnetic fields do not exhibit a plane-wave relationship, and the power does not decrease with the square of distance from the source but varies considerably from point to point. The near-field region is subdivided into the *reactive* near-field zone, which is closest to the radiating structure and contains most or nearly all of the stored energy, and the radiating near-field zone (Rayleigh), where the radiating field predominates over the reactive field but lacks substantial plane-wave character and is complicated in structure.

Far-field zone: It is the region far enough from the antenna that radiated power per unit area decreases with the square of the distance from the source. In the far-field environment, the EM field propagates away from the source of radiation. The radiated energy is stored alternately in the electric and magnetic field of the propagating EM wave. The electric field vector and the magnetic field vector are perpendicular to each other in a plane wave condition. Both of these vectors are perpendicular to the power vector, which points in the direction of the radiation (each of these vectors is mutually perpendicular to the other two). In the far-field zone, the ratio between **E** and **H** is equal to a constant known as the impedance of free space (Z_o) and has a value of approximately 377 Ω. This value is derived from the permittivity and permeability of free space. The distance R_{NF} from the antenna to the far-field zone is defined as

$$R_{NF} = 2\frac{D^2}{\lambda}$$
(6.3)

where D is the greatest distance of the radiating structure in meters (m), and λ is the wavelength in meters (m). In the case of a circular dish, D is just the diameter. While in the case of a rectangular horn, it is the diagonal distance across the mouth. At this point, the maximum phase difference of EM waves coming from various points on the antenna is 22.5 degrees [3]. However, larger phase difference and therefore shorter distance to the far-field zone could be marked while performing hazard assessment. The new distance is defined as

$$R_{NF} = 0.5\frac{D^2}{\lambda}$$
(6.4)

Plane wave: This is an electromagnetic wave characterized by mutually orthogonal electric and magnetic fields that are related by the impedance of free space. For the plane waves P and E, exhibit the following relationship: $P = E^2/377$.

Types of Antennas

Antennas are made in different shapes and sizes [Figure 6-6]. They are used in radio and TV broadcasting, radar systems, radio communications, cellular communications, and many other applications.

Isotropic antenna: This is a hypothetical source radiating power equally in all directions. It is used as a reference radiator when describing the radiation properties of real antennas.

Wire antenna:	Any wire acts like an antenna. The wire need not be straight. Usually, wire antennas are designed to operate between 2-30 MHz. These are physically long since they operate at low frequencies.
Half-wave antenna:	This is an antenna whose electrical length is half the wavelength of the radio signal, or half the distance the radio wave travels during one cycle.
Loop antenna:	Basically, a loop antenna is used for AM broadcasting at the long wave band. There are two types of loop antennas, one is the ferrite bar (as in AM radio), and the other is wound on an air core form. The loop antenna is very directional, and need not to be circular. There can be more than one turn also.
Aperture antenna:	This is the part of a plane surface of a directional antenna, which is very near to the antenna and normal to the direction of maximum radiant intensity through which the major part of the radiation passes. An example of aperture is the waveguide horn.
Slot antenna:	A radiating element (hole) created by a slot in a conducting surface or in the wall of a waveguide or cavity.
Dish antenna:	Parabolic dishes are used for the reception and transmission of radio waves to satellites and terrestrial links. They receive waves and focus them through the parabolic focal point where the receiving antenna is placed.
Helical antenna:	This is a wire wound in the form of a helix. Helical antenna can easily generate circular-polarized waves. They operate in a wide frequency bandwidth. When the helix circumference is one wavelength, maximum radiation is generated along the helix axis.
Microstrip antenna:	The microstrip antenna is very low profile and has mechanical strength. Such an antenna is becoming popular for microwave applications, as it is small and easily fabricated. To fabricate a microstrip antenna, an

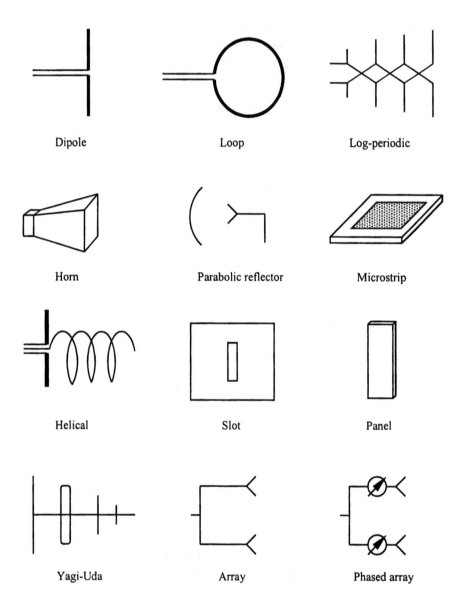

Figure 6-6 Various types of antennas.

area of conductor is printed on the surface of a thin dielectric substrate with a ground plane (almost any shape is possible).

Antenna array: When several antennas are connected together, the combination is called antenna array and the array as a whole behaves as if it is a single antenna. Active arrays have each element individually driven by their own feeds, whereas passive arrays have a principal radiator passing energy to parasitic elements.

Yagi-Uda antenna:

The Yag-Uda antenna is familiar to everyone as it is commonly used for television reception. This is a passive array, with a single driven element, and the other elements are driven parasitically. It consists of a folded dipole-radiating element with a number of parasitic elements.

Log-periodic antenna:

This is a wide-band antenna consisting of dipoles of successively diminishing length connected in parallel across the feed. Only that dipole which is very close to a half-wavelength long loads the feed; the dipole behind and in front acts as reflector and director to give the array a little gain.

Line antenna:

This is a leaky transmission line whose wave velocity is close to that of waves in free space. The resulting "phase matching" condition allows resonant transfer from the transmission line to the free space wave.

Whip antenna:

This is cylindrical in shape. The size varies according to the frequency and gain for which it is designed. The whip antenna is also called *stick* or *pipe* antenna, and is usually omnidirectional.

Panel antenna:

Panel antenna (also called directional) is an antenna or array of antennas designed to concentrate the radiation in a particular area. Panel antenna is typically flat, rectangular device. This antenna is used for cellular base stations in cities and suburban areas where greater customer capacity is needed.

Phased array antenna:

Several antennas can be arrayed in space to make a desired directional pattern. By controlling the phase shift between successive elements in an array antenna, the direction can be steered electronically without physically moving the antenna structure.

6.3 RADIO AND TELEVISION TRANSMITTERS

Radio and television broadcast stations transmit their signals via AM and FM broadcasting antennas. The strength of these signals to which a worker or member of the public can be exposed is determined by the frequency of radiation. Broadcast antennas transmit at various frequencies, depending on the channel ranging. Usually, broadcasters operate in the 535-1705 kHz band for AM radio and in the 2-806 MHz band for FM radio, and in the VHF and UHF bands for television channels.

6.3.1 AM Radio Stations

Amplitude modulation (AM) is a simple, effective process for transmitting information. AM operates on a specific frequency known as a carrier. This signal never changes in power. The operating power of a broadcasting station is the carrier power. The audio signal is added to the carrier creating modulation.

At AM radio stations, monopole antennas are usually used for medium and long wave broadcasting. Due to the relatively long wavelength in the AM frequency band, it is important to consider the strength of both electric and magnetic fields in the vicinity of transmitting antennas. Fields from such antennas decrease sharply with distance. Consequently, safety limits for such stations are not as prohibitive as those are for other frequencies.

Radio broadcasting in the high frequency (short-wave) spectrum generally employs high-transmitter power, commonly in the 50-500 kW range, or greater, with either curtain antenna arrays or rhombic antennas fed with open-wire transmission lines from the transmitter. Figure 6-7 shows a schematic diagram of a curtain antenna array.

At high frequencies (3-30 MHz), broadcast stations use multiple transmitters and multiple antennas. An antenna switch room (matrix room) provides the necessary relays to interconnect any transmitter to any antenna. Because transmission lines are all open structures, high RF fields are present within the room and in such case, both electric and magnetic fields must be measured to properly evaluate the exposure.

A significant aspect of these high frequency facilities is the presence of vertically polarized electric fields beneath the large, horizontally polarized antenna array. These vertically polarized fields come about because of the high RF potential between the elements and the ground. This phenomenon leads to the existence of electric fields that may induce substantial currents in a standing person. In some cases, these induced body currents may exceed the exposure limits well before either electric or magnetic fields exceed their corresponding exposure limits.

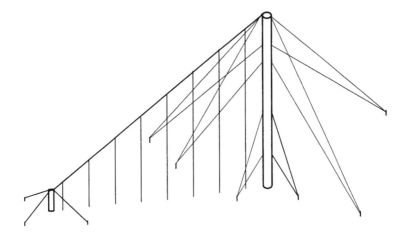

Figure 6-7 A curtain antenna array.

6.3.2 FM Radio Stations

The concept of frequency modulation (FM) was practically introduced as an alternative to AM in 1931. FM operates by superimposing the intelligence (audio or video) signal on a high-frequency carrier. So, the carrier's signal departs from its reference value by an amount proportional to the intelligence amplitude.

FM radio stations transmit in the 88-108 MHz band. Antennas applied for FM radio stations usually consist of an array of elements built-up vertically and side-mounted on a tower or tower-top pole. In some cases, FM radio antennas may have a relatively large number of elements. The elements are usually spaced about one wavelength apart (around 3 meters) and are fed in phase with power distributed equally among the elements. Sometimes the spacing is one-half wavelength to eliminate the end-fire mode of phase addition, lessening downward radiation. Such antennas are omnidirectional, producing a circular coverage pattern.

6.3.3 FM Television Stations

FM TV channels operate in the 54-88/174-220 MHz band for VHF and 470-806 MHz for UHF. Antennas used for television broadcasting usually consist of an array of radiating elements mounted on a tower. Compared to many FM antennas, the elements used for television broadcasting are generally of more complex design and radiate less energy downward. Also television broadcast antennas are often mounted on higher towers than those used for FM radio broadcasting.

6.4 RADAR SYSTEMS

The word *radar* is an acronym, used by the United States Navy in 1942, which stands for *radio detecting and ranging*. The radar was developed for military purposes during the 1940s. In addition to its usual application for military detection, navigation, and weather, police traffic radar devices are widely used.

Typical radar measures the strength and round-trip time of the RFR signals (short pulses) that are emitted by a radar antenna and reflected off a distant surface or object. About 1500 high-power pulses per second are transmitted toward the target, with each pulse having a pulse width of typically 10-50 μs. The pulse normally covers a small band of frequencies, centered on the operating frequency of the radar. The radar antenna alternately transmits and receives pulses at particular wavelengths (in the range 1 cm to 1 m, which corresponds to the frequency range of about 300 MHz to 30 GHz) and polarization (waves polarized in a single vertical or horizontal plane).

The radar detects the reflected pulses and, from the time delay between the emission of the pulse and the arrival of its reflection, it calculates the distance of the obstacle. This process is repeated in every direction as the antenna scans the horizon. The resulting information is displayed on a fluorescent screen as a presentation of the area surrounding the target.

6.4.1 Stationary Radar

Radar and navigational aids are fixed sources of RFR used to control, assist, or provide information concerning traffic on land, at sea, or in the air. Some examples of stationary radar and navigational aid sources include air route surveillance radars, air traffic control radars, height-finder radars, instrument landing systems, VHF omnidirectional range (VOR) navigational aids, marker beacons, and radars used for weather prediction; also included in this category are radars used in meteorological or research activities. The majority of these sources are located at land or along the coast.

A phased array antenna can electronically steer the direction of the antenna beam instantaneously as shown in Figure 6-8. In multifunction radar, this capability is utilized to allow the system to multiplex its time between different functions. The main functions are surveillance and multiple target tracking.

The intensity of the radiation from these sources depends on several factors, including frequency of the radiation, characteristics, of the source, power transmitted to the source, pulse width, repetition rate, and the distance from the source. Airport workers incur most cases of overexposure if they are standing near one of these sources while it is operating. It is possible also that the public may get close to one of these sources and be exposed to hazardous levels of RFR.

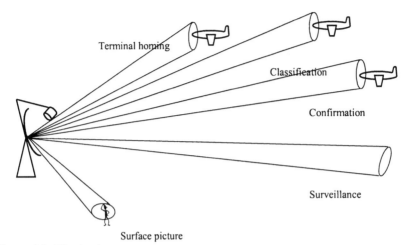

Terminal homing

Classification

Confirmation

Surveillance

Surface picture

Figure 6-8 Fixed radar.

In addition to the above radars, many small marine vessels such as police launches, fishing boats, or pleasure crafts are equipped with navigational radars of power up to 10 kW. Due to the small size of these vessels, the radar antenna is sometimes mounted in close proximity to areas nearby to persons either on the vehicle itself or on nearby structures.

6.4.2 Traffic Radar Devices

Police use radar for traffic speed measurement, although their use was not popular until 1970s. Early traffic radar was large and suitable only for stationary application. During the 1970s, radar speed measuring devices evolved from the original bulky stationary models to the present sophisticated models capable of monitoring vehicle speeds in both stationary and moving modes. A large number of police officers began to have radar units at their disposal for daily use.

The early traffic radar was designed to operate at the range of 10.525 GHz. Therefore, such devices used to be known as X-band radars. In 1975, 24.15 GHz, which lies in the k-band, was introduced as a second traffic radar frequency. During the 1990s, a third frequency of traffic radar was introduced that operates at 33.7-36 GHz, which lies at the ka-band of the electromagnetic spectrum.

All traffic radar units operate by transmitting a low-power signal, detecting a portion of energy reflected from a moving target, and comparing the frequency of the received signal with that of the transmitted signal. This difference in frequency is directly proportional to the speed of the target vehicle with respect to the radar unit, a phenomenon known as the *Doppler effect*. Doppler radar emits continuous wave (CW) rather than pulses. Traffic radar emits power in the range

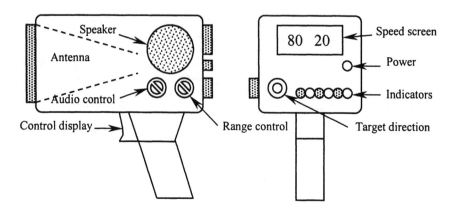

Figure 6-9 Moving traffic radar.

of 10 to 100 mW, with 15 mW being a fairly typical value, an amount considered to be rather low. Compared to any other type of stationary radar, the power level of the traffic radar is very low. This power is also low compared to other RF-emitting devices used in close proximity to persons such as cellular phones.

Traffic radar devices are used in two basic modes, *stationary* or *moving*. Stationary mode radar had to be used by an officer in a fixed position. In the moving mode, the patrol vehicle must be in motion and can monitor the speed of target vehicle approaching from the opposite direction. The radar unit measures the speed of the two vehicles. The two speeds are added to each other. The patrol vehicle speed is subtracted from the total of the two therefore giving the target speed. The readout is usually obtained in a fraction of a second.

The radar range depends upon two things: power of the radar and reflectivity of the target. The amount of power is determined by the design of the radar. The reflectivity of the target, however, varies with each vehicle and is therefore of great importance to each motorist. For highway vehicles, radar reflectivity is generally a matter of size and shape. The smaller the vehicle, the lesser its reflection, and therefore the shorter the range. Some vehicles are out of range on some radar until they drive within 200 meters of the antenna, while big, flat surfaces perpendicular to the beam make fine reflectors. Figure 6-9 shows an illustration of moving traffic radar.

Radiation levels associated with radar vary according to the particular make and model. Usually radiation intensity drops to safe levels at distances of several meters from the antenna. Exposure to radiation from radar above the safety limits is most likely in the immediate vicinity of the antenna when it is stationary. Average power exposure goes below the recommended limits when the antenna is rotating, as for normal operation of the radar. Operating procedures should be imposed to block radiation except when the antenna is rotating.

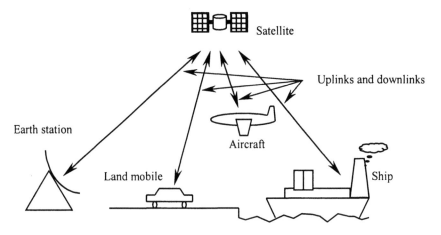

Satellite

Uplinks and downlinks

Earth station

Aircraft

Land mobile

Ship

Figure 6-10 Components of a satellite communication network.

6.5 SATELLITE EARTH STATIONS

A satellite is a special wireless receiver/transmitter that is launched by a rocket and placed in orbit around the Earth under gravitational attraction. Currently, there are hundreds of satellites in operation. Satellites serve a variety of functions: globally relaying telephone signals, weather forecasting, remote sensing of the earth and the environment, television broadcasting, and as platforms for the global positioning system (GPS).

Satellites operate through very sophisticated communication networks that provide a wide range of voice, data, and video services to both fixed and mobile terminals. The viability of the network is in large attributed to the use of orbiting satellite services. The main components of a satellite network are the earth stations and spaceships, which act as relay stations with wide area coverage of the earth as shown in Figure 6-10.

Satellite earth stations, which are of public concern regarding their RFR, consist of large parabolic dishlike antennas that are used to transmit or receive signals via satellites. Satellites receive the signals beamed up to them and, in turn, retransmit the signal back down to earthbound receiving stations. Since earth station antennas are directed toward the satellites above the earth, the transmitted beams point skyward at various angles of inclination, depending on the satellite being used. Because of the longer distances involved (for example, 36,000 km for geostationary satellites), the power levels used to transmit these signals are relatively high when compared to those used for microwave point-to-point links. The diameter of the beam used for transmission is narrow and highly directional. Therefore, it is unlikely that a member of the public would access the main beam.

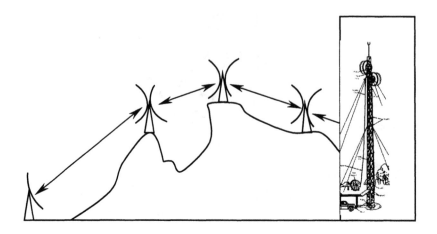

Figure 6-11   Microwave transmission link and a site.

Radiation levels on the ground vary, depending upon the angle of inclination of the antenna, the antenna pattern itself, and the intensity of the transmitted signal. A worker who needs to gain access to one of these antennas may easily be exposed to hazardous RFR levels if proper precautions are not taken. Moreover, not all earth station antennas transmit signals. Some antennas are only used to receive information and therefore, do not pose any health hazard. Included in this group would be the type of satellite dish that can be purchased by the general public for the purpose of viewing television programs.

6.6   MICROWAVE COMMUNICATIONS

A point-to-point microwave relay system is a high capacity facility that provides line-of-sight radio communications and must not be obstructed. Microwave communication antennas transmit and receive low power signals across relatively short distances as shown in Figure 6-11. These antennas are usually rectangular or circular in shape (dishes) and have a variety of applications such as transmitting telephone and telegraph messages and serving as links between broadcast or cable TV studios and broadcast antennas. These dishes receive the signal and focus it through the parabolic focal point where the receiving antenna is placed. Microwave signals from these antennas travel in a directed, narrow beam from a transmitting to a receiving antenna and the dispersion of microwave energy outside the beam path is minimal or insignificant. Under certain geographic or atmospheric surroundings, the beam may be bent from the actual line-of-sight path.

In general, receiving and transmitting dishes must be accurately aligned for maximum performance. Based on current research findings, it is not expected that any harmful effect would result from exposure to radiation from microwave links.

6.7 MOBILE RADIO EQUIPMENT

Mobile (not cellular) radio is the oldest form of wireless communications. It has been developing for decades. Starting in 1921 in the United States, mobile radios began operating at 2 MHz, just above the present AM radio broadcast band. These were mainly experimental police department radios, with practical systems not implemented until the 1940s.

The first mobile telephone service was introduced on 17 June 1946 in Saint Louis, Missouri. AT&T and Southwestern Bell introduced the first American commercial mobile radiotelephone service. This early system used a wide-area architecture, where a single base station atop a high building managed a few radio channels connecting users to the public switched telephone network (PSTN). They operated on six channels in the 150-MHz band with 60 kHz channel spacing. A centrally located transceiver served a wide area with a few frequencies transmitting a large amount of RF power to distances about 100 km away. Within a few years, the mobile radio was serving airports, taxi operators, fire stations, police departments, security personnel, truck fleets, and many other applications. It is a good service for areas not well served by cellular communications.

Simple mobile radio systems use a single channel where all users share this channel and only one person at a time can use the channel. More sophisticated mobile radio systems are trunked with multiple channels. Trunking systems can support quite a bit more traffic than can a system with as many radio channels available but without trunking aids. Users would meet at that channel and agree to switch to one of the free channels to carry out their conversation.

Mobile radio uses vertical polarization, which allows the vertical antenna to be used and an omnidirectional coverage achieved irrespective of the direction of the vehicle. The vertical mobile antennas fitted to vehicles are of various lengths (related to the wavelength). Such antennas, however, require the body of the vehicle to provide the missing portion of the antenna in order to achieve good transmission and reception. The vehicle provides the ground plane for the antenna, therefore, it is better to fix the antenna in the middle of the roof where a large metallic plate is available. The simplest and most common type of antenna is a quarter-wave ($\lambda/4$) antenna. Larger antennas with higher gain, such as a half-wave ($\lambda/2$) antenna and a $5\lambda/8$ antenna, are also used. A collinear antenna consisting of a $\lambda/2$ antenna on the top and a $\lambda/4$ antenna at the bottom joined by a coil is also used [4]. Figure 6-12 shows many common mobile radio antennas.

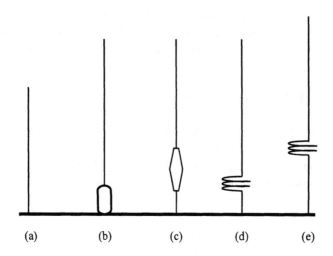

Figure 6-12   (a) A simple λ/4 antenna. (b) A radiator with spring. (c) A radiator with encapsulated coil. (d) An open coil radiator. (e) A half wave mounted over λ/4 antenna.

6.8 PAGING SYSTEMS

The beginning of the paging industry in the United States is traced back to the first land-mobile radio systems pioneered by the Detroit Police Department as early as 1921 when the concept of one-way information broadcasting was introduced [4]. In 1956, the first radio paging system was installed in St. Thomas Hospital in London [5]. Since that time, the commercial paging market has been widely used as a quick, convenient, and reliable method of communication, despite the wide use of cellular phones in recent years.

6.8.1 Pagers

Pagers are designed to listen to one frequency channel. Information contained on this channel may be tone, voice, or digital data. When the pager receives the identification signal, it beeps, vibrates, or flashes a light to inform the subscriber that a paging message has been received. The pager has a small liquid crystal display (LCD) for displaying up to 20 numeric digits, typically the caller's phone number, prices, product numbers, etc.

The first pager was analog only, and each pager was assigned a separate frequency. Later, digital technology allowed many pagers to share one frequency. A single frequency could be coded in such a way that thousands or even millions of pagers could share the same frequency without interfering with each other.

Two-way paging systems are now being released, where the receipt of messages can be acknowledged, and the subscriber can transmit a programmed reply to a received message.

Paging services come in several forms: tone-only, tone and voice, numeric, alphanumeric, and computer interface. Tone-only paging is the simplest and cheapest to hire and can alert the subscriber that someone wants to communicate. This type of service is most useful when the subscriber only needs to call one place, such as an office.

Tone-and-voice paging, the follow-up of tone-only, allows the subscriber to receive a voice message. However, the voice message may be missed if the subscriber has the pager turned off or is out of transmitter range.

Numeric paging is liked in the market today. A caller dials the phone number assigned to the pager and then, using a touch-tone phone, enters the number of the phone for a reply. With the arrival of numeric display pagers during 1980s, the alert tone is followed by a display of the phone number to call back. For example, the numeric pager notifies the subscriber about receiving a call, and the subscriber can retrieve the phone number of the caller from the pager display.

Alphanumeric pagers display alphabetic or numeric messages entered by the calling party or operator using a computer/modem combination or a custom page-entry device designed to enter alphanumeric pages. The alphanumeric pager requires the caller to have access to an alphanumeric terminal or a message center that can send alphanumeric messages to the pager. This type of service is relatively expensive, but it might be valuable if the pager subscriber benefits by having instant information rather than having to call someone for it.

6.8.2 Types of Paging Systems

Paging information is sent to a pager via a paging network. The paging network begins at the connection to the PSTN. For example, the caller accesses one of three things: a voice mail, a paging operator, or touch-tone telephone dial. The resulting paging messages are assembled in the paging terminal and sent to the network controller where they are combined into batches, based on their final destination. All billing and management services are also controlled at this point.

There are many types of paging formats currently in use. Analog formats use a multitone (two, five, or six tones) pager signaling sequence. These formats can transmit numeric information, such as phone numbers, or voice. In addition to the analog formats, several digital formats are in use. The most common, and the worldwide standard at this time, is the post office code standardization advisory group (POCSAG). The POCSAG is a synchronous paging format that allows pages to be transmitted in a single-batch structure.

Paging systems are divided into two types due to geographical area [5]: on-site radio paging, and wide-area paging.

On-Site Radio Paging

This type of paging is used within certain site premises and is designed to alert and inform people by using voice, data, or beeps. Four types are in use:

1. Induction loop paging (16-150 kHz): This paging system is suitable for sites up to about 4 hectares. A leaky coaxial cable connects buildings within the site from which energy radiates.
2. HF (26-31 MHz) and VHF on-site paging (49 MHz): All the licenses are for nonspeech paging only and must consist of data or beeps.
3. UHF (459 MHz) on-site paging: The system is implemented in heavily reinforced buildings and factories.
4. Local communications (459 MHz): It may replace the existing HF and UHF two-way paging. It allows users to acknowledge a paging call by speech.

Wide-Area Paging Systems

These systems allow the transmission of one-way calls via a base station. The coverage for paging systems may vary significantly in extent. For a small city or country, one paging transmitter site may be adequate, but when the area to be covered is extensive it may be necessary to have multiple transmitter sites. When more than one transmitter is used for the purpose of improving coverage, the technique of simultaneous transmission (simulcasting) from all the transmitters usually needs to be employed. Simulcast is a reliable technique of achieving wide-area coverage. This technique involves sending the paging signal from multiple paging transmitters at precisely the same time. Larger coverage area arises from combining the individual transmitter coverage.

The coverage area varies from about 5 to 20 km from the base station depending on the transmitting power, geographical area, and type of antenna. Many paging companies cover more than just one geographical area. For example, the company may serve an entire state or country. The network controller specifies the site controller(s) for which the batched messages are intended and sends them out. Each site, covering a particular geographical location, may contain one or more paging transmitter. Once the site controller receives the batch of pages, it uplinks them to the paging transmitter(s), which then transmit the batch of messages at the same time on the same frequency using a simulcast technique. Typically, transmitters are located at the top of tall buildings, hills, or towers to gain additional height, and therefore coverage.

6.9 CELLULAR COMMUNICATIONS

The cellular scenario is really different from the mobile radio. It is a kind of band-limited analog or digital transmission in which a subscriber has a wireless connection from a mobile telephone to a relatively nearby base station. Cellular communication is presently the fastest growing part of the telecommunication industry. It is adding customers at the rate 30-40% a year, and promises to become the preferred medium of telecommunications in the near future. To keep up with the increasing demand for available radio channels and to secure quality of services, there is a continual need for extra cells in metropolitan areas and their suburbs.

AT&T Bell Laboratories proposed the cellular concept as the advanced mobile phone system (AMPS) in 1971 [6]. The idea started by replacing the single base station high above the center of a city with many low-powered base stations, distributed over the coverage area on sites placed closer to ground. The low-power cell sites were linked through a central switching and control center.

Cellular communication systems started to spread out all over the world in the early 1980s. It was a turning point in telecommunications, adding radio access and mobility to the telephone network for the first time in history. AMPS appeared in North America, Australia, and parts of Asia. Other first-generation analog systems followed: NMT-450 and NMT-900 appeared in Scandinavia, and the rest of Europe, and parts of Asia: C-Netz in Germany, Austria, Portugal, and South Africa; RC 2000 in France; TACS and ETACS in the United Kingdom, Ireland, and parts of Asia; RTMS in Italy; and MCSL1 and JTACS in Japan.

First-generation (1G) analog cellular systems were followed in the early 1990s by second-generation (2G) digital systems offering a larger number of mobile subscribers better service quality and a wide range of value-added services, such as data. 2G celular systems use digital modulation and processing techniques. These digital systems ensure greater call clarity and security, prevent cloning fraud, and have several standards. The digital cellular has become a success, with hundred millions of subscribers worldwide. The majority is in Global System for Mobile Communication (GSM).

Today, standardization is moving toward 3G cellular systems in the European Telecommunication Standardization Institute (ETSI), under a project called Universal Mobile Telecommunication System (UMTS) and in the International Telecommunication Union (ITU), where it is called IMT2000. The 2-GHz frequency band (1920-1980 MHz band and 2110-2170 MHz band) has been allocated in Europe and Asia for the 3G systems. With the enlargement of GSM networks, it seems that the UMTS/IMT2000 will draw on GSM network technology. Yet, the UMTS should arrive sometime after the year 2002. The 3G system allows even additional services so that applications at high bit rates can be

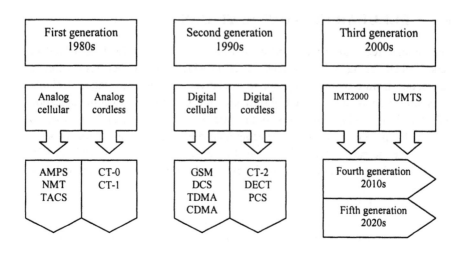

Figure 6-13 Current and future mobile systems.

delivered. This means that the wireless terminal is becoming a generic platform for the whole range of communications involving voice, data, video, and images. Such terminals are more interesting to people since they offer more services rather than simple voice connections.

However, demands for higher access speeds for multimedia communications will continue to include the fourth generation (4G) and fifth generation (5G). The 4G is used, in a broad sense, to include several systems; not only cellular systems, but also many new types of communication systems such as broadband wireless access systems, millimeter-wave LANs, intelligent transport systems (ITSs), and high altitude stratospheric platform station (HAPS) systems. When 4G systems are used in a narrow sense as cellular systems, they will be known as 4G-cellular [7, 8].

Figure 6-13 shows the current and future mobile systems. It is important to specify that cordless phone does not constitute a service in the strict sense, but rather a wireless consumer product. No license is required for the operation of the phone but the product must be manufactured in conformance with standards.

6.9.1   Overview of the Cellular System

Cellular communication theory is simple while the operation is extremely complex. The cellular system uses enormous number of low-power wireless transmitters to create cells, which are the primary geographic service areas of the cellular system. Variable power levels allow cells to be sized according to the subscriber density and demand within a certain region. As subscribers move from cell to cell, their conversations are handed off between cells to maintain seamless services. Channels (frequencies) used in one cell may be reused in another cell some distance away. Cells may be added to accommodate growth, creating new cells in uncovered areas or overlaying cells in existing areas. Each subscriber uses a separate, temporary radio channel to talk to the cell site. The cell site communicates with many subscribers at once, using one channel per subscriber. The radio path can be identified for both the *downlink* path, the path from a cell site to the subscriber, and for *uplink* path from the subscriber to the cell site.

The basic structure of the cellular network includes telephone systems and radio services. Where mobile radio operates in a closed network and has no access to the telephone system, cellular system allows interconnection to the telephone network. Figure 6-14 shows a typical topology for the cellular system. The main parts of the cellular system are radio link, switching system, database, processing center, and external network. The mobile connection of the cellular subscriber and fixed network is realized with radio links. The mobile station (MS) is usually a small handset. It corresponds with the base transceiver station (BTS). Each cell site has a BTS with a transceiver and antenna system.

The BTS plays a key role in the cellular system by acting as a radio relay station. The signal strength declines or increases as the subscriber moves toward or away from the BTS. Each BTS uses carefully chosen frequencies to reduce interference with neighboring cells. BTS equipment by itself is nothing without a means to manage it. In the GSM and PCS 1900, this is accomplished by the use of a base station controller (BSC). The BSC is a high-capacity switch, which provides control of radio functions, such as handover, management of radio network resources and handling of cell configuration data. The BSC coordinates with the mobile telecommunication switching office (MTSO), also called mobile switching center (MSC). With AMPS, however, the mobile switch controls the whole network and interacts with distant databases and the PSTN.

The switching utility is a combination of computing platforms and transmission facilities that route user information and signaling among nodes throughout the mobile network. The MSC is the control unit for the cellular system. It switches the calls to the cells. It provides the interfacing with telephone networks and monitors the traffic for charging and billing. Also, the MSC provides overall network management. The BTS is connected to the MSC with conventional trunks (microwave link or fiber optic). In addition, the MSC is connected to both local and distant switches.

A database is required to provide services to mobile subscribers. For example, in the GSM, the home location register (HLR) stores subscriber data relative to network intelligence. The visitor location register (VLR) maintains temporary working copies of active subscribers in the network. While, the authentication center (AC) performs functions that validate a mobile station's identity.

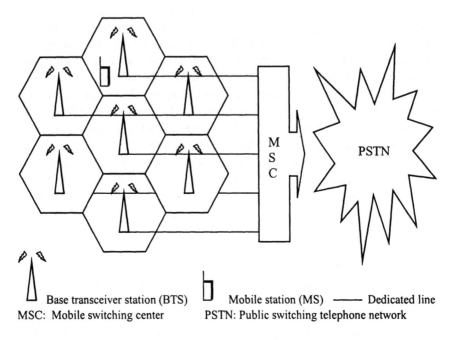

Base transceiver station (BTS)   Mobile station (MS) ——— Dedicated line
MSC: Mobile switching center   PSTN: Public switching telephone network

Figure 6-14 A typical cellular system.

6.9.2 Cellular Technologies

Cellular phones transmit either analog or digital signals, depending on the type of instrument and the service available. An analog signal has a continuous nature rather than a pulsed or discrete nature, while the digital signal is discrete. Analog cellular systems are 1G systems. Several analog standards have been developed worldwide. The analog system uses FM radio waves to transmit voice grade signals.

Cellular systems use several ways to transmit information. Several competing technologies of multiplexing transmission schemes are common in use for the cellular systems. They are frequency division multiple access (FDMA); time division multiple access (TDMA); and code division multiple access (CDMA).

FDMA

FDMA is division of the frequency band allocated for wireless cellular communication into several channels, each of which can carry a voice conversation or, with digital service, carry digital data. The FDMA architecture is also known as narrowband mobile radio as the bandwidth of the individual data or digitized analog signal is relatively narrow compared with TDMA and CDMA applications. FDMA is a basic technology in analog cellular systems like AMPS, which is the most widely installed cellular phone system in North America. With FDMA, each channel can be assigned to only one user at a time. FDMA is also used in the total access communications system (TACS).

TDMA

TDMA was first used experimentally in Japan in 1982. It was found as a possibility to reduce the cost of base stations, since many users could share the same transceiver. Under TDMA, subscribers share the radio spectrum in time domain. Each subscriber is allocated a time slot. Eventually, TDMA has better spectrum efficiency performance than FDMA. Usually, the subscriber accesses the entire frequency band allocated to the system (wide-band TDMA) or only certain part of the band (narrow-band TDMA). In TDMA, transmission takes place in bursts from the mobile to the BTS (uplink), with only one user transmitting to the base station at any given time. In the downlink, the BTS transmits continuously, with the subscriber listening only during the assigned time slot.

The TDMA technique serves all 2G systems. In 1987, narrow-band TDMA with 200-kHz channel spacing was chosen for the GSM standard. Each 200-kHz TDMA carrier can handle eight full-rate voice calls at 13 kbps each or 16 half-rate voice calls.

In 1989, narrow-band TDMA was also selected as the digital standard for the AMPS with a 30-kHz bandwidth and is called digital (d)-AMPS. Each 30-kHz carrier can handle three voice calls, each at 8 kbps. However, a 25-kHz channel was selected for the personal digital cellular (PDC) Japanese system.

CDMA

An alternative multiplexing scheme to FDMA and TDMA is CDMA, which uses the entire spectrum of bandwidth for all users in the cell. It transmits all the subscribers' signals onto the channel at the same time. CDMA system, pioneered by Qualcomm, Inc., of San Diego, was standardized and is known as the IS-95 standard of the Electronic Industries Association (EIAIS-95).

In CDMA, messages are transmitted in sequences of ones and zeroes with a special code attached so that only the intended receivers can decode the messages. CDMA segregates users not on the basis of frequency bands or time slots, but by certain high-speed spreading codes applied to transmission as secondary modulation. CDMA assigns a unique code to each bit of information, transmitting these little pieces over the spectrum. All transmissions share the same bandwidth at the same time, but each is modulated by its own spreading code, which is orthogonal to all of the system's other spreading codes. As a result, every user looks like random interference (background noise) to all other users and can be easily suppressed as long as the received signal to noise ratio is high enough [9, 10].

In 1998, ETSI decided to base the UMTS standard on a new wide-band W-CDMA technology using 5-MHz wide-band radio carrier. This technology can support access to wireless multimedia applications. The W-CDMA is different from the narrow-band CDMA system such as IS-95, which was principally designed for voice communications. Improved capacity and coverage are additional advantages of W-CDMA [8].

6.9.3   Base Transceiver Stations

The combination of antennas and associated electronic equipment is referred to as BTS or cell site. BTSs vary everywhere in appearance, but every BTS has a set of transmitting and receiving antennas, which often look like vertical whips or panels. Principal antennas for cellular transmission are generally located on towers, water tanks, and other support structures such as rooftops and the sides of buildings. Since the cellular radio is a duplex system, good performance is required in both transmitting and receiving directions. Such performance depends on many variables over which the designer or the operator has control, such as type of antenna, gain, bandwidth, height, input impedance, mechanical rigidity, ground plane, coverage pattern, available power to drive it, application of simple or multiple antenna configuration, and polarization. Other variables where the designer has no control are topography between the BTS and MS as well as speed and direction of the MS if on vehicle.

Typical heights for BTS structures are 10-75 meters. Usually, a BTS utilizes either several omnidirectional antennas that look like poles, 3 to 5 meters in height, or a number of sector antennas that look like rectangular panels. Since a vertical dipole has an omnidirectional pattern, many dipoles can be stacked together to produce high gain omidirectional antenna.

A typical BTS antenna will have four half-wave dipoles spaced by 1 wavelength vertically and fed in phase [11]. Another type of BTS antenna is the high-gain sector antenna. Sectorizing technique divides the cell into 3 or 6 distinct areas (120 and 60 degrees around the site respectively). Each sector gets its own frequencies to operate on. The number of antennas depends on the service area, e.g., in a high density service area six transmitting antennas, each with up to sixteen radio channels, could be used. The antenna height is critical, it must be high enough to secure good coverage and at the same time low enough to prevent interfering with remote cells. Figure 6-15 shows three types of BTS antennas.

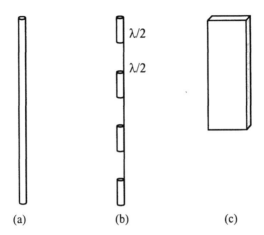

$\lambda/2$

$\lambda/2$

(a)   (b)   (c)

Figure 6-15 (a) Low-gain (whip) antenna. (b) Intermediate-gain stacked vertical dipoles. (c) High-gain (sector) antenna.

The effective radiated power (ERP) of the cellular system depends on the number of channels authorized at a cell site. However, all channels would not be expected to be operating together, therefore reducing overall emission levels. The majority of BTSs in urban areas operate at an ERP of 100 watts per channel or even less. An ERP of 100 watts corresponds to an actual radiated power of 5-10 watts (ERP referenced to a half-wave dipole is a cellular way of expressing the signal power emitted from a BTS antenna and depends on the directional characteristics of the antenna). With the expansion of the cellular system capacity by dividing cells (adding more BTSs), lower ERP can be used. ERP, antenna height, and number of channels depend on the traffic load. When traffic is low, a typical BTS might have a 75-meter tower, 10 to 20 active channels, and about 100 watts per channel of ERP. The greater the number of BTS, the heavier the controlling of the distributed BTS is. As the traffic increases, the preclusive effect of BTS becomes too great. Several changes must occur as the BTS evolves into a higher capacity facility to cope with growing demand without also precluding channel reuse nearby. First, antenna heights must drop to 30-50 meters. Second, ERP must decrease to about 20 to 50 watts per channel. Omnidirectional antennas give way to directional antennas aimed to serve just a slice of the overall coverage area. The radiation from these antennas is beamed horizontally at the horizon with a slightly downward tilt. Number of active channels within the entire service area increases, to perhaps 40-50, but the number in any one-sector lessons. In some cases, the BTS will have an ERP below 10 watts per channel, and with a more number of channels.

Table 6-2   Maximum Power for Mobile and Portable Stations

Class	Maximum RF Power (W)
I	20
II	8
III	5
IV	2
V	0.8

6.9.4   Mobile and Portable Stations

Mobile and portable wireless transmitting stations include those devices operating in wireless, cellular, personal, and satellite communication services.

A mobile station (MS) is defined as transmitting/receiving device used in an unfixed position. Examples include cellular telephones, devices using vehicle-mounted antennas, and wireless devices used with personal computers.

A portable station (PS) is defined as a transmitting/receiving device used with its radiating structure in direct contact with the user's body. Examples include handheld cellular and PCS phones that incorporate the antenna into the handset.

The power classes for mobile and portable stations are shown in Table 6-2 [11]. The most commonly used power levels are 5 W, 2 W, and 0.8 W for the handheld units and 20 W or 8 W for the vehicle mounted and portable units.

Today, there is a strong trend toward the use of handheld cellular phones. The early models of these communication devices included large battery packs and carrying cases. Cellular phones are becoming even smaller than a package of cigarettes, and some models are capable of transmitting computer files, paging, e-mailing, and even surfing the Internet. More value-added wireless services and features will be added to cellular phones of the 21st century such as video and digital cameras, gaming consoles, and personal stereos. The market for the new generation of cellular phones is expected to reach one billion consumers in the next five years. Due to this accelerated growth, drastically changes in the demographics of cellular phone users have taken place. The change moved from middle-aged businessmen to all age group users to become integral part of personal lives.

The cellular phone consists of front and back covers that sandwich two printed circuit boards, which run along the entire length of the phone. The top board (LCD/keypad board) is regularly responsible for input/output functions and contains the keypad, LCD module, and microphone (a loudspeaker is attached to the inside of the front cover). The lower or main board contains most of the RF and digital processing components.

Presently, there are two types of cellular phones in common use: analog and digital. The 2G phones have appeared alongside of, and in some places have replaced, their analog predecessors. Analog cellular phones transmit and receive voice carrying RF signals continuously, whereas digital phones code voice into packets of RF signals, which are then transmitted in regular pulses. Analog phones have larger capacity and require less frequent battery charging.

A digital cellular phone (GSM, for example) can be divided into two parts. The first part contains the hardware and software to support radio functions. It is the device available at retail shops to buy or rent. The second part contains terminal/user-specific data in the form of a smart card called subscriber identification module (SIM card), which can be considered a sort of logical terminal. The SIM card plugs into the first part of the phone and remains in it for the period of use. The service provider usually issues the SIM card after subscription.

6.10 PERSONAL COMMUNICATION SYSTEMS

The concept of personal communication system (PCS) or personal communications network (PCN) aims at providing two way communication services, speech and data to individual users, indoors or outdoors. PCS and PCN appear to synonymous, with Americans preferring former and Europeans preferring the latter nomenclature.

6.10.1 PCS/PCN Standards

PCS/PCN started as another choice to the cellular concept and possibly as an improvement to it. Basic needs for these systems include low-power technology to provide voice and quite fast-rate data to small, lightweight, economical, pocket-sized personal handsets that can be used for long time without attention to batteries. The aim is to provide telecommunication services economically over wide areas, including indoors and outdoors.

Examples of PCS/PCN standards are: IS-54; IS-95; DCS; PACS; W-CDMA; CDMA/TDMA/FDMA; and DECT. The IS-54 PCS standard works easily with the IS-54 cellular standard. It is relatively easy to build handsets and base stations that can handle both standards. This applies to the IS-95 PCS standard and IS-95 cellular with the DCS standard and GSM cellular network. The W-CDMA and CDMA/TDMA/FDMA standards use the full 5-MHz bandwidth of small PCS allocations. The DECT standard is well suited for indoor communications.

The power for IS-54, IS-95, and DCS is in the range of 100 to 200 mW, while the power for PACS, W-CDMA, CDMA/TDMA/FDMA, and DECT is in the range of 20 to 500 MW.

Like cellular, PCS/PCN suits mobile users and requires a number of antennas to cover a certain area (a cell radius less than 1 km in a dense urban environment to 5 km in the rural environment). It generally requires more cells (microcells) for coverage, but has the advantage of fewer blind spots. Microcells are smaller than cellular cells and, therefore, require a greater number of smaller, lower-powered antennas in the initial deployment than a cellular service would to cover the same territory. Radio coverage and system characteristics are optimal for low-power handsets. The phone itself is slightly smaller than a cellular phone.

6.10.2 Wireless Multimedia Communicators

In recent years, efforts have been dedicated to the investigation of wireless systems able to provide interactive and multimedia services to users in different contexts, such as the mobile environment [12, 13]. The advancement in high-speed networking, wireless communications, integrated circuit technology, and multimedia-based applications caused multimedia communications to emerge, propelled by the strong vision of being able to communicate from anywhere at any time with any type of data.

The hindering to reading large amounts of text on a computer screen, instead of paper, is due in large part to the inconvenience of the usual fixed desktop placement of the screen. An electronic viewing device should have the convenience of paper, but should maintain the capabilities of an advanced multimedia desktop unit. This implies the portable device should be light and allow convenient observation, and have a long battery life, while providing color video and audio output, pen, and microphone inputs.

The most demanding requirement of the communicator is that full motion video be transmitted properly over a wireless downlink from a base station, which performs the interface between a high bandwidth network backbone and the communicator. Video quality equivalent to present day television may be compressed to rates on the order of 1-2 Mbps, which sets the minimum data rate for this link. The data on the uplink (from the portable to the base station) is audio and pen data, which can be adequately transferred by a rate of 64 kbps [14].

Current communicators are low-power, portable devices that can transmit and receive multimedia data through the wireless network. The communicator is equipped with a bird's-eye camera, microphone, and LCD screen, serving as both a video-telephone screen and a computer screen. The conventional keyboard is likely to be replaced by the pressure-sensitive writing tablet, providing optical handwriting recognition, signature verification, etc.

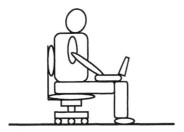

Figure 6-17 A user with wireless multimedia communicator.

Wireless communicators may pose risk of human exposure to RFR since the users most probably use them for long periods. Exposure is increased because the equipment rests on the user's lap at the genital level. An example of such situation is shown in Figure 6-17.

6.11 NONCOMMUNICATION SOURCES

Equipment or appliances designed to generate and locally use RF energy for industrial, domestic or similar purposes, excluding applications in the field of telecommunications, are another sources of RFR. A major application is the production of a physical effect, such as heating.

6.11.1 Sealers and Dielectric Heaters

RF energy in the frequency range 3 to 300 MHz is used in industry for a variety of heating processes. To generate heat, the signal must penetrate the material and transmit energy. The level of energy transmitted depends on the material's conductivity. The term "RF heat sealing" is often used interchangeably with dielectric heat sealing or welding. When a dielectric material comes into contact with EM energy, part of the energy will go through a change of state and be dissipated as heat with the dielectric. The dissipation depends on the atomic and molecular structure of the material, the frequency, and the field strength.

The term "dielectric heating" describes this phenomenon at any frequency while RF or HF heating describes this process over a limited frequency range (1-200 MHz). In the case of RF or HF welding of thermoplastics, the mechanism producing heat in the dielectric is *dipolar* and *interfacial* polarization. The term *dipolar polarization* is related to molecules that are permanently polarized by chemical forces and realigned when in contact with the EM field. *Interfacial polarization* means the accretion of charges at discontinuity within the material due to the migration of electrons under the influence of field. The field may cause

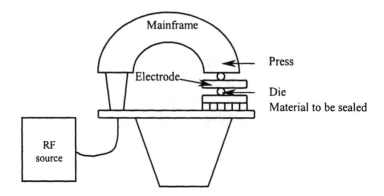

Figure 6-18 Schematic diagram of a RF sealer.

oscillatory displacement of the polarized components as realignment with the positive and negative oscillations occurs. This phenomenon is the source of the heat generated in the dielectric.

RF heaters and sealers operate at 13.56, 27.12, 40.68, 100, and even up to 300 MHz. These devices are also known as RF solders fusers, molders, fasteners, or embossers. Heat sealers have the potential of creating extremely strong EM fields because of their design. A high-power RF generator applies voltage to the sealing electrode that is brought into contact with the material being sealed, typically some form of vinyl, such that the dielectric losses in the material lead to rapid heating and melting of the material. Changing the dies to suit the material may seal objects of different shapes.

Application of heaters and sealers include the manufacture of many plastic products such as toys, life jackets, rain apparel, packaging materials, wood laminations, embossing and drying operations in the textile, paper, plastic and leather industries, and the curing of various materials. Sealers of this type provide very strong and comprehensive seals without the need for solvents. Figure 6-18 shows a schematic diagram of a RF sealer.

6.11.2 Microwave Ovens

RF energy has the ability to penetrate deeply into food material and to produce heat instantaneously as it penetrates; this is in sharp contrast to conventional heating, which depends on the conduction of heat from the food surface to the inside. This property led to the invention of the microwave oven. Raytheon invented the microwave oven shortly after World War II, but their sales did not become notable until late 1960s. Since that time, the market for microwave ovens has grown to become one of today's most popular home appliances.

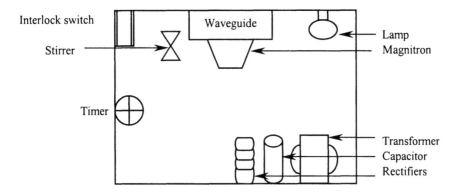

Figure 6-19 A simplified schematic of a microwave oven.

A microwave oven contains a magnetron that produces microwave energy; a high-voltage direct current power supply (a high-voltage transformer, a set of rectifiers, and a capacitor) that provides power to the magnetron; and a computerized control system that turns the power supply and magnetron on and off. The microwave energy is transmitted into a waveguide, which feeds the energy into the cooking area. Some models use a type of rotating antenna, while others rotate the food through energy on a revolving carousel; both of which scatter the energy throughout the cooking compartment. This is minimized by the use of a mode-stirring fan and rotating carousel [15, 16]. Figure 6-19 shows a simplified schematic of microwave oven.

The microwaves penetrate the food and cause water molecules within the food to vibrate at the operating frequency (2.45 GHz). While most microwave ovens operate at 2.45 GHz, that frequency is not a resonant frequency for water molecules. Using a frequency that water molecules respond to strongly (as in a resonance) would be a mistake because water molecules at the surface of the food would absorb all the microwaves and the center of the food would remain raw. Instead, 2.45 GHz was chosen because it is absorbed weakly enough in liquid water (not free water molecules) that the waves maintain good strength even deep inside a typical piece of food. Higher frequencies would penetrate less well and cook less evenly. Lower frequencies would penetrate better, but would be absorbed so weakly that they would not cook well.

There are two quantities present in the microwave oven: electric and magnetic fields (emitted from the transformer) and EM waves (radiated by the magnetron). Metal walls of the oven easily stop the electric fields and EM waves, while the magnetic fields, however, are not stopped, and propagate through the walls into the user's body. In addition, the waves see the screen in the front as a wall, and hit the little holes in the screen propagating in all directions from the holes.

REFERENCES

[1] Corazza, G. C., Marconi's History, *Proceedings of the IEEE*, pp. 1307-1311, 1998.

[2] Radiofrequency Radiation: Health Effects and Interference Status of Current Research and Regulation, A Report to the General Assembly, Technical Report No. 38, 1996.

[3] Dayem, R. A., (ed.), *PCS & Digital Cellular Technologies: Assessing Your Option*, Prentice Hall, Upper Saddle River, NJ, 1997.

[4] White, G., *Mobile Radio Technology*, BH Newnes, London, UK, 1994.

[5] Hon, A. S., *An Introduction To Paging-What It Is And How It Works*, Motorola Electronics Pte Ltd, Singapore, 1993.

[6] Peterson, A. C., Jr., Vehicle Radiotelephony Becomes a Bell System Practice, *Bell Laboratories Record* 137, 1947.

[7] Uddenfeldt, J., Digital Cellular: Its Roots and its Future, *Proceedings of the IEEE* 86, pp. 1319-1324, 1998.

[8] Ohmori, S., The Future Generations of Mobile Communications Based on Broadband Access Technologies, *IEEE Communications* 38 (12), pp. 134-142, 2000.

[9] Feher, K., *Wireless Digital Communications: Modulation & Spread Spectrum Applications*, Prentice Hall, Englewood Cliffs, NJ, 1995.

[10] Malcolm, W. O., The Mobile Phone Meets the Internet, *IEEE Spectrum* 36, pp. 20-28, 1999.

[11] Garg, V. K., and J. E. Wilkes, *Wireless and Personal Communications Systems*, Prentice Hall, Upper Saddle River, NJ, 1996.

[12] Andrisano, O., V. Tralli, and R. Verdone, Millimeter Waves for Short-Range Multimedia Communication Systems, *Proceedings of the IEEE* 86, pp. 1383-1401, 1998.

[13] Barringer, B., T. Burd, F. Burghardt, A. Burstein, A. Chandrakasan, R. Doering, S. Narayanaswamy, T. Pering, B. Richards, T. Truman, J. Rabaey, and R. Brodersen, Infopad: A System Design for Portable Multimedia Access, *Calgary Wireless Conference*, July 1994.

[14] Hanzo, L., Bandwidth-Efficient Wireless Multimedia Communications, *Proceedings of the IEEE* 86, pp. 1342-1382, 1998.

[15] Bloomfield, L. A., Microwave Oven, How Things Work, The University of Virginia, Charlottesville, Virginia, 2000.

[16] Gallawa, J. C., How Does a Microwave Oven Work? Basic Theory of Operation, Internet Document at http://www.gallawa.com/microtech/how_work.html, 1999.

7

Introduction to Bioelectromagnetics

7.1 GENERAL

Bioeletromagnetics is a vast interdisciplinary field that incorporates physics, engineering, and life sciences to understand the interaction of electromagnetic fields with biological systems. This field has become very important due to the rapid development of electromagnetic applications through the tremendous increase in use of various devices employing EM energy in the workplace and home. The mechanism by which EM fields produce biological effects is being investigated. Substantial advances have been made, and scientists in this field have written many comprehensive papers, which are considered a good source of information, especially for engineers and life scientists. Lin [1] gives a good introduction to the role of EM theory in biology and medicine. Stuchly [2] outlines the biophysical basis for interaction of RF fields with living systems. In 1999, Durney and Christensen [3] published an introductory book to bioelectromagnetics, as an effort to fulfill the need of readers in this specialization. Their book explains in detail the basic concepts, principles, and characteristic behaviors of electric and magnetic fields as they pertain to biological systems. It is a good resource for life scientists, engineers, and physicists collaborating in work involving bioeffects of EM fields.

7.2 EM PROPERTIES OF BIOLOGICAL MATERIALS

A basic knowledge of biological material properties, their uniqueness, and their variability among living systems may provide a basis for the exploitation of EM interaction mechanisms. When compared to nonliving materials such as copper, relatively little is known about the physical properties of biological materials. In general, the EM properties of matter have been given in terms of permittivity ε, permeability μ, and conductivity σ [4]. These quantities express the macroscopic properties of a substance without giving any thought to the microscopic (atomic and molecular) structure, which is responsible for the macroscopic behavior.

Scientists and engineers need to have some understanding of how these properties function inside living systems and need to consider the interaction of EM fields with biological materials at the microscopic as well as macroscopic level.

7.2.1 Microscopic Model

General Model

Electric charges play a very important role in the makeup of matter. According to the *Bohr* model of an atom, negative charges (electrons) move around a nucleus consisting of positive charges (protons) and uncharged neutrons. All materials are made up of atoms, which contribute to their electrical properties, including their ability to conduct or resist electrical current. In the Bohr model, the attractive force between opposite charges is balanced by the outward centrifugal force to maintain the electrons in stable orbits.

Since matter is made up of a large number of charged particles, external electric and magnetic fields must exert some kind of effect on matter. This effect will exist whether the electrons are free to move or tightly bound to the atoms. Every charged particle in matter is subject to the fields of other particles, including the long-range fields of charged particles and the short-range fields of neutral particles. The manner in which charged particles respond to the application of electric and magnetic fields should be utilized while considering interaction of EM fields with biological systems.

Biological Model

Microscopic anatomy covers cell biology, tissue biology, and organ/system histology, with the structure and function of cells, tissues, and organs reviewed at the light and electron microscope level. Microscopic anatomy is an important biological model and is the approach widely considered by life scientists. Nevertheless, it may be essential also for engineering professionals working in the field of life science. For understanding the microscopic model, it is useful first to consider the interaction of exogenous field (external field) with the cell components and, secondly, the consequent modification of cellular activity [5].

At the microscopic level, all tissues are composed of cells and extracellular fluids. The cell has two distinct parts: the outer, insulating membrane and the inner cytoplasm and nucleus which, such as the extracellular fluid, has high conductivity. Because of the membrane, the cell appears to be an insulator. Accordingly, almost all the current induced in tissues by low-frequency electric field flows around the cells. The insulating membrane, which completely surrounds the conducting core, makes the cell itself a series combination of the membrane capacitance and the cytoplasmic resistance.

7.2.2 Macroscopic Model

The macroscopic approach deals with the whole biological material exposed to EM fields generated by the exogenous fields. This approach requires complete knowledge of the EM properties of the material. Ability to solve Maxwell's equations with the appropriate boundary conditions is also required.

Two basic quantities characterize the electrical properties of any material [5]: one that describes energy *dissipation* and another that describes energy *storage*. Electrical dissipation is the result of charge motion (or transport) called *conduction*. Conductivity (σ) is the ability of material to transport a charge through the process of conduction, normalized by geometry to describe the material property. Dissipation (or energy loss) results from the conversion of electrical energy into thermal energy through momentum transfer during collision as the charges move.

Electrical storage is the result of a charge storing energy when an external force moves the charge from some equilibrium position opposed by a restoring force trying to move the charge back. The above process is called dielectric polarization; it is normalized by geometry to create a material property called permittivity. When polarization occurs, it causes charges to move, the charge motion is also dissipative.

The electrical properties of biological materials are summarized by the following two parameters:

1. Conductivity σ, which relates the in-phase movement of charges (conduction currents) to the electric field.
2. Permittivity ε, which relates the out-of-phase movement of charges (displacement currents) to the electric field.

In connection with the interaction mechanisms, RFR travels through the following three types of biological materials [5, 6]:

1. Suspensions of cells and protein molecules.

2. Similar suspensions in a condensed state such as muscle and body organ tissues like liver, kidney, and heart. These tissues have a high water content (about 70%) and a macromolecular content of about 25% by weight.
3. Tissues of lower water content such as fatty tissues, bone, and bone marrow.

The electrical properties of biological materials and the operating frequency determine the EM interaction mechanisms. Biological materials are regarded as a lossy dielectric, which is frequently macroscopically or microscopically heterogeneous [7, 8]. It is defined as

$$\varepsilon'' = \frac{\sigma}{\omega\varepsilon_o} \tag{7.1}$$

where $\omega = 2\pi f$ is the radian frequency of the applied field.

For time harmonic (steady-state sinusoidal time dependence) fields, the loss is taken into account by considering the permittivity ε to be complex. It is represented by

$$\varepsilon^* = \varepsilon_o (\varepsilon' - j\varepsilon'') \tag{7.2}$$

where $\varepsilon' - j\varepsilon''$ is the complex relative permittivity, ε' is the real part of the complex relative permittivity, also called the dielectric constant, and ε'' is the imaginary part of the complex relative permittivity. Physically, ε' is a measure of the relative amount of polarization that occurs for a given applied electric fields, and ε'' is a measure of both the friction associated with changing polarization and drift of conduction charges. The values of both dielectric constant and conductivity vary substantially with frequency as illustrated in Figure 7-1 [9].

The permittivity of biological tissues depends on the type of tissue (e.g. skin, fat, or muscle), water content, temperature, and frequency. The permittivity and frequency may also determine how far the EM wave penetrates into the body. The term *depth of penetration* (D_p) usually quantifies this. For objects with homogeneous properties and with RFR incident at right angles to the surface, depth of penetration is defined as the distance at which the power density is decreased by absorption to about 0.13534 of the body's surface value. However, the magnitude of the electric and the magnetic field reduces by a factor of 0.36788. Depth of penetration is defined as

$$D_p = \frac{1}{\alpha} \tag{7.3}$$

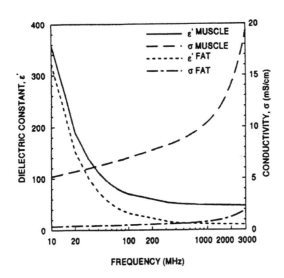

Figure 7-1 The variation of electrical properties of muscle and fat with frequency.

where α is the attenuation constant of the material in nepers per meter. Values of D_p varies from a small fraction of a millimeter at the upper frequencies of RFR range, to a few centimeters for high water content tissues at frequencies of few megahertz and to more depths for low water content tissues. Tables 7-1 to 7-5 give details of electrical properties of muscle, fat, tumor, water, and blood as a function of frequency [10-21].

Another technique aimed to calculate the dielectric properties of biological tissues in the frequency range 10 Hz to 100 GHz using the parametric model is implemented by Gabriel and colleagues [22-25]. It is based on a client-server approach. The server program runs in background on a centralized system, which manages the parameter's database (14 parameters for each of the 50 defined tissues) for finding the dielectric properties of tissues at various frequencies.

7.3 WAVES AND MATTER

When EM radiation contacts matter, it interacts with atoms in the medium and behaves like a particle in a way and like a wave in another way. Particle-like behaviors include *reflection*, *scattering*, and *absorption*. The wavelike behaviors include *reflection*, *refraction*, *transmission*, *diffraction*, and *absorption*. The end effect of the radiation on matter depends on many factors including wavelength components of the radiation, the sending medium, the receiving medium, the polarization components of the radiation, and the angle of incidence.

Table 7-1   Electrical Properties of Muscle

f(MHz)	λ_o(cm)	ε'	ε''	σ(mho/m)	λ(cm)	D_p(cm)
13	2307.69	160.0	864.0	0.62	101.26	19.65
27	1111.11	113.0	339.0	0.51	72.45	16.22
100	300.00	72.0	159.0	0.88	27.02	6.76
200	150.00	57.0	90.0	1.00	16.59	4.86
300	100.00	54.0	72.2	1.20	11.78	3.80
433	69.28	53.0	42.5	1.22	8.91	4.09
750	40.00	52.0	36.9	1.54	5.26	2.66
915	32.79	51.0	31.5	1.60	4.40	2.50
1500	20.00	49.0	21.2	1.77	2.80	2.18
2000	15.00	48.1	18.3	2.03	2.13	1.87
2450	12.24	47.0	16.2	2.20	1.76	1.70
3000	10.00	46.0	13.6	2.27	1.46	1.63

Table 7-2   Electrical Properties of Fat

f(MHz)	λ_o(cm)	ε'	ε''	σ(mho/m)	λ(cm)	D_p(cm)
13	2307.69	25.00	8.4	0.01	455.33	449.40
27	1111.11	20.00	3.4	0.01	247.57	473.40
100	300.00	7.50	3.4	0.02	106.96	79.88
200	150.00	6.00	2.3	0.03	60.18	52.47
300	100.00	5.70	1.9	0.03	41.28	39.29
433	69.28	5.60	1.6	0.04	28.99	33.40
750	40.00	5.60	1.3	0.05	16.79	23.66
915	32.79	5.60	1.1	0.06	13.79	22.87
1500	20.00	5.55	0.9	0.07	8.46	16.95
2000	15.00	5.55	0.8	0.09	6.35	14.29
2450	12.24	5.50	0.7	0.10	5.21	13.27
3000	10.00	5.40	0.6	0.10	4.30	12.52

Table 7-3 Electrical Properties of Tumor

f(MHz)	λ₀(cm)	ε′	ε″	σ(mho/m)	λ(cm)	Dₚ(cm)
13	2307.69	205.0	1273.85	0.92	84.40	15.99
27	1111.11	180.0	606.67	0.91	55.12	11.92
100	300.00	101.0	196.38	1.09	23.65	6.25
200	150.00	78.0	109.80	1.22	14.55	4.55
300	100.00	74.0	78.60	1.31	10.48	3.92
433	69.28	63.0	64.02	1.54	7.93	3.05
750	40.00	61.0	47.04	1.96	4.81	2.28
915	32.79	60.0	39.93	2.03	4.03	2.15
1500	20.00	59.0	26.04	2.17	2.55	1.95
2000	15.00	57.0	22.77	2.53	1.95	1.64
2450	12.24	56.0	20.72	2.82	1.61	1.45
3000	10.00	55.0	17.88	2.98	1.33	1.36

Table 7-4 Electrical Properties of Water

f(MHz)	λ₀(cm)	ε′	ε″	σ(mho/m)	λ(cm)	Dₚ(cm)
13	2307.69	78.3	0.32	0.00	260.79	20596.53
27	1111.11	78.3	0.34	0.00	125.57	9333.50
100	300.00	78.3	0.40	0.00	33.90	2142.04
200	150.00	78.3	0.90	0.01	16.95	476.02
300	100.00	78.3	1.19	0.02	11.30	240.01
433	69.28	78.3	1.55	0.04	7.83	127.67
750	40.00	78.3	2.84	0.12	4.52	40.23
915	32.79	78.1	3.80	0.19	3.71	24.62
1500	20.00	77.9	5.70	0.47	2.26	10.00
2000	15.00	77.9	7.20	0.80	1.70	5.94
2450	12.24	76.6	8.80	1.20	1.40	3.94
3000	10.00	75.8	11.00	1.83	1.15	2.56

Table 7-5 Electrical Properties of Blood

f(MHz)	λ_0(cm)	ε'	ε''	σ(mho/m)	λ(cm)	D_p(cm)
13	2307.69	200.0	1523.08	1.10	78.32	14.41
100	300.00	73.0	216.00	1.20	24.45	5.50
300	100.00	63.0	72.00	1.20	11.23	3.99
433	69.28	62.0	52.13	1.25	8.19	3.63
915	32.79	60.0	27.54	1.40	4.13	3.05
2450	12.24	58.0	15.65	2.13	1.59	1.94

7.3.1 Reflection

Waves generally travel through space in a straight line. When a RF wave encounters a boundary between two media, some of the energy is reflected by the boundary while the remaining portion is transmitted in the other medium. The reflection from a smooth surface is shown in Figure 7-2. Reflection depends on the smoothness of the material's surface relative to the wavelength of the radiation. A rough surface will affect both the relative direction and the phase coherency of the reflected wave. This characteristic determines both the amount of radiation that is reflected back to the first medium and the purity of the information that is preserved in the reflected wave.

7.3.2 Refraction

Refraction is the deflection or bending of EM waves when they pass from one kind of transparent medium into another as shown in Figure 7-3. The medium's *index of refraction* determines the speed of waves through specific material. It is the ratio between the speed of the wave in a vacuum and the speed of the wave in the substance of the observed medium. The refraction exists in the earth's atmosphere. It alters the trajectory of radio waves, but can change with time.

7.3.3 Scattering

Scattering is the redirection of EM radiation due to its interaction with matter. The scattering mechanism depends on the size of the particles composing the medium and the wavelength of the radiation. The radiation expresses Rayleigh

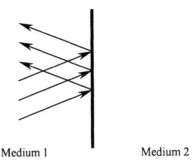

Medium 1   Medium 2

Figure 7-2   Reflection at a boundary.

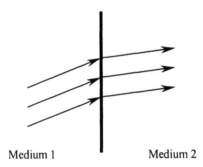

Medium 1   Medium 2

Figure 7-3   Refraction of a wave.

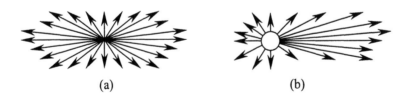

(a)   (b)

Figure 7-4   (a) Rayleigh scattering. (b) Mie scattering.

scattering, which is nondirectional when the size of the particles is on the order of the radiation wavelength. The diffusion by larger particles is called *Mie* scattering, which is not as wavelength-dependent as Rayleigh scattering. This scattering profile is dependent on particle size and can produce forward and backward scattering. Figure 7-4 illustrates both Rayleigh scattering and Mie scattering.

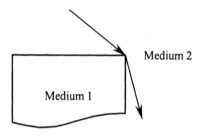

Figure 7-5 Diffraction.

7.3.4   Diffraction

A phenomenon called diffraction allows EM radiation to bend, pass through small apertures, and move around small particles of matter. The smaller the aperture or particles, the more the radiation rays will bend. This bending is quantitatively referred to as diffraction as shown in Figure 7-5. Because stars are so distant from earth, their light is almost entirely collimated. However, what we on earth see is actually the star's diffraction patterns, which occur when starlight passes through galactic dust.

7.3.5   Transmission and Absorption

The wavelength of the EM radiation greatly influences transmission and absorption because a given material can be transmissive at one wavelength and absorptive at another. For instance, red glass transmits light with wavelengths near 650 nm; it absorbs the complementary color green, which has wavelengths near 550 nm. Transmission of radiation occurs when materials lack the properties necessary for absorption.

Absorption is both particle-like and wavelike behavior. When EM radiation interacts with matter, it can be absorbed, transferring the energy to the medium. For a particle, this interaction is an inelastic collision. For a wave, the energy is transferred from the EM energy into energy modes in the absorbing medium.

The absorption process is divided into certain categories that correspond to modes of molecular energy storage. These categories include *thermal*, *vibrational*, *rotational*, and *electronic* modes. The thermal mode of energy storage consists of translational movement modes, in which atoms move horizontally and vertically about their lattice points in a medium. This is commonly referred to as heat.

The vibrational energy mode consists of intramolecular vibrations between component atoms.

The rotational energy mode includes inertial energy stored in the orientation of spinning polarized molecules in local electric fields that are found within some materials and can be stimulated by RFR.

Electronic modes consist of the different orbital energy states to which electrons can be excited. These modes produce new radiation energies as the excited electrons drop back to their original orbitals. RFR may stimulate both electronic and vibrational modes.

The amount of energy that a material will absorb from radiation depends on the frequency of radiation, intensity of beam, and the duration of exposure. The most important of these parameters is the frequency. RFR can excite translational and vibrational modes and generate heat. The intensity of the beam is also a factor in determining how much energy is absorbed. The larger the intensity of the beam, the more energy is available to be transferred. Also, the longer the duration of exposure, the more energy will be absorbed.

7.4 INTERACTION MECHANISMS

The entire EM spectrum can interact with living matter; however, the mechanisms of interaction are not the same. For wavelengths shorter than 250 μm, biological molecules are ionized by ionizing radiation. At longer wavelengths, the photon energy of the wave is insufficient for ionizing the molecules. The waves propagate within tissues with reduced velocities, and are refracted, diffracted, and reflected when encountering inhomogeneities. The specific electrical properties of each tissue govern the reduction of velocity, refraction, and diffraction. These properties, as well as the geometry of the inhomogeneities, determine the fraction of energy absorbed by tissues. The main parameters that describe nonionizing waves are the frequency of oscillation, the amplitude of the **E** or **H** field, and the phase angle, which defines the instantaneous state of the oscillation.

E and **H** fields interact with materials in two ways. First, **E** and **H** exert forces on the charged particles in the material, changing the charge pattern that originally existed. Second, the altered charged pattern in the material produces additional **E** and **H** fields. Materials are usually classified as being either magnetic or nonmagnetic. Magnetic materials have magnetic dipoles that are strongly affected by applied fields, while nonmagnetic materials do not. However, biological materials are considered nonmagnetic materials.

As discussed in Section 7.2, the interaction of EM fields with biological materials is considered through either microscopic or macroscopic models. Considering the interaction on a microscopic level with charges in the material is practically difficult. Therefore, we will describe it macroscopically through the following three ways [5, 20]:

1. The polarization of bound charges
2. The orientation of permanent electric dipoles
3. The drift of conduction charges (both electronic and ionic)

Materials mainly affected by the first two ways are dielectrics, such as biological tissues, while conductors are affected by the third way.

7.4.1   Polarization of Bound Charges

Bound charges are strongly constrained by restoring forces in a material that may move only very slightly. Without the application of an **E** field, positive and negative bound charges in an atom or molecule are superimposed upon each other and effectively cancel out. When an **E** field is applied, the forces on the positive and negative charges are in opposite directions and the charges separate, resulting in induced *electric dipole*. A dipole is a combination of positive and negative charges separated by a small distance. Such a dipole is said to be an induced dipole because it is created by the induction of an **E** field. The creation of an electric dipole by separation of charge is called induced polarization.

7.4.2   Orientation of Permanent Electric Dipoles

Permanent dipoles, which are randomly oriented in a material with no **E** field applied, tend to align with an applied **E** field as shown in Figure 7-6. Since the field is reversing polarity, the molecules try to flip back and forth in order to maintain the minimum energy configuration. The net alignment of permanent dipoles produces new fields. The drift of conduction charges in an applied **E** field occurs because these charges are free to move substantial distances in response to **E** fields. The movement of conduction charges is called *drift*. A large drift means high conductivity.

7.4.3   Drift of Conduction Charges

The third effect of an applied **E** field is illustrated in Figure 7-7. Some charges in biological material are free because they are loosely bound and can be moved by an applied **E** field. These charges can move a short distance, collide with other particles, and then move in a different direction, resulting in a small macroscopic average velocity in the direction of the applied **E** field.

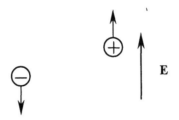

Figure 7-6 The orientation of permanent electric dipoles.

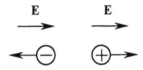

Figure 7-7 The drift of conduction charges.

7.5 WAVELENGTH AND OBJECT SIZE

The characteristics of EM fields are different for different wavelength ranges. More precisely, the characteristics depend on the size of the object as compared to the frequency. Assume that d is the largest dimension of the object when compared to the wavelength λ of the EM field. The characteristics of EM fields can be categorized into three terms: $\lambda >> d$ [Figure 7-8]; $\lambda \approx d$ [Figure 7-9]; and $\lambda << d$ [Figure 7-10] [3].

7.5.1 Wavelength Larger Than the Object Size

Certain approximations may be applied when the wavelength is very large compared to the size of the radiated object ($\lambda >> d$). These approximations are called *low-frequency approximations* because the frequency is low when the wavelength is very large compared to the object. One primary approximation approach is the *electric circuit theory*, where current and voltage are the main parameters. It involves two time-varying scalar functions: current and voltage.

7.5.2 Wavelength Equivalent to the Object Size

Another approximation is called *quasi-static EM field theory*. This approximation is used to find **E** or **H** field at frequencies below 30 MHz. Owing to the theory, **E**

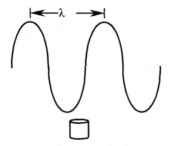

Figure 7-8 The wavelength is large compared to the size of the object.

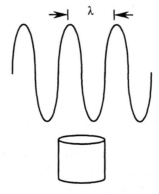

Figure 7-9 The wavelength is comparable with the size of the object.

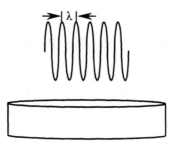

Figure 7-10 The wavelength is small compared to the body.

and **H** exist independently. When the wavelength is approximately in the same order of the radiated object ($\lambda \approx d$), EM field theory should be used. **E** and **H** fields are coupled and may be expressed in terms of propagation. In the 30 MHz-10 GHz range, Maxwell's equations must be solved without approximation.

7.5.3 Wavelength Smaller Than the Object Size

When the wavelength is very small compared to the size of the radiated object ($\lambda \ll d$), *geometrical optical theory* can be applied (in frequencies above 10 GHz), except for very high frequency, where special theories are used, for example, *X-ray theory*. The propagation effect is significant in this range of frequencies. Here **E** and **H** fields are strongly coupled with each other.

7.5.4 Resonance

In human body, RF energy is absorbed more efficiently at frequencies near the body's natural resonant frequency and therefore maximum heating occurs. At very low frequency range (< 1MHz), a human-size biological object absorbs very little RF energy. The absorption can be appreciable at the resonant frequency near 70-80 MHz if the person's body is insulated from the ground (for an average man about 160-170 cm tall where the long dimension of the body is approximately 0.4 wavelengths) [26]. This frequency is about 35-40 MHz if the person is grounded. Likewise, the resonant frequency for an average woman about 160 cm tall (insulated from ground), is about 80 MHz. For the model of a 5-year-old child, the resonant frequency is even higher than those of adults are, and the resonant SAR is about 0.3 W/kg per 1 mW/cm^2 [27].

In addition to the whole body, body parts can also be resonant. The adult head, for example, is resonant at around 400 MHz, while a baby's smaller head resonates at near 700 MHz. Accordingly, body size determines the frequency at which most RF energy is absorbed. As the frequency increases above resonance, less RF heating generally occurs. However, additional longitudinal resonance occurs at about 1 GHz near the body surface.

7.6 PROPAGATION THROUGH BIOLOGICAL MEDIA

The propagation of EM waves in a biological medium [Figure 7-11] is studied mathematically by solving Maxwell's equations under appropriate boundary conditions. These equations are very powerful, but complicated and difficult to solve. For simplicity, let us assume that a biological medium is infinite in extent, source-free, isotropic, and homogeneous. The medium is isotropic if ε is a scalar constant, so **D** and **E** are the same in every direction. A homogeneous medium is one for which ε, μ, and σ are constant. For this case, Maxwell's equations become

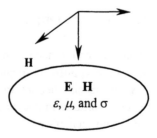

Figure 7-11 A biological body under EM radiation.

$$\nabla \times \mathbf{E} = -\frac{\partial \mathbf{B}}{\partial t} \tag{7.4}$$

$$\nabla \times \mathbf{H} = \mathbf{J} + \frac{\partial \mathbf{D}}{\partial t} \tag{7.5}$$

$$\nabla \cdot \mathbf{B} = 0 \tag{7.6}$$

$$\nabla \cdot \mathbf{D} = 0 \tag{7.7}$$

Further, since the medium is assumed to be isotropic, its permittivity, permeability, and conductivity are scalars. In case the medium is homogeneous, these parameters are constants.

In order to solve this set of simultaneous equations for the vectors **E** and **H**, the vector **H** may be eliminated from the equation in the following way:

$$\nabla \times (\nabla \times \mathbf{E}) = -\mu \frac{\partial}{\partial t} (\nabla \times \mathbf{H})$$

$$= -\mu \frac{\partial}{\partial t} (\sigma \mathbf{E} + \varepsilon \frac{\partial \mathbf{E}}{\partial t})$$

$$= -\mu \sigma \frac{\partial \mathbf{E}}{\partial t} - \varepsilon \mu \frac{\partial^2 \mathbf{E}}{\partial t^2} \tag{7.8}$$

Using the vector identity, the equation determining the vector **E** comes out to be

$$\nabla \times \nabla \times \mathbf{E} = \nabla(\nabla \cdot \mathbf{E}) - \nabla^2 \mathbf{E} \tag{7.9}$$

and using Equation (7.7)

$$(\nabla^2 - \mu\sigma \frac{\partial}{\partial t} - \mu\varepsilon \frac{\partial^2}{\partial t^2}) \mathbf{E} = 0 \qquad (7.10)$$

Similarly, by eliminating **E** from the Maxwell's equations, it may shown that **H** satisfies the equation

$$(\nabla^2 - \mu\sigma \frac{\partial}{\partial t} - \mu\varepsilon \frac{\partial^2}{\partial t^2}) \mathbf{H} = 0 \qquad (7.11)$$

That is, both **E** and **H** satisfy the equation (called the *wave equation*):

$$(\nabla^2 - \mu\sigma \frac{\partial}{\partial t} - \mu\varepsilon \frac{\partial^2}{\partial t^2}) \begin{pmatrix} \mathbf{E} \\ \mathbf{H} \end{pmatrix} = \begin{pmatrix} 0 \\ 0 \end{pmatrix} \qquad (7.12)$$

In view of the fact that equations governing **E** and **H** in the biological material (Maxwell's equations) are linear and keeping in mind that any arbitrarily time-varying function can be expressed as a sum of number of sinusoidal functions, time dependence of the fields, **E** and **H**, can be given by the factor $e^{j\omega t}$ so that

$$\frac{\partial}{\partial t} \equiv j\omega$$

$$\frac{\partial^2}{\partial t^2} \equiv -\omega^2$$

Using both relationships in Equation (7.10), the wave equation becomes

$$\nabla^2 \mathbf{E} + \gamma^2 \mathbf{E} = 0 \qquad (7.13)$$

where

$$\gamma^2 = \omega^2 \mu\varepsilon - j\omega\mu\sigma$$
$$= \omega^2 \mu\varepsilon_0 \left(\varepsilon' - j\frac{\sigma}{\omega\varepsilon}\right)$$
$$= \frac{\omega^2}{c^2}(\varepsilon' - j\varepsilon'') \qquad (7.14)$$

where c is the free space velocity (3×10^8 m/s) and γ is the propagation constant. This is, in general, a complex quantity and may be written in the form

$$\gamma = \alpha + j\beta \tag{7.15}$$

where the attenuation constant is

$$\alpha = \frac{\sqrt{2}c}{\omega\sqrt{\varepsilon'}\left(\sqrt{1+\left(\dfrac{\varepsilon''}{\varepsilon'}\right)^2}+1\right)^{1/2}} \tag{7.16}$$

for $\dfrac{\varepsilon''}{\varepsilon'} \leq 1$

$$\alpha = \frac{\omega\sqrt{\mu\varepsilon}}{\sqrt{2}}\left(\frac{\varepsilon''}{\varepsilon'}\right) \tag{7.17}$$

and the phase constant in radians per meter is

$$\beta = \frac{\sqrt{2}c}{\omega\sqrt{\varepsilon'}\left(\sqrt{1+\left(\dfrac{\varepsilon''}{\varepsilon'}\right)^2}-1\right)^{1/}} \tag{7.18}$$

for $\dfrac{\varepsilon''}{\varepsilon'} \leq 1$

$$\beta = \omega\sqrt{\mu\varepsilon}\left[1+0.125\left(\frac{\varepsilon''}{\varepsilon'}\right)^2\right] \tag{7.19}$$

Using Equation (7.19), the wavelength λ can be determined by

$$\lambda = \frac{2\pi}{\beta} \tag{7.20}$$

If the incident wave is a linearly polarized uniform plane wave traveling along the z-direction, then Equations (7.10) and (7.11) are of the form

$$\mathbf{E} = E_i e^{-\alpha z} e^{j(wt-\beta z)} i_x \tag{7.21}$$

$$\mathbf{H} = H_i e^{-\alpha z} e^{j(wt-\beta z)} i_y \tag{7.22}$$

where $E_i = \eta H_i$

The intrinsic impedance of biological material η is given by

$$\eta = \sqrt{\frac{\mu}{\varepsilon}} \left[1 - 0.378 \left(\frac{\varepsilon''}{\varepsilon'} \right)^2 + j0.5 \left(\frac{\varepsilon''}{\varepsilon'} \right) \right]$$

(7.23)

The Poynting vector, that is, the power flowing per unit area of cross section (W/m2), gives the power density associated with an EM wave

$$P_i = E_i \times H_i$$

(7.24)

For a uniform plane wave, time-average power flowing is given by

$$P_i = \frac{|E_i|^2}{2\eta} = \frac{1}{2} \eta |H_i|^2$$

(7.25)

7.7 ABSORPTION IN BIOLOGICAL MATERIALS

At radio frequencies, biological tissues behave like solutions of electrolytes that contain polar molecules. RFR interacts with biological systems by way of ionic conduction (oscillation of free charges) and rotation of polar molecules of water and protein relaxation. Absorbed RF energy is transformed into kinetic energy of molecules, which is associated with a rise in temperature of the irradiated tissues.

In order to understand the factors influencing the rise in body temperature due to RF absorption, it is useful to study the different heat pathways within the body. The heat may be transferred to the environment only after it is first transferred to the body surface. This heat transfer may be accomplished by three mechanisms: *thermal conduction, thermal radiation, convection*, and *sweat evaporation*.

Thermal conduction is the process in which heat transfer takes place by molecular diffusion. The amount of heat energy flowing per second per unit area is proportional to the temperature gradient. Body tissues are quite poor thermal conductors with values of conductivity between 2-10 cal/min/m/°C.

Thermal radiation is the heat loss due to radiation from the surface of the human body.

Convection is the process in which heat is transferred by the simultaneous action of molecular diffusion and mixing motion.

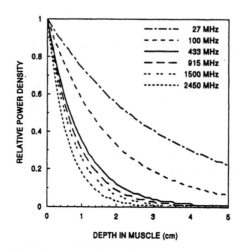

Figure 7-12 Power absorption in muscle as a function of depth at different frequencies.

Evaporation is the heat loss due to evaporation at the surface per unit area (including sweat and insensible perspiration), and it depends on the arterial blood flow, the wind speed, and the humidity.

Sweating is controlled by the central neural integrative mechanism, which receives signals from the thermosensitive sites within the body.

Temperature differences, which would exist in the absence of blood flow, are equalized by the blood flow. The blood flow also controls the effective body insulation through constriction expansion of the cutaneous capillaries, so that the distance the heat has to flow through the superficial layer to the superficial epidermis increases or decreases accordingly.

A nonuniform distribution of absorbed power is a well-established fact, which may lead to involved interactions. In some exposure situations, only certain parts of the body are absorbing RF power causing nonuniform heating, which is generally referred to as hot spots.

It is observed from Equation (7.21) and (7.22) that the wave gets attenuated as it propagates in the biological material along the z-axis. As shown from Figure 7-12, at a given depth uses of lower frequency results in a higher power density. It is also clear that a given power density is achieved at a greater depths in the muscle than that for a higher frequency. Not shown in Figure 7-12 is that penetration depth at about 30 GHz and higher is largely confined to the outer layers of the skin (much like for sunlight).

The energy is transferred from the applied **E** field to the material in the form of kinetic energy of charged particles. The rate of change of the energy transferred to the material is called the absorbed power. This power is also called power transferred, but from the bioelectromagnetics point of view, the term *specific absorption rate* (SAR) is the preferred one. SAR is a quantity properly averaged in time and space and expressed in watts per kilogram (W/kg). SAR values are of key importance when validating possible health hazards and setting safety standards [see Chapter 13 for details].

For steady-state sinusoidal fields, the time-averaged absorbed power per unit volume is given by

$$P_a = \sigma |E|^2 \qquad (7.26)$$

where $|E|$ is the root-mean-square (RMS) magnitude of the **E**-field at certain point in the material. To find the total absorbed power in a material, the power calculated from Equation (7.26) must be calculated at each point inside the body and integrated over the volume of the body. Figure 7-12 shows power absorption in muscle by a plane wave as a function of depth at different frequencies.

REFERENCES

[1] Lin, J. C., (ed.), *Electromagnetics in Biology and Medicine, Review of Radio Science 1993-1996*, Oxford University Press, London, UK, 1996.

[2] Stuchly, M. A., Biological Effects of Radiofrequency Fields, *Proceedings of the International Non-Ionizing Radiation Workshop*, Melbourne, Australia, 5-9 April, 1988.

[3] Durney, H. D., and D. A. Christensen, *Basic Introduction to Bioelectromagnetics*, CRC Press, Boca Raton, FL, 1999.

[4] Jordan, E. C., and K. G. Balmain, *Electromagnetic Waves and Radiating Systems*, Prentice Hall, Englewood Cliffs, NJ, 1968.

[5] Robert, P., *Electrical and Magnetic Properties of Materials*, Artech House, Norwood, MA, 1988.

[6] Hand, J. W., Electromagnetic Techniques in Cancer Therapy by Hyperthermia, *IEE Proceedings* 128, pp. 593-601, 1981.

[7] Schwan, H. P., Interaction of Microwave and Radio Frequency Radiation with Biological Systems, *IEEE Transactions on Microwave Theory and Techniques* 19, pp. 146-152, 1971.

[8] Roberts, J. E., and H. F. Cook, Microwave in Medical and Biological Research, *British Journal of Applied Physics* 3, pp. 33-40, 1952.

[9] Pressman, A. S., *Electromagnetic Fields and Life*, Plenum Press, New York, NY, 1970.

[10] Habash, R. W. Y., Non-Invasive Microwave Hyperthermia, Ph.D Thesis, Indian Institute of Science, Bangalore, India, 1994.

[11] Schepps, J. L., and K. R. Foster, The UHF and Microwave Dielectric Properties of Normal and Tumour Tissues: Variations in Dielectric Properties with Tissue Water Content, *Physics in Medicine and Biology* 25, pp. 1149-1158, 1980.

[12] Foster, K. R., and J. L. Schepps, Dielectric Properties of Tumour and Normal Tissues at Radio Through Microwave Frequencies, *Journal of Microwave Power* 16, pp. 108-119, 1981.

[13] Cook, H., The Dielectric Behaviour of Some Types of Human Tissues at Microwave Frequencies, *British Journal of Applied Physics* 2, pp. 295-300, 1951.

[14] Schwan, H. P., Electrical Properties of Tissues and Cells, *Advances in Biological and Medical Physics* 5, pp. 147-209, 1957.

[15] Sheppard, R. J., and E. H. Grant, Complex Permittivity of Water at 25°C, *The Journal of Chemical Physics* 64, pp. 2257-2258, 1976.

[16] Stuchly, M. A., and S. S. Stuchly, Dielectric Properties of Biological Substances-Tabulated, *Journal of Microwave Power* 15, pp. 19-26, 1980.

[17] Stuchly, M. A., A. Kraszewiski, S. S. Stuchly, and A. M. Smith, Dielectric Properties of Animal Tissues *In Vivo* at Radio and Microwave Frequencies: Comparison between Species, *Physics in Medicine and Biology* 27, pp. 927-936, 1982.

[18] Gabriel, C., R. J. Sheppard, and E. H. Grant, Dielectric Properties of Ocular Tissues at 37°C, *Physics in Medicine and Biology* 28, pp. 43-49, 1983.

[19] Peloso, R., D. T. Tuma, and R. K. Jain, Dielectric Properties of Solid Tumours During Normothermia and Hyperthermia, *IEEE Transactions on Biomedical Engineering* 31, pp. 725-728, 1984.

[20] Hurt, W. D., Multiterm Debye Dispersion Relations for Permittivity of Muscle, *IEEE Transactions on Biomedical Engineering* 32, pp. 60-64, 1985.

[21] Durney, C. H., H. Massoudi, and M. F. Iskander, *Radiofrequency Radiation Dosimetry Handbook*, Electrical Engineering Department, The University of Utah, Salt Lake City, Utah, 1986.

[22] Gabriel, C., Compilation of the Dielectric Properties of Body Tissues at RF and Microwave Frequencies, Report N.AL/OE-TR-1996-0037, Occupational and Environmental Health Directorate, Radiofrequency Radiation Division, Brooks Air Force Base, Texas, 1996.

[23] Gabriel, C., S. Gabriel, and E. Corthout, The Dielectric Properties of Biological Tissues: I. Literature Survey, *Physics in Medicine and Biology* 41, pp. 2231-2249, 1996.

[24] Gabriel, S., R. W. Lau, and C. Gabriel, The Dielectric Properties of Biological Tissues: II. Measurements in the Frequency Range 10 Hz to 20 GHz, *Physics in Medicine and Biology* 41, pp. 2251-2269, 1996.

[25] Gabriel, S., R. W. Lau, and C. Gabriel, The Dielectric Properties of Biological Tissues: III. Parametric Models for the Dielectric Spectrum of Tissues, *Physics in Medicine and Biology* 41, pp. 2271-2293, 1996.

[26] Durney, C. H., C. C. Johnson, P. W. Barber, H. Massoudi, M. F. Iskander, J. L. Lords, K. K. Ryser, S. J. Allen, and J. C. Mitchell, *Radiofrequency Radiation Dosimetry Handbook*, USAF School on Aerospace Medicine, Brooks AFB, Texas, 1978.

[27] Heynick, L. N., Radiofrequency Electromagnetic Fields (RFEMF) and Cancer: A Comprehensive Review of the Literature Pertinent to Air Force Operations, Air Force Research Laboratory Final Report, 1996.

8

Bioeffects of Radio Frequency Radiation

8.1 INTRODUCTION

As stated in Chapter 6, there are several useful applications of radio frequency technology for society, but there are also concerns about possible adverse health effects associated with human exposure to radio frequency radiation (RFR) emitted by various facilities and devices used in daily life.

RFR has the potential to interact with biological systems; however, the outcome is dependent on the radiation level. RFR can cause visible biological injuries if exposure intensity is sufficient. Meanwhile low-level RFR may have harmful effects, or may not have any at all! It is not possible to verify that such effects will occur. This is due to the fact that several factors are involved, especially ones related to life-based sciences.

A significant number of studies have been carried out to date to explore the relationship between exposure to RFR and illnesses including cancer, but it will be a long time before we have the results of most of these studies. These studies describe various experimental investigations with laboratory animals, tissue preparations, and cells, with detailed information on the bioeffects of RFR.

8.2 BIOLOGICAL EFFECTS

The interaction of RF fields with living systems and, consequently, their related bioeffects, can be considered at various levels including the molecular, subcellular, organ, or system level, or the entire body.

Repacholi [1] and Pakhomov et al. [2] published comprehensive literature reviews on the current state of research on biological effects and health

223

implications of RFR. According to Repacholi [1], bioeffects due to RFR are classified as follows:

1. High-level (thermal) effects.
2. Intermediate-level (athermal) effects.
3. Low-level (nonthermal) effects.

8.2.1 Thermal Effects

An obvious outcome of RFR absorption by the human body is heating (thermal effect), where the core temperature of the body rises a few degrees despite the process of *thermoregulation* by the body. Thermal effects have been known since investigations into therapeutic applications of electricity were developed by theoretical studies in electromagnetics by Faraday, Ampere, Gauss, and Maxwell, in addition to the development of AC sources by d'Arsonval and Tesla.

Many of the biological effects of RFR that have significant implications on human health are related to induced heating or induced current. Heating is the primary interaction of RF fields at high frequencies especially above about 1 MHz. Below about 1 MHz, the induction of currents in the body is the dominant action of RFR. Heating from RFR best relates to SAR rather than to incident power density to account for differences in coupling.

Biological systems alter their functions as a result of a change in temperature. It is worth mentioning that most adverse health effects due to RF exposure between 1 MHz and 10 GHz are consistent with responses to induced heating, resulting in raising tissue temperatures higher than 1°C. Elevated temperatures have obvious effects on humans such as cataracts, increased blood pressure, dizziness, weakness, disorientation, and nausea.

During the 1940s, researchers reported cataracts in animals exposed to RF energy. Testicular degeneration in some animals was also observed. During the same period, physicians reported cases of bleeding among radar equipment workers at the Hughes Aircraft Plant [3]. This raised the issue of possible danger to workers and civilians due to exposure to RF energy from radar and telecommunication transmitters.

Thermal effects can be defined as energy deposition higher than the thermoregulatory capacity of the human body. Usually, the human body generates heat due to food consumption, which is known as the *basal metabolic rate* (BMR). The BMR is defined as the heat production of a human in a thermoneutral environment (33°C or 91°F) at rest mentally and physically more than 12 hours after the last meal. The standard BMR for a 70-kg man is approximately 1.2 W/kg, but it can be altered by changes in active body mass, diets, and endocrine levels [4]. If a human is subjected to heating from an external source at a much greater rate, thermal damage can occur. However, exposure levels comparable to the BMR might produce thermal effects due to thermoregulation.

Thermal effects imposed on the body by a given SAR are strongly affected by ambient temperature, relative humidity, and airflow. The induced heating increases with increasing body mass, at least in small animals. The human body attempts to regulate temperature increase due to thermal effect through perspiration and heat exchange via blood circulation. Certain areas with limited blood circulatory ability, such as the lens of the eye and the testes, run a particularly high risk of being damaged by the induction of cataracts (opacity) and burns. Other thermal effects may show up around electrically conducting objects, either implanted (nails, screws, artificial hip joints, etc.) or external (watches, bows of spectacles, etc.). For adverse health effects, such as eye cataracts and skin burns, to occur from exposure to RF fields at high frequencies, power densities above 1000 W/m^2 are needed. Such densities are not found near conventional RF sources but they do exist in close proximity to powerful transmitters such as radars.

8.2.2 Athermal and Nonthermal Effects

Controversy surrounds two issues regarding biological effects of intermediate- and low-level RFR. First, whether RFR at such levels can even cause harmful biological changes in the absence of demonstrable thermal effects. Second, whether effects can occur from RFR when thermoregulation maintains the body temperature at the normal level despite the EM energy deposition, or when thermoregulation is not challenged and there is no significant temperature change. In response to the first issue, investigations on the extremely low-level RFR have been established and some results confirmed but knowledge is yet inconclusive.

Regarding the second issue, there can be two meanings to the term "effect." It may mean an effect that occurs under circumstance of no evident change in temperature or the exposure level is low enough not to trigger thermoregulation in the biological body under irradiation, suggesting that physiological mechanisms maintain the exposed body at a constant temperature. Such case is related to nonthermal effect where the effect occurs through mechanisms other than those due to macroscopic heating. The second meaning is that RFR causes biological effects, without the involvement of heat. This is sometimes referred to as athermal effect. In this case, the thermoregulatory system maintains the irradiated body at its normal temperature. Meanwhile, the macroscopic behavior of the body emerges out of quantum dynamics producing the physics of living matter to a point where biochemistry has to be considered [5].

A review of the literature on the effects of intermediate- and low-level RFR shows that exposure at relatively low SAR (less than 2 W/kg) under certain conditions could affect the nervous system [6-10]. This includes effects on blood-brain barrier (BBB), morphology, electrophysiology, neurotransmitter activity, and metabolism. Also, RFR at such levels might affect the immune system, gene and chromosomal morphology, enzyme activity, neurological function, cell morphology, membrane ion permeability, intracellular ion concentration, mutation rates, tumor promotion, endocrine secretion rates, etc. A few of the above effects are contradicted by other research findings, leaving our understanding unclear. In most cases the mechanisms of the effects are not understood.

Enormous caution should be taken in applying the existing research results to evaluate the effect of RFR during cellular phone use. It is apparent that as yet not enough research data is available to conclude whether exposure to RFR during the normal use of cellular phones can lead to any adverse health effect. Since the parameters of RFR, such as frequency, intensity, duration, waveform, etc., are important determinants of biological responses, more research is needed to investigate the interaction of such parameters under normal pattern of phone use.

Many researchers see the biological effects from RFR at intermediate- and low-level exposures as scientifically established. For example, Dr. Ross Adey at the Department of Biochemistry, University of California, Riverside, defends the possibility of such effects. He states [11] "microwave bioeffects at the cellular level support the concepts of athermal responses not mediated by tissue heating. A spectrum of these biological responses shows dependence on ELF amplitude- or pulse modulation of the imposed fields. Cell membranes have been identified as the site of transduction of many of these responses, with initiation of enzyme cascades that chemically couple cell surface RF signals to intracellular systems, including some that reach cell nuclei and regulate processes of cell growth and division."

Meanwhile, Dr. Kenneth Foster at the Department of Bioengineering, University of Pennsylvania does not confirm Adey's conclusion. He states that "from the perspective of health and safety, the question should be: Does evidence exist for some overlooked hazard from weak EM fields? Many research groups have examined the scientific literature, and so far the answer is a resounding no." Dr. Foster identifies membrane excitation, electric field-charge interactions, permanent dipole interactions, induced dipole interactions, magnetic field effects, free radical effects, and effects on the BBB. He argues that either there is no connection to a permanent hazardous result or the effects only occur at field strengths much higher than those found in communications applications. He sees the identification of hazardous nonthermal effects as highly speculative and the result of less-than-careful research. The views of scientists who do not find nonthermal effects are examined in *Phantom Risk*: *Scientific Interpretation and the Law* [12]. Dr. Foster is a coauthor of the book.

8.3 LABORATORY INVESTIGATIONS

As discussed in the previous section, RF fields may induce nonthermal effects in addition to thermal effects. Nonthermal effects are not yet taken into consideration for the establishment of protection guidelines because there is still too little scientific evidence about their presence and importance. They are, if present, usually thought to be responsible for cancer induction, although cancer can be related to thermal effects.

An important point to recognize first is how RF energy propagates through a biological body. How do reflection, refraction, and differential absorption take place within the body? How does the power get distributed and for how long it is there, especially in low exposure situation where the temperature is not measurable? What are the consequences? Importantly, RF field is sometimes utilized with a strength that alternates with a low frequency, ELF through the process of modulation (a high-frequency carrier wave and a low-frequency modulated signal). The effect of the RF component may therefore be difficult to distinguish from the effect of the low-frequency component. A considerable body of research has focused on low-frequency magnetic fields, or on RF fields that are keyed, pulsed or modulated at a low-audio frequency (often below 100 Hz). Several studies suggest that humans and animals might adapt to the presence of a steady RF carrier more readily than to an intermittent or modulated RF source.

Adey [11] recognized the modulation frequency-dependent bioeffects to raise significant questions about the validity of continued use of the thermally based SAR as a universally valid predictor of bioeffects attributable to RFR.

The overview of literature in the rest of this chapter will only be indicative, without absolute guarantees for possible adverse health effects. It could be a guideline for high-quality research rather than probable scientific findings (sometimes even biased) in the future.

8.3.1 Genetic Effects

Agents that can damage the DNA of cells are assumed to have carcinogenic potential [15, 16]. They are called genotoxins, or are referred to as having genotoxic activity. The concept of DNA damage as a whole and as a basis for cancer formation (genotoxic carcinogenesis) is challenged by evidence that cancer may result from factors not acting directly on nuclear DNA (epigenetic carcinogenesis). If RF fields are not directly mutagenic, there is always the question of whether they can enhance the development of malignant cells, or alter the repair processes that deal with changes in genetic material resulting from other spontaneous alterations. Related to this question is a concern over the effect on health of prolonged or repeated exposure to low-level RFR. Many literature reviews treat this subject extensively [15-17]. The reviewers believed that genetic changes observed in RFR studies only occurred in the presence of a substantial temperature rise [18]. In general, these observations are consistent with the interpretation that RFR, because of the low amount of energy in photons, does not cause direct damage to the DNA.

Cellular Studies

Nonionizing radiation is not known to damage DNA in the way ionizing radiation does. However, it is likely that RF exposure can alter certain cellular processes. This may indirectly affect the structure of the DNA. Since a very large number of cellular components, cellular processes, and cellular systems can conceivably be affected by EM waves, cellular studies are essential to explain and lead the experimental work. The basis of current critical studies on RFR biological effects is the reported presence (mostly not replicated) of effects on the cellular DNA.

A pilot study [19] was conducted to assess chromosomal damage in a group of workers believed to be heavily exposed to RFR. Thirty-eight telecom employees who had worked for at least five years as radio linesmen had been exposed to estimated RFR levels of between 400 kHz to 20 GHz. They were matched with 38 control subjects (clerical workers). Two hundred cells from each member of each pair were assessed for damage using standard testing methods. The result showed no significant difference between the radio linesmen and the control subjects.

Investigations of Dhahi et al. [20], Habash [21], Dhahi et al. [22], Kerbacher et al. [23], Meltz [24], Ciaravino et al. [25], and Gos et al. [26] on different cell systems provided evidence for a lack of direct genotoxic and mutagenic effects of continuous and pulsed RFR at different power densities. Also, no synergistic effect was found between the applied field and mitomycin C, adriamycin, and proflavin.

Gene transcription (the way in which genes are activated to form different types of protein, for example that specific for liver or skin) appears to be affected by RFR. Some DNA expression is turned on and some turned off as a result of exposure. The shape of cells, their secretion, and growth rates has been shown to change from exposure. French [27] indicates that exposure to 835 MHz using cells grown in the laboratory causes changes to genetic makeup.

A synergistic effect was found with mitomycin C (MMC) in an investigation of 954-MHz waves emitted by the antenna of a GSM base station on blood samples [28], followed by lymphocyte cultivation in the presence of MMC. A highly reproducible synergistic effect was observed as based on the frequencies of sister chromatid exchanges in metaphase figures.

In 1995, Lai and Singh [29] at the University of Washington, Seattle, assayed levels of DNA single-strand breaks in brain cells from rats being exposed to 2.45-GHz microwaves using an alkaline microgel electrophoresis method. No significant effect was found after 2 hours of exposure to pulsed (2 μs width, 500 pps) microwaves. However, they noticed an increase in single-strand DNA at whole-body SAR values of 0.6 and 1.2 W/kg at 4-hours postexposure. In rats exposed for 2 hours to CW 2.45 GHz microwaves (SAR = 1.2 W/kg), increases in brain cell DNA single-strand breaks were observed immediately as well as at 4-hours postexposure. The findings of this study are of specific importance with regard to the possible, but to date totally unproven, link between RFR and brain cancer. Moreover, the results obtained from other studies in the same laboratory show some kind of effects of RFR on DNA [30, 31]. The publication of these studies created a controversy in the cellular communication industry because they appeared to confirm suspicions rose by a few other researchers that radiation from cellular phones might be promoting tumor formation, especially for customers who use such equipment for long periods of time.

Following the publication by Lai and Singh [29], Malyapa et al. [32] found through their research study that they could not detect the effect reported by Lai and Singh. Nevertheless, there were some differences between the two studies.

Phillips et al. [33], through a study funded by Motorola, explored the possibility of DNA damage (single-strand breaks) in Molt-4 T-lymphoblastoid cells exposed to pulsed 813.5625-MHz or 836.35-MHz (TDMA) cellular telephone signals at SAR range of 0.0024-0.024 W/kg. They reported increases as well as decreases in DNA damage depending on exposure duration and signal type. They concluded that further studies were warranted to distinguish possible direct RFR effects on DNA damage from effects on DNA repair.

In 2000, Vijayalaxmi et al. [34] found no evidence for induction of DNA single-strand breaks and alkali-labile lesions in human peripheral blood samples collected from three healthy human volunteers exposed in vitro to pulsed-wave 2450-MHz RFR, either immediately or at 4 hours after exposure.

An increased frequency of chromosome aberrations was found in experiments involving other cell types, RFR, and cytogenetic endpoints [35-37].

Goswami et al. [38] studied the possible effects of FM CW analog (835.62-MHz) or CDMA digital (847.74-MHz) signals on gene expression and other changes in mouse fibroblast cells. Exposure of serum-deprived cells to 835.62-MHz FMCW or 847.74-MHz CDMA RFR at an average SAR of 0.6 W/kg did not significantly change the kinetics of proto-oncogene expression after serum stimulation. In exponential growth phase only, there was a slight (1.4- to twofold) statistically significant increase in c-fos expression levels, which suggests that expression of specific genes could be affected by RF exposure.

Animal Studies

While exposure parameters can be better controlled by cellular studies, animal studies may provide a more convincing indication of possible health consequences. Manikowska et al. [39] observed *in vivo* changes in metaphase counts and translocation numbers even at low-exposure levels. This was found in mice that were exposed for two weeks to pulsed 9.4-GHz microwaves, one hour a day for 5 days a week. Also, Manikowska et al. [40] exposed male CBA/CAY mice to 2.45-GHz microwaves. They observed increased chromosome exchanges and other cytogenetic abnormalities in germ cells exposed as spermatocytes.

A further investigation of possible RF-induced DNA (strand breaks) continued. In a study sponsored by Motorola, Malyapa et al. [41] could not detect RF-induced DNA damage in the exposed versus unexposed animals.

Summary of Genetic Studies

As discussed in Chapter 3, agents that can damage the genetic material are understood to have carcinogenic capability. Experimental studies, especially cellular, of RF exposure have not found evidence for genotoxicity unless the incident power density and SAR were high enough to cause thermal injury.

There are few positive findings for genetic effects of RFR at low intensity, however, those findings were either not replicated, or could not be confirmed while replicated by others.

Two large reviews [42, 43] published in 1998 reached a conclusion indicating that RFR is not directly genotoxic. This means that RFR does not induce genetic effects, at least under low-level conditions, but there may be some indirect effects on the replication and/or transcription of genes under relatively restricted exposure conditions.

8.3.2 Cell Proliferation

Disturbance of the normal cell cycle is a possible sign of uncontrolled growth of cancer cells. Czerska et al. [44] reported an increased proliferation of cells exposed to 2.45-GHz RFR at SAR of 1 W/kg when the radiation was pulsed. However, CW RFR increased proliferation only when absorbed energy was high enough to induce heating.

Increased and decreased cell proliferation rates were reported by Cleary et al.

[45, 46] after applying 27 MHz and 2.45 GHz (CW and pulsed) at SARs between 5 and 196 W/kg. The temperature was kept constant throughout the irradiation by usage of a temperature control system.

Kwee and Raskmark [47, 48] found that exposure to low-level RFR (0.021-2.1 mW/kg) from a GSM phone caused a decrease in cell proliferation *in vitro*.

Velizarov et al. [49] performed on the same cell line and with the same exposure system as in [47]. The field was generated by signal simulation of the GSM at 960 MHz. Cell cultures were exposed in a specially constructed chamber. The corresponding sham experiments were performed under the same experimental conditions. The results showed a significant change in cell proliferation in the exposed cells in comparison to the nonexposed (control) cells.

In contrast, Stagg et al. [50] found no dependable effects on cell numbers while making test of proliferation in the C6 glioma cell exposed to a TDMA signal at incident power densities: 0.1; 1.0; and 10 mW/cm^2.

8.3.3 Cell Transformation

The study of carcinogenesis was greatly facilitated by the discovery of the morphological transformation of mammalian cells in culture. The occurrence of morphological cell transformation involves changes in the growth control of cultured cells.

Balcer-Kubiczek and Harrison [51-53] exposed cells to 120-Hz-modulated microwaves (SAR from 0.1 to 4.4 W/kg) followed by treatment with a phorbol ester tumor promoter. Cell transformation was induced in a dose-dependent way (increasing with increasing SAR value).

Malyapa et al. [54] explored the possible effect of analog (835.62 MHz) or digital (847.74 MHz CDMA) cellular telephone signals on promotion of neoplastic transformation. They found no statistical difference in neoplastic transformation frequencies in exposed versus unexposed cells.

8.3.4 Enzymes

It is believed that low-level modulated RFR can affect intracellular activities of enzymes. Byus et al. [55, 56] reported, for example, evidence of effects on the activity of ornithine decarboxylase (ODC), as well as ODC messenger RNA levels and polyamine export in a number of cultured cell lines after exposure to 450 MHz sinusoidally modulated at 16-Hz (1 mW/cm^2) RFR. The effect was noted for certain modulations of the carrier wave illustrating the window effect.

Cain et al. [57] explored whether ELF-modulated RF (TDMA) fields influence induced activity of the ODC enzyme in cells. They first found evidence of inhibited ODC activity at three and four hours after irradiation at 8.4 mW/cm^2 (SAR of 7.8 mW/kg), but no such effect at other times of exposures.

Penafiel et al. [58] reported an increase in ODC activity in L929 cells after irradiation to 835 MHz RFR at SAR between 1-3 W/kg. They noticed a rise in the ODC activity when the wave was sinusoidally modulated at 16 or 50 Hz.

Raj et al. [59] exposed developing rats to 2.45 GHz RFR (2 hours per day for 35 days at incident power density 0.334 mW/cm^2). A 1.5-fold increase in brain ODC was observed in the exposed group compared to control.

In a Motorola-funded study, Cain et al. [60] explored the possible effects of 1.6-GHz (IRIDIUM) digital signals on ODC and polyamine levels in the brain tissues of fetal Fisher 344 rats exposed *in utero*. The animals were exposed in a tail-first manner in a carrousel arrangement at 0.16, 1.6, or 5 W/kg brain average SAR. In the cerebrum, ODC decreased in the exposed versus unexposed animals with no change in putricine, spermine, or spermidine levels.

8.3.5 Hormones

The influence of ELF fields on hormones, such as melatonin, has been extensively discussed in Chapter 3, however, RFR is also known to influence the concentration of some hormones, including melatonin, in the blood. Burch et al. [61] suggested that the association of occupational cellular telephone use reduced daytime melatonin production.

Stark et al. [62] conducted a pilot study to investigate the influence of RFR at 3-30 MHz on salivary melatonin concentration in dairy cattle. Two commercial dairy herds at two farms were compared; one located at a distance of 500 meters (exposed), the other at a distance of 4 km (unexposed) from a RF transmitter. At each farm, five cows were monitored with respect to their salivary melatonin concentrations over a period of ten consecutive days. The transmitter was switched off during three of the ten days. The average nightly field strength readings were 21-fold greater on the exposed farm (1.59 mA/m) than on the control farm (0.076 mA/m). The mean values of the two initial nights did not show a significant difference between exposed and unexposed cows. Hence, a chronic melatonin reduction effect seemed unlikely. However, on the first night of reexposure after the transmitter had been off for three days, the difference in salivary melatonin concentration between the two farms was statistically significant, indicating a two- to sevenfold increase of melatonin concentration in the exposed cows.

In a related study, Lai and Singh [63] indicated that treatment of rats immediately before and after RF exposure with either melatonin or the spin-trap compound N-tert-butyl-alpha-phenylnitrone blocks the effects of RFR.

8.3.6 Immune Activities

Because of the essential role of the immune system for survival, many investigators have sought to determine the potential impact of RFR on the immune system. Lyle et al. [64] showed that exposure to sinusoidal amplitude-modulated RFR at nonthermal levels can reduce immune functions in cells. A 450-MHz RFR was modulated with a 60-Hz ELF field. Tests indicated that a modulated carrier wave of 450 MHz by itself had no effect, and modulation frequencies of 40,. 16, and 3 Hz had a progressively smaller effect than 60 Hz. Peak suppression of the lymphocyte effectiveness (immune function effectiveness) was observed at 60-Hz modulation.

Changes in the immunological functions of mice were, for example, observed by Veyret et al. [65] after a 5-day exposure to low-level RFR (0.015 W/kg) 9.4-GHz amplitude-modulated signal at around 20 MHz.

Elekes et al. [66] tested the effect of continuous 2.45 GHz, 50 Hz amplitude-modulated square waves (SAR of 0.14 W/kg) on the immune response. CW exposures (6 days, 3 hours/day) induced elevations of the number of antibody-producing cells in the spleen of male mice. Also, AM RFR induced elevation of the spleen index (+15%) and antibody-producing cell number (+55%) in the spleen of male mice. No changes were observed in female mice. In conclusion, both types of exposure conditions induced moderate elevation of antibody production in male mice, but not at all in female mice.

Fesenko et al. [67] indicated that whole body microwave sinusoidal irradiation of male NMRI mice with 8.15-18 GHz (1 Hz within) at a power density of 1 μW/cm^2 causes a significant enhancement of tumor necrosis factor (TNF) production in peritoneal macrophages and splenic T lymphocytes. RFR affected T cells, facilitating their capacity to proliferate in response to mitogenic stimulation. The exposure duration necessary for the stimulation of cellular immunity ranged from 5 hours to 3 days. Chronic irradiation of mice for 7 days produced the decreasing of TNF production in peritoneal macrophages. The exposure of mice for 24 hours increased the TNF production and immune proliferative response, and these stimulatory effects persisted over 3 days after the termination of exposure.

The effect of 8.15-18-GHz (1 Hz within) RFR at a power density of 1 μW/cm^2 on the TNF production and immune response was tested by Novoselova et al. [68]. A single 5-hour whole-body exposure induced a significant increase in TNF production in peritoneal macrophages and splenic T cells. The mitogenic response in T lymphocytes increased after RF exposure. The activation of cellular immunity was observed within 3 days after exposure. These results demonstrate that irradiation with low-power density RFR stimulates the immune potential of macrophages and T cells, and that antioxidant treatment enhances the effect of RFR, in particular at later terms, when the effect of irradiation is reduced.

8.3.7 Membrane Functions

Cells have voltage across their membranes and voltage-gated ion channels through their membranes. They use ions (e.g., Ca2$^+$) for many cell regulatory processes including signal transduction and gap junction gate regulation. Altering the electric field on the surface of cells changes the receptor efficiency and interferes with the voltage-gated ion channels [69]. Intervention with membrane-mediated signal detection, transduction, or amplification processes may cause various biological nonthermal effects. The movement of cellular calcium ion (Ca^{2+}) by RFR is a significant response in the order of cellular activities.

There have been a number of studies on enhanced calcium efflux using ELF-modulated RFR; however, it was demonstrated that the significant component was the ELF signal and not the high-frequency carrier signal. Meanwhile, investigations on acetylcholinesterase activity using the same types of RFR might be related to calcium transport [70]. According to Saunders et al. [71], "Some studies confirmed alterations of membrane transport of ions and transient inhibition of energy-delivering systems by RFR."

An effect of low-power 10.750-GHz RFR on the function of acetylcholine receptors was also observed by Tarricone et al. [72]. It was shown that the opening frequency of these ion channels decreased during irradiation. The relevance of most of these membrane effects for human health remains unclear.

Linz et al. [73] studied the influence of RF fields of 180, 900, and 1800 MHz on the membrane potential, action potential, L-type Ca2$^+$ current and potassium currents of isolated ventricular myocytes. The study was based on 90 guinea-pig myocytes and 20 rat myocytes. The fields were applied in rectangular waveguides (1800 MHz at 80, 480, 600, 720, or 880 mW/kg, and 900 MHz, 250 mW/kg) or in a TEM-cell (180 MHz at 80 mW/kg and 900 MHz at 15 mW/kg). Fields of 1800 and 900 MHz were pulsed according to the GSM standard. None of the tested electrophysiological parameters were changed significantly by RF exposure.

8.4 ANIMAL CANCER STUDIES

As RF exposure is not considered to be directly carcinogenic, research should be aimed particularly toward possible promotional and copromotional effects. Juutilainen [74] reviewed the scientific literature of animal studies on cancer-related effects focusing on the effects of weak RFR.

8.4.1   Normal Animal Studies

An interesting study was performed by Guy et al. [75] who exposed 100 rats from 2 to 27 months of age to pulsed microwaves at SAR of 0.4 W/kg. The exposed group had a notable increase in primary malignant lesions compared to the control group when lesions were pooled regardless of their location in the body.

A notable study regarding cancer and prolonged exposure was the one done at the University of Washington with laboratory rats [76]. One hundred rats were exposed to 2.45-GHz RFR pulse modulated at 800 Hz for 21.5 hours per day for 25 months at SARs between 0.15 and 0.4 W/kg depending on animal weight. The exposed rats had a significantly larger number of primary malignant tumors at the end of the two-year exposure. However, there were no differences between the exposed and sham-exposed animals for any specific type of tumor, or when benign tumors were added to the count.

In a Motorola-funded study, Adey et al. [77] exposed Fisher 244 rats to pulse-modulated RFR signal at 837 MHz. Exposure started with whole-body exposure of pregnant rats and continued with whole-body exposure of the litter through weaning. Starting at 7 weeks of age, the rats were given RFR to the head that continued for 22 months. Brain SAR ranged from 0.7 to 1.6 W/kg, and whole-body SAR ranged from 0.2 to 0.7 W/kg. The number of brain tumors was not significantly reduced in the groups exposed to RFR. The same group reported a similar negative finding when they exposed Fisher 244 rats to analog FM signal, comparable to those used in the TDMA cellular system [78].

In another Motorola-funded study, Morrissey et al. [79] examined expression levels of stress response and cancer-associated genes in the brains of mice exposed to one hour of RFR at 1.6 GHz. No effects were observed at low levels of exposure. Meanwhile, an increase in c-fos mRNA (preliminary cancer-causing gene) levels in the brain in a pattern was observed only at SAR levels equal to or greater than six times the maximum peak dose and 30 times the maximum whole-body average dose from an actual wireless telephone.

A few other animal experimental studies [80, 81] have specifically studied the influence of RFR on tumor development, but these are not definitive either.

8.4.2   Cancer-Prone Animal Studies

Repacholi et al. [82] exposed 100 mice to 900 MHz RFR for 60 minutes per day for 18 months. Depending upon the size of the mice and their orientation in the field, the power density ranged from 0.26 to 1.3 mW/cm^2 (SAR between 0.008 to 4.2 W/kg). They examined the possibility that long-term RF exposure would enhance the incidence of lymphomas in mice that were genetically predisposed to develop lymphomas. The incidence of lymphoma in the exposed mice was significantly higher than in the controls.

Toler et al. [83] carried out an investigation into 200 female mammary-tumor-prone mice exposed to pulsed 435-MHz RFR at 1.0 mW/cm^2 (0.32 W/kg). The pulse frequency was 1 kHz. Exposure continued for 22 hours per day, 7 days per week for 21 months. Under the circumstances of the study, there were no differences in mammary tumor incidence between the exposed mice and sham-exposed mice; and there were no differences between the groups in the numbers of malignant, metastatic, or benign tumors.

The above finding was confirmed by Frei et al. [84, 85] under similar exposure conditions, except that the mammary tumor-prone mice were exposed at 2.45 GHz for 18 months at SAR of 0.3 W/kg or 1.0 W/kg. One hundred animals per group were exposed or sham-exposed for 20 hours per day, 7 days per week for 18 months. As a result, no significant differences were observed in mammary tumor incidence or in the number of malignant, metastatic, or benign tumors.

8.4.3   Studies of Animals Treated with Chemical Carcinogens

Szmigielski et al. [86] exposed mice to 2.45 GHz RFR for up to 10 months to investigate the ability of RFR to promote various types of cancer. Exposures were at 5 or 15 mW/cm^2 (SAR of 2-3 and 6-8 W/kg). Controls included both normal animals and animals subject to confinement stress. A carcinogen (benzopyrene) was painted on the backs of the mice, and the animals were exposed to RFR. Both RF exposure and confinement stress significantly accelerated the appearance of the chemically induced skin tumors. Also, the investigators injected tumor cells into mice and looked for lung metastases and again both RF exposure and confinement stress increased the number of metastases.

Wu et al. [87] exposed 26 mice to a chemical carcinogen plus 2.45 GHz RFR at 10 mW/cm^2 (SAR of 10-12 W/kg). Exposure continued for 3 hours per day, 6 days per week for 5 months. The chemical carcinogen used is known to cause colon cancer. No difference in colon cancer rates were seen between animals treated with the carcinogen alone and the animals treated with the carcinogen plus RFR.

Chagnaud et al. [88] exposed rats injected with benzo(a)pyrene and tumors to far-field GSM signal at 900 MHz with power density of 200 μW/cm^2 (SAR of 0.27 W/kg) for 10 days (2 hours/day, 5 days/week). There were 10 animals in each of the exposed groups. No difference between the groups in any of the parameters was observed.

Imaida et al. [89] examined the possibility that exposure to RFR could promote chemically induced liver cancer in rats. They subjected 48 male F344 rats per group to a single dose of diethylnitrosamine (DEN) and later to a partial hepatectomy. They were then exposed to 929 MHz at SAR of 0.6-0.9 W/kg. Exposure was for 90 minutes per day, 5 days per week for 6 weeks. No difference in liver cancer rates was seen between RF-exposed rats and rats given only the chemical carcinogen.

Also, Imaida et al. [90] reported a lack of liver cancer promotion in rats exposed to 1.439 GHz at SAR of 2.0 W/kg. TDMA signals for the Personal Digital Cellular (PDC) Japanese cellular standard were directed to rats through a quarter-wavelength monopole antenna. Numerical dosimetry showed that the peak SARs within the liver were 1.91 to 0.937 W/kg, while the whole-body average SARs were 0.680 to 0.453 W/kg, when the time-averaged radiation power was 0.33 W. The exposure was for 90 minutes a day, 5 days a week, over 6 weeks, to male F344 rats given a single dose of DEN.

In a Motorola-funded study, Adey et al. [91] exposed Fischer 344 rats to FM signal (836.55 MHz +/- 12.5 kHz deviation) simulating exposures in the head of cellular phone users. They tested for effects on spontaneous tumorigenicity of CNS tumors in the offspring of pregnant rats and also for modified incidence of primary CNS tumors in rats treated with a single dose of the neurocarcinogen ethylnitrosourea (ENU) in *utero*. An ENU dosage (4 mg/kg) was selected to give an expected brain tumor incidence of 10-15% over the mean life span of 26 months. There were no effects on survival attributable to RFR in either ENU-treated or in sham-treated groups. No RFR-mediated changes were observed in number, incidence, or histological type of either spontaneous or ENU-induced brain tumors, nor were gender differences detected in tumor numbers.

8.5 ANIMAL STUDIES—NONCANCER

Most of experimental studies focus on carcinogenesis, tumor promotion, and mutagenic effects. Other noncancer effects are also considered. Sienkiewicz [92] reviewed the recent noncancer animal studies. He concluded that well-conducted studies targeted at specific endpoints using established animal models would help to provide better standards and guidelines for human exposure.

8.5.1 Morphology of the Brain

RFR can induce morphological changes in the CNS only under relatively high intensity or prolonged exposure [93-95]. Irradiation of animals with RFR at SAR greater than 2 W/kg may produce morphological alterations in the CNS [96].

Oldendorf [97] performed one of the earliest studies on the effect of RFR on the CNS. The results showed that focal coagulation necrosis could be produced in the brain of rabbits exposed to 2.45 GHz by the generated thermal energy.

According to Adey [98] and Adey et al. [99], RF carriers sinusoidally modulated at ELF frequencies can cause CNS changes.

Wu et al. [100] explored the effects of EM pulse exposure on the CNS of Wistar rats. The exposure results in changes of the content of neurotransmitters in different cerebral areas of rats, lowering their ability of learning.

In 1997, Vorobyov et al. [101] studied averaged EEG frequency spectra in eight adult male rats with chronically implanted carbon electrodes in symmetrical somesthetic areas when a weak (0.1-0.2 mW/cm^2) RFR at 945 MHz, amplitude-modulated at 4 Hz, was applied. Intermittent (1 minute on, and 1 minute off) field exposure for 10 minutes duration was used. No difference between control and exposure experiments was observed under these routines of data averaging. Significant elevations of EEG asymmetry in 10-14 Hz range were observed during the first 20 seconds after four from five onsets of the RFR, when averaged spectra was obtained for every 10 seconds.

Tsurita et al. [102] investigated the effect of exposing rats to a 1439 MHz TDMA on the morphological changes of the brain. The exposure period was two or four weeks. The energy dose rate peaked at 2 W/kg in the brain; the average over the whole body was 0.25 W/kg. No significant changes were observed in the groups of rats exposed to RFR.

8.5.2 Morphology of the Eye

RFR was found cataractogenic if the exposure intensity and the duration are sufficient. Richardson et al. [103] were able to induce lenticular opacities in the eyes of rabbits and dogs exposed to RFR at a distance of 5 cm.

Lesions in the cornea, degenerative changes in cells of the iris and retina, and changed visual functions were reported by Kues and Monahan [104] and Kues et al. [105] in nonhuman primates after frequent RF exposures (CW 2.45-GHz RFR at SAR of 0.26 W/kg). Simultaneous treatment with certain drugs irritated ocular responses to RFR.

In a study funded by Hewlett Packard Laboratories, Kues et al. [106] examined ocular effects associated with exposure to millimeter waves at 60 GHz and power density of 10 mW/cm^2. To confirm the results of the rabbit experiments in higher species, the second phase of the study used nonhuman primates (*Macaca Mulatta*). Acute exposure of both rabbits and nonhuman primates consisted of a single 8-hour irradiation, and the repeated exposure protocol consisted of five separate 4-hour irradiations on consecutive days. One eye in each animal was exposed and the contralateral eye served as the sham-exposed control. They concluded that single or repeated exposure to 60-GHz CW RFR at 10 mW/cm^2 did not result in any detectable ocular damage.

8.5.3 Behavioral Changes

Changes in behavior occurred after RF exposure at SAR of 1.2 W/kg [107]. Behavioral changes were observed also at SAR of 2.5 W/kg [108].

Lai et al. [109] found that RF exposure showed retarded learning of a task. Rats were exposed to pulsed 2.45 GHz (2 μs pulses, 500 pps) at an average whole-body SAR of 0.6 W/kg in a cylindrical waveguide system for 45 minutes each day before being tested in a 12-arm maze.

Kemerov et al. [110] carried out experiments on 24 Wistar rats divided into 4 groups (1 control and 3 experimental). The rats were exposed to RFR on the head area at a power density of 10 mW/cm². The results suggested that RF exposure could slow down the formation of conditioned responses. Behavioral effects were mild at athermal dosages and the animals adapted easily to exposure conditions.

In a study funded by Deutsche Teklekom, Bornhausen and Scheingraber [111] exposed Wistar rats during pregnancy to a low-level (0.1 mW/cm²) 900 MHz, 217 Hz pulse-modulated RFR. Whole-body SAR values for the freely roaming, pregnant animals ranged between 17.5 and 75 mW/kg. Analyses of performance scores and of inter-response intervals (IRI) patterns showed that exposure *in utero* to the GSM field did not induce any measurable cognitive deficits.

8.5.4 Blood-Brain Barrier

The blood-brain barrier (BBB) is a physiologically complex system. It separates the brain and cerebral spinal fluid of the CNS from the blood. It primarily consists of an essentially continuous layer of cells lining the blood vessels of the brain. It protects sensitive brain tissues from ordinary variations in the composition of blood while allowing transport of nutrients into the brain. But the BBB is not an absolute barrier between the blood and the brain; rather it retards the rate at which substances cross between the blood stream and the brain.

Any disruption to the BBB has serious consequences on health. The BBB may break down following brain trauma or brain heating. The BBB breakdown is risky if it allows enough concentrations of blood borne neurotoxins (such as urea) to enter the brain. Substances needed by the brain i.e., glucose, cross the BBB either by passive transport or may be transported across in small bubbles of fluids.

RFR-induced breakdown of the BBB was produced experimentally and reported in the literature for more than 25 years [112-117]. However, other studies have not found RFR-induced disruption of the BBB [118, 119]. Most of the studies conclude that high-intensity RFR is required to alter the permeability of the BBB.

8.6 CONCLUDING REMARKS

A significant uncertainty is in the interpretation of the experimental studies since many of them have supplied insufficient details about the exposure conditions. However, the evidence for other effects is the moderate experimental research, which need more independent replication in order to verify the suggestions of health effects in epidemiological studies. Also, that most of the effects do not directly relate to illnesses in humans or their significance is doubtful due to the lack of explanation of the interaction mechanisms. In that sense, lack of evidence for possible adverse health effects does not equate with evidence of no effect.

The balance of research evidence available does not propose that environmental RFR causes cancer or other diseases. But there is now some evidence that effects on biological functions, including those of the brain, may be induced by RFR at levels comparable to those associated with the use of cellular phones for instance. There is, as yet, no evidence that these biological effects develop health hazards but currently only limited data is available.

No one, so far, knows for sure what the long-term effects of RFR are and whether they are cumulative. The outcome of a cumulative effect is especially substantial in considering the health effect. The long-term cumulative exposure is the product of time and mean personal exposure. In fact, the effect of ionizing radiation, such as from X-rays, is cumulative. This matter was raised after a number of studies reported effects after prolonged (or repeated) exposure.

It is important to note that modulated or pulsed RFR seems to be more effective in producing an effect. It can also elicit a different effect, especially on brain function, when compared with CW radiation of the same characteristics. Many studies supporting this fact have been summarized throughout this chapter. Juutilainen and de Seze [120] reviewed this matter extensively.

Well-conducted, independent, and unbiased research is required. Such independence finds its path clearly through a) the advancement in research that extends foundation for better understanding of living systems; b) the government sponsorship for organized experimental investigations at certain lines of research; and c) openness and full divulgence of facts regarding emissions from potential RF sources. This means more money, time, and precise assessment and intermittent exposure schedules resembling the normal pattern of controversial sources, such as cellular phones is needed to fully investigate the effects.

In conclusion, effects of RFR are only a threat if the dosage of radiation is very high. In the case of most environmental RFR, especially cellular phones, the dose is not very high, but it needs detection. The detection of biological responses to low-level exposure requires the design of sophisticated sensitive research procedure. The sensitivity creates a greater possibility of producing contradictory results. Such research depends critically on the skill and experience of the researcher and it is necessary that results be compared with prudent investigation in properly structured and independent research laboratories with equal expertise.

REFERENCES

[1] Repacholi, M. H., Low-Level Exposure to Radiofrequency Electromagnetic Fields: Health Effects and Research Needs, *Bioelectromagnetics* 19, pp. 20-32, 1998.

[2] Pakhomov, A. G., Y. Akyel, O. N. Pakhomova, B. E. Stuck, and M. R. Murphy, Current State and Implications of Research on Biological Effects of Millimeter Waves: A Review of the Literature, *Bioelectromagnetics* 19, pp. 393-414, 1998.

[3] Albert Bren, S. P., Historical Introduction to EMF Health Effects, *IEEE Engineering in Medicine and Biology Magazine* 15, 1996.

[4] Polk, C., and E. Postow, (eds.), *Handbook of Biological Effects of Electromagnetic Fields*, CRC Press, Boca Raton, FL, 1996.

[5] Vorst, A. V., Microwave Bioelectromagnetics in Europe, *IEEE MTT-S Digest*, pp. 1137-1140, 1993.

[6] Lai, H., Research on the Neurological Effects of Nonionizing Radiation at the University of Washington, *Bioelectromagnetics* 13, pp. 513-526, 1992.

[7] Dimbylow, P. J., FDTD Calculations of SAR for a Dipole Closely Coupled to the Head at 900 MHz and 1.9 GHz, *Physics in Medicine and Biology* 38, pp. 361-368, 1993.

[8] Dimbylow, P. J., and J. M. Mann, SAR Calculations in an Anatomically Realistic Model of the Head for Mobile Communication Transceivers at 900 MHz and 1.8 GHz, *Physics in Medicine and Biology* 39, pp. 1527-1553, 1994.

[9] Martens, L., J. DeMoerloose, C. DeWagter, and D. DeZutter, Calculation of the Electromagnetic Fields Induced in the Head of an Operator of a Cordless Telephone, *Radio Science* 30, pp. 415-420, 1995.

[10] Lai, H., Neurological Effects of Microwave Irradiation, In *Advances in Electromagnetic Fields in Living Systems* 1 (ed. Lin, J. C.), pp. 27-80, Plenum Press, New York, NY, 1994.

[11] Adey, W. R., Cell and Molecular Biology Associated with Radiation Fields of Mobile Telephones, *Bioelectromagnetics Research*, University of California, Riverside, CA, 1999.

[12] Foster, K., D. Bernstein, and P. Huber, (eds.), *Phantom Risk: Scientific Interpretation and the Law*, The MIT Press, Cambridge, MA, 1996.

[13] Moulder, J. E., and K. R. Foster, Biological Effects of Power-Frequency Fields as They Relate to Carcinogenesis, *Proceedings of Society for Experimental Biology and Medicine* 209, pp. 309-324, 1995.

[14] Moulder, J. E., Power-Frequency Fields and Cancer, *Critical Reviews in Biomedical Engineering* 26, pp. 1-116, 1998.

[15] Biological Effects and Exposure Criteria for Radiofrequency Electromagnetic Fields, Report No. 86, National Council on Radiation Protection and Measurement, Bethesda, Maryland, 1986.

[16] Elder, J. A., Radiofrequency Radiation Activities and Issues: A 1986 Perspective,

Health Physics 53, pp. 607-611, 1987.

[17] Michaelson, S. M., and J. C. Lin, *Biological Effects and Health Implications of Radiofrequency Radiation*, Plenum Press, New York, NY, 1987.

[18] Blackman, C. F., Genetic and Mutagenesis, In *Biological Effects of Radiofrequency Radiation* (eds. Elder, J. A., and D. F. Cahill), US Environmental Protection Agency, Washington, DC, 1984.

[19] Garson, O. M., T. L. McRobert, L. J. Campbell, B. Hocking, and I. Gordon, A Chromosomal Study with Long Term Exposure to Radio Frequency Radiation, *Medical Journal of Australia* 155, pp. 289-292, 1991.

[20] Dhahi, S. J., R. W. Y. Habash, and H. T. Alhafid, Lack of Mutagenic Effects on Conidia of Aspergillus Amstelodami Irradiated by 8.7175 GHz Microwaves, *Journal of Microwave Power* 17, pp. 346-351, 1982.

[21] Habash, R. W. Y., Bio-Effects of the Non-Ionizing Electromagnetic Fields: Genetic Effect of Some Microwave Frequencies, M.Sc Thesis, University of Mosul, Iraq, 1983.

[22] Dhahi, S. J., R. W. Y. Habash, and H. T. Alhafid, Mutagenic Effects of Some Microwave Frequencies on Conidia of Aspergillus Amstelodami, *Second National Radio Science Conference*, pp. 423-429, Cairo, Egypt, 1984.

[23] Kerbacher, J. J., M. L. Meltz, and D. N. Erwin, Influence of Radiofrequency Radiation on Chromosome Aberrations in CHO Cells and its Interaction with DNA-Damaging Agents, *Radiation Research* 123, pp. 311-319, 1990.

[24] Meltz, M. L., P. Eagan, and D. N. Erwin, Proflavin and Microwave Radiation: Absence of a Mutagenic Interaction, *Bioelectromagnetics* 11, pp. 149-157, 1990.

[25] Ciaravino, V., M. L. Meltz, and D. N. Erwin, Absence of a Synergistic Effect between Moderate-Power Radiofrequency Electromagnetic Radiation and Adriamycin on Cell-Cyle Progression and Sister Chromatid Exchange, *Bioelectromagnetics* 12, pp. 289-298, 1991.

[26] Gos, P., B. Eicher, J. Kohli, W. –D. Heyer, No Mutagenic or Recombinogenic Effects of Mobile Phone Fields at 900 MHz in the Yeast Saccharomyces Cerevisiae, *Bioelectromagnetics* 21, pp. 515-523, 2000.

[27] French, P., Australian Research Shows Electromagnetic Radiation Causes Changes to Genetic Makup, *Electromagnetics Forum* 1, 1996.

[28] Maes, A., M. Collier, D. Slaets, and L. Verschaeve, 954 MHz Microwaves Enhance the Mutagenic Properties of Mitomycin, *Environmental and Molecular Mutagenesis* 28, pp. 26-30, 1996.

[29] Lai, H., and N. P. Singh, Acute Low-Intensity Microwave Exposure Increases DNA Single-Strand Breaks in Rat Brain Cells, *Bioelectromagnetics* 16, pp. 207-210, 1995.

[30] Lai, H., and N. P. Singh, Single and Double Strand DNA Breaks in Rat Brain Cells After Acute Exposure to Radiofrequency Electromagnetic Radiation, *International Journal of Radiation Biology* 69, pp. 513-521, 1996.

[31] Lai, H., M. A. Carino, and N. P. Singh, Naltrexone Blocks RFR-Induced DNA Double Strand Breaks in Rat Brain Cells, *Wireless Networks* 3, pp. 471-476, 1997.

[32] Malyapa, R. S., E. W. Ahern, W. L. Straube, E. G. Moros, W. F. Pickard, and J. L. Roti Roti, Measurement of DNA Damage After Exposure to 2450 MHz Electromagnetic Radiation, *Radiation Research* 148, pp. 608-617, 1997.

[33] Phillips, J. L., O. Ivaschuk, T. Oshida-Jones, R. A. Jones, M. Campbell-Beacler, and

W. Haggreu, DNA Damage in Molt-4 T-Lymphoblastoid Cells Exposed to Cellular Telephone RFs *In Vitro, Bioelectrochemistry and Bioenergetics* 45, pp. 103-110 1998.

[34] Vijayalaxmi, B. Z. Leal, M. Szilagyi, T. J. Prihoda, and M. L. Meltz, Primary DNA Damage in Human Blood Lymphocytes Exposed *In Vitro* to 2450 MHz Radiofrequency, *Radiation Research* 153, pp. 479-486, 2000.

[35] Garaj-Vrhovac, V., D. Horvat, and Z. Koren, The Effect of Microwave Radiation on the Cell Genome, *Mutation Research* 243, pp. 87-93, 1990.

[36] D'Ambrosio, G., M. B. Lioi, R. Massa, M. R. Scarfi, and O. Zeni, Genotoxicity of Microwaves (Abs.), *1st World Congress on Electricity and Magnetism in Biology and Medicine*, p. 59, Orlando, FL, 1992.

[37] Maes, A., L. Verschaeve, A. Arroyo, C. Dewagter, and L. Vercruyssen, *In Vitro* Cytogenetic Effects of 2450 MHz Waves on Human Peripheral Blood Lymphocytes, *Bioelectromagnetics* 14, pp. 495-501, 1993.

[38] Goswami, P. C., L. D. Albee, A. J. Parsian, J. D. Baty, E. G. Moros, W. F. Pickard, J. L. Roti-Roti, and C. R. Hunt, Proto-Oncogene mRNA Levels and Activities of Multiple Transcription Factors in C3H10T1/2 Murine Embryonic Fibroblasts Exposed to 835.62 and 847.74 MHz Cellular Phone Communication Frequency Radiation, *Radiation Research* 151, pp. 300-309, 1999.

[39] Manikowska, E., J. M. Luciani, B. Servantie, P. Czerski, J. Obrenovitch, and A. Stahl, Effects of 9.4 GHz Microwave Exposure on Meiosis in Mice, *Experientia* 35, pp. 388-389, 1979.

[40] Manikowska, E., P. Czerski, and W. M. Leach, Effects of 2.45 GHz Microwaves on Meiotic Chromosomes of Male CBA/CAY Mice, *Journal of Heredity* 76, pp. 71-73, 1985.

[41] Malyapa, R. S., E. W. Ahern, C. Bi, W. L. Straube, M. LaRegina, W. F. Pickard, and J. L. Roti Roti, DNA Damage in Rat Brain Cells After *In Vivo* Exposure to 2450 MHz Electromagnetic Radiation and Various Methods of Euthanasia, *Radiation Research* 149, pp. 637-645, 1998.

[42] Verschaeve, L., and A. Maes, Genetic, Carcinogenic and Teratogenic Effects of Radiofrequency Fields, *Mutation Research* 410, pp. 141-165, 1998.

[43] Brusick, D., R. Albertini, D. McRee, D. Peterson, G. Williams, P. Hanawalt, and J. Preston, Genotoxicity of Radiofrequency Radiation, *Environmental and Molecular Mutagenesis* 32, pp. 1-16, 1998.

[44] Czerska, E. M., E. C. Elson, C. C. Davis, M. L. Swicord, and P. Czerski, Effects of Continuos and Pulsed 2450-MHZ Radiation on Spontaneous Lymphoblastoid Tranformation of Human Lymphocytes *In Vitro, Bioelectromagnetics* 13, pp. 247-259, 1992.

[45] Cleary, S. F., L. M. Liu, and R. E. Merchant, *In Vitro* Lymphcyte Proliferation Induced by Radiofrequency Electromagnetic Radiation Under Isothermal Conditions, *Bioelectromagnetics* 11, pp. 47-56, 1990.

[46] Cleary, S. F., Z. Du, G. Cao, L. M. Liu, and C. McCrady, Effect of Radiofrequency Radiation on Cytolytic T Lymphocytes, *The Federation of American Societies for Experimental Biology Journal* 10, pp. 913-919, 1996.

[47] Kwee, S., and P. Raskmark, Radiofrequency Electromagnetic Fields and Cell Proliferation, *Second World Congress for Electricity and Magnetism in Biology and*

Medicine, Bologna, Italy, 1997.

[48] Kwee, S., and P. Raskmark, Changes in Cell Proliferation Due to Environmental Non-Ionizing Radiation: 2. Microwave Radiation, *Bioelectrochemistry and Bioenergetics* 44, pp. 251-255, 1998.

[49] Velizarov, S., P. Raskmark, and S. Kwee, The Effects of Radiofrequency Fields on Cell Proliferation are Non-Thermal, *Bioelectrochemistry and Bioenergetics* 48, pp. 177-180, 1999.

[50] Stagg, R. B., W. J. Thomas, R. A. Jones, and W. R. Adey, Cell Proliferation in C6 Glioma Cells Exposed to a 836.55 MHz Frequency Modulated Radiofrequency Field, pp. 45-46, *The Bioelectromagnetics Society Meeting*, Boston, MA, 1995.

[51] Balcer-Kubiczek, E. K., and G. H. Harrison, Evidence for Microwave Carcinogenesis *In Vitro*, *Carcinogenesis* 6, pp. 859-864, 1985.

[52] Balcer-Kubiczek, E. K., and G. H. Harrison, Induction of Neoplastic Transformation in C3H/10T1/2 Cells by 2.45 GHz Microwaves and Phorbol Ester, *Radiation Research* 117, pp. 531-537, 1989.

[53] Balcer-Kubiczek, E. K., and G. H. Harrison, Neoplastic Transformation of C3H/10T1/2 Cells Following Exposure to 120 Hz Modulated 2.45 GHz Microwaves and Phorbol Ester Tumor Promotor, *Radiation Research* 126, pp. 65-72, 1991.

[54] Malyapa, R. S., E. W. Aher, E. G. Moros, W. L. Strube, W. F. Pickard, and J. L. Roti Roti, Lack of Neoplastic Transformation in C3H10T1/2 Cells Following Exposure to Cellular Phone Communications Frequencies, *The Bioelectromagnetics Society Meeting*, Petersburg, FL, 1998.

[55] Byus, C. V., K. Kartum, S. Pieper, and W. R. Adey, Increased Ornithine Decarboxylase Activity in Cultured Cells Exposed to Low Energy Modulated Microwave Fields and Phorbol Ester Tumor Promoters, *Cancer Research* 48, pp. 4222-4226, 1988.

[56] Byus, C. V., and L. Hawel, Additional Considerations About the Bioeffects of Mobile Communications, In *Mobile Communications Safety* (eds. Kuster, N., Q. Balzano, and J. C. Lin), Chapman & Hall, London, UK, 1997.

[57] Cain, C. D., D. L. Thomas, M. Ghaffari, and W. R. Adey, 837 MHz Digital Cellular Telephone RF Fields and Induced ODC Activity in C3H10T1/2 Cells, *The Bioelectromagnetics Society Meeting*, Victoria, BC, Canada, 1996.

[58] Penafiel, M. L., T. Litovitz, D. Krause, A. Desta, and J. M. Mullins, Role of Modulation on the Effect of Microwaves on Ornithine Decarboxylase in L929 Cells, *Bioelectromagnetics* 18, pp. 132-141, 1997.

[59] Paul Raj, R., J. Behari, and A. R. Rao, Effects of Low Level 2.45 GHz Microwave Radiation on Ca2+ Efflux and ODC Activity in Chronically Exposed Developing Rat Brain, *National Seminar on Low-Level Electromagnetic Field Phenomena in Biological Systems*, New Delhi, India, 1999.

[60] Cain, C. D., M. Ghaffari, R. A. Jones, C. V. Byus, and W. R. Adey, Digital Cellphone Field Exposures, *In Utero*, Alter ODC and Polyamine Levels in Fetal Rat Brains, *The Bioelectromagnetics Society Meeting*, Long Beach, CA, 1999.

[61] Burch, J. B., J. S. Reif, C. A. Pitrat, T. J. Keele, and M. G. Yost, Cellular Telephone Use and Excreton of a Urinary Melatonin Metabolite, *Abstract of the Annual Review of Research on Biological Effects of Electric and Magnetic Fields from the Generation, Delivery and Use of Electricity*, San Diego, CA, 1997.

[62] Stark, K. D., T. Krebs, E. Altpeter, B. Manz, C. Griot, and T. Abelin, Absence of Chronic Effect of Exposure to Short-Wave Radio Broadcast Signal on Salivary Melatonin Concentrations in Dairy Cattle, *Journal of Pineal Research* 22, pp. 171-176, 1997.

[63] Lai, H., and N. P. Singh, Melatonin and a Spin-Trap Compound Block Radiofrequency Electromagnetic Radiation-Induced DNA Strand Breaks in Rat Brain Cells, *Bioelectromagnetics* 18, pp. 446-454, 1997.

[64] Lyle, D. B., P. Schechter, W. R. Adey, and R. L. Lundak, Suppression of T-Lymphocyte Cytotoxicity Following Exposure to Sinusoidally Amplitude-Modulated Fields, *Bioelectromagnetics* 4, pp. 281-92, 1983.

[65] Veyret, B., C. Bouthet, P. Deschaud, R. de Seze, M. Geffara, J. Joussot-Dubien, M. le Diraison, J. M. Moreau, and A. Caristan, Antibody Response of Mice Exposed to Low-Power Microwaves Under Combined Pulse and Amplitude Modulation, *Bioelectromagnetics* 12, pp. 47-56, 1991.

[66] Elekes, E., G. Thuroczy, and L. D. Szabo, Effect on the Immune System of Mice Exposed Chronically to 50 Hz Amplitude-Modulated 2.45 GHz Microwaves, *Bioelectromagnetics* 17, pp.246-248, 1996.

[67] Fesenko, E. E., V. R. Makar, E. G. Novoselova, and V. B. Sadovnikov, Microwaves and Cellular Immunity. I. Effect of Whole Body Microwave irradiation on Tumor Necrosis Factor Production in Mouse Cells, *Bioelectrochemistry and Bioenergetics* 49, pp. 29-35, 1999.

[68] Novoselova, E. G., E. E. Fesenko, V. R. Makar, and V. B. Sadovnikov, Microwaves and Cellular Immunity. II. Immunostimulating Effects of Microwaves and Naturally Occurring Antioxidant Nutrients, *Bioelectrochemistry and Bioenergetics* 49, pp. 37-41, 1999.

[69] Cherry, N., Criticism of the Health Assessment in the ICNIRP Guidelines for Radiofrequency and Microwave Radiation (100 kHz-300 GHz), Lincoln University, New Zealand, 2000.

[70] Dutta, S. K., K. Das, B. Ghosh, and R. Parshad, Dose Dependence of Acetylcholinesterase Activity in Neuroblastoma Cells Exposed to Modulated Radio-Frequency Electromagnetic Radiation, *Bioelectromagnetics* 13, pp. 317-322, 1992.

[71] Saunders, R. D., C. I. Kowalczuk, and Z. J. Sienkiewicz, Biological Effects of Exposure to Non-Ionizing Electromagnetic Fields and Radiation. III, Radiofrequency and Microwave Radiation, NRPB-R240, Chilton, Didcot, Oxfordshire, UK, 1991.

[72] Tarricone, L., C. Cito, and D. D'Inzeo, ACh Receptor Channel's Interaction with MW Fields, *Bioelectrochemistry and Bioenergetics* 30, pp. 275-285, 1993.

[73] Linz, K. W., C. von Westphalen, J. Streckert, V. Hansen, and R. Meyer, Membrane Potential and Currents of Isolated Heart Muscle Cells Exposed to Pulsed Radio Frequency Fields, *Bioelectromagnetics* 20, pp. 497-511, 1999.

[74] Juutilainen, J., Review of Animal Studies on Cancer-Related Effects of RF Exposure, *COST 244 bis Project: Forum on Future European Research on Mobile Communications and Health*, pp. 25-30, 19-20 April 1999.

[75] Guy, A. W., C. -K. Chou, L. L. Kunz, J. Crowley, and J. Krupp, Effects of Long-Term Low-Level Radiofrequency Radiation Exposure on Rats, (USFSAM-TR-85-11), Brooks Air Force Base, USAF School of Aerospace Medicine, Texas, 1985.

[76] Chou, C. –K., A. W. Guy, L. L. Kunz, R. B. Johnson, J. J. Crowley, and J. H. Krupp, Long-Term, Low-Level Microwave Irradiation of Rats, *Bioelectromagnetics* 13, pp. 469-496, 1992.

[77] Adey, W. R., C. V. Byus, C. D. Cain, R. J. Higgins, R. A. Jones, C. J. Kean, N. Kuster, A. MacMurray, R. B. Stagg, G. Zimmerman, J. L. Phillips, and N. Haggren, Spontaneous and Nitrosourea-Induced Primary Tumors of the Central Nervous System in Fischer 344 Rats Chronically Exposed to 836 MHz Modulated Microwaves, *Radiation Research* 152, pp. 293-302, 1999.

[78] Adey, W. R., C. V. Byus, C. D. Cain, R. J. Higgins, R. A. Jones, C. J. Kean, N. Kuster, A. MacMurray, R. B. Stagg, G. Zimmerman, J. L. Phillips, and N. Haggren, Incidence of Spontaneous and Nitrosourea-Induced Primary Tumors in the Central Nervous System, *Second World Congress for Electricity and Magnetism in Biology and Medicine*, Bologna, Italy, 1997.

[79] Morrissey, J. J., S. Rauey, E. Heasley, P. Rathinavelua, M. Dauphinee, and J. H. Fallon, Iridium Exposure Increase C-fos Expression in the Mouse Brain, *Neuroscience* 92, pp. 1539-1546, 1999.

[80] Byus, C. V., K. Kartun, S. Pieper, and W. R. Adey, Increased Ornithine Decarboxylase Activity in Cultured Cells Exposed to Low Energy Modulated Microwave Fields and Phorbol Ester Tumor Promoters, *Cancer Research* 48, pp. 4222-4226, 1988.

[81] Szmigielski, S, A. Szudzinski, A. Pietraszek, M. Bielec, M. Janiak, and J. K. Wrembel, Accelerated Development of Spontaneous and Benzopyrene-Induced Skin Cancer in Mice Exposed to 2450-MHz Microwave Radiation, *Bioelectromagnetics* 3, pp. 179-191, 1982.

[82] Repacholi, M. H., A. Basten, V. Gebski, D. Noonan, J. Finnie, and A. W. Harris, Lymphomas in Eμ-Piml Transgenic Mice Exposed to Pulsed 900 MHz Electromagnetic Fields, *Radiation Research* 147, pp. 631-640 1997.

[83] Toler, J. C., W. W. Shelton, M. R. Frei, J. H. Merritt, and M. A. Stedham, Long-Term Low-Level Exposure of Mice Prone to Mammary Tumors to 435 MHz Radiofrequency Radiation, *Radiation Research* 148, pp. 227-234, 1997.

[84] Frei, M. R., R. E. Berger, S. J. Dusch, V. Guel, J. R. Jauchem, J. H. Merritt, and M. A. Stedham, Chronic Exposure of Cancer-Prone Mice to Low-Level 2450 MHz Radiofrequency Radiation, *Bioelectromagnetic* 19, pp. 20-31, 1998.

[85] Frei, M. R., J. R. Jauchem, S. J. Dusch, J. H. Merritt, R. E. Berger, and, and M. A. Stedham, Chronic Low-Level (1.0 W/Kg) Exposure of Mammary Cancer-Prone Mice to 2450 MHz Microwaves, *Radiation Research* 150, pp. 568-576, 1998.

[86] Szmigielski, S., A. Szudzinski, A. Pietraszek, M. Bielec, M. Janiak, and J. K. Wrembel, Accelerated development of Spontaneous and Benzopyrene-Induced Skin Cancer in Mice Exposed to 2450 MHz Microwave Radiation, *Bioelectromagnetics* 3, pp. 179-191, 1982.

[87] Wu, R. W., H. Chiang, B. J. Shao, N. G. Li, and Y. D. Fu, Effects of 2.45 GHz Microwave Radiation and Phorbol Ester 12-O-Tetradecanoylphorbol-13-Acetate on Dimethylhydrazine-Induced Colon Cancer in Mice, *Bioelectromagnetics* 15, pp. 531-538, 1994.

[88] Chagnaud, J. -L., B. Veyret, and B. Despres, Effects of Pulsed Microwaves on Chemically-Induced Tumors, *The Bioelectromagnetics Society Meeting*, p. 28,

Boston, MA, 1995.

[89] Imaida, K., M. Taki, T. Yamaguchi, T. Ito, S. Watanabe, K. Wake, A. Aimoto, Y. Kamimura, N. Ito, and T. Shirai, Lack of Promoting Effects of the Electromagnetic Near-Field Used for Cellular Phones (929.2 MHz) on Rat Liver Carcinogenesis in a Medium-Term Liver Bioassay, *Carcinogenesis* 19, pp. 311-314, 1998.

[90] Imaida, K., M. Taki, S. Watanabe, Y. Kamimura, T. Ito, T. Yamaguchi, N. Ito, and T. Shirai, The 1.5 GHz Electromagnetic Near-Field Used for Cellular Phones Does not Promote Rat Liver Carcinogenesis in a Medium-Term Liver Bioassay, *Japanese Journal of Cancer Research* 89, pp. 995-1002, 1998.

[91] Adey, W. R, C. V. Byus, C. D. Cain, R. J. Higgins, R. A. Jones, C. J. Kean, N. Kuster, A. MacMurray, R. B. Stagg, and G. Zimmerman, Spontaneous and Nitrosourea-Induced Primary Tumors of the Central Nervous System in Fischer 344 Rats Exposed to Frequency-Modulated Microwave Fields, *Cancer Research* 60, pp. 1857-1863, 2000.

[92] Sienkiewicz, Z., Non-Cancer Animal Studies, *COST 244 bis Project: Forum on Future European Research on Mobile Communications and Health*, pp. 31-37, 19-20 April 1999.

[93] Gordon, Z. V., Biological Effects of Microwaves in Occupational Hygiene, Israel Program for Scientific Translations, Jerusalem, Israel, 1970.

[94] Tolgskaya, M. S., and Z. V. Gordon, Pathological Effects of Radiowaves, (Translated from Russian), Consultants Bureau, New York, NY, 1973.

[95] Albert, E. N., and M. DeSantis, Do Microwaves Alter Nervous System Structure? *Annals of the New York Academy of Sciences* 247, pp. 87-108, 1975.

[96] *Nonionizing Radiation Protection*, WHO Publications, European Series 25, 1989.

[97] Oldendorf, W. H., Focal Neurological Lesions Produced by Microwave Irradiations, *Proceedings of Society for Experimental Biology and Medicine* 72, pp. 432-434, 1949.

[98] Adey, W. R., Tissue Interactions with Nonionizing Electromagnetic Fields, *Physiological Reviews* 61, pp. 435-514, 1981.

[99] Adey, W. R., S. M. Bawin, and A. F. Lawrence, Effects of Weak Amplitude Modulated Microwave Fields on Calcium Efflux from Awake Cat Cerebral Cortex, *Bioelectromagnetics* 3, pp. 295-307, 1982.

[100] Wu, Y., Y. Jia, Y. Guo, and Z. Zheng, Influence of EMP on the Nervous System of Rats, *ACTA Biophysica Sinica* 15, pp. 152-157, 1999.

[101] Vorobyov, V. V., A. A. Galchenko, N. I. Kukushkin, and I. G. Akoev, Effects of Weak Microwave Fields Amplitude Modulated at ELF on EEG of Symmetric Brain Areas in Rats, *Bioelectromagnetics* 18, pp. 293-298, 1997.

[102] Tsurita, G., H. Nagawa, S. Ueno, S. Watanabe, and M. Taki, Biological and Morphological Effects on the Brain After Exposure of Rats to a 1439 MHz TDMA Field, *Bioelectromagnetics* 21, pp. 364-371, 2000.

[103] Richardson, A. W., T. D. Dauve, and H. M. Hines, Experimental Lenticular Opacities Produced by Microwave Radiations, *Arch physics Medical Rehabilitation* 29, pp. 765-769, 1948.

[104] Kues, H. A., and J. C. Monahan, Microwave-Induced Changes to the Primate Eye, *Johns Hopkins APL Tech Digest* 13, pp. 244-254, 1992.

[105] Kues, H. A., J. C. Monahan, S. A. D'Anna, D. S. McLeod, G. A. Lutty, and S.

Koslov, Increased Sensitivity of the Non-Human Primate Eye to Microwave Radiation Following Ophthalmic Drug Pretreatment, *Bioelectromagnetics* 13, pp. 379-393, 1992.

[106] Kues, H. A., S. A. D'Anna, R. Osiander, W. R. Green, and J. C. Monahan, Absence of Ocular Effects After Either Single or Repeated Exposure to 10 mW/cm^2 from a 60 GHz CW Source, *Bioelectromagnetics* 20, pp. 463-473, 1999.

[107] D'Andrea, J. A., O. P. Gandhi, J. L. Lords, C. H. Durney, C. C. Johnson, and L. Astle, Physiological and Behavioral Effects of Exposure to 2450 MHz Microwaves, *Journal of Microwave Power* 14, pp. 351-362, 1980.

[108] De Lorge, J. O., and C. S. Ezell, Observing Responses of Rats Exposed to 1.28- and 5.62 GHz Microwaves, *Bioelectromagnetics* 1, pp. 183-198, 1980.

[109] Lai, H., A. Horita, and A. W. Guy, Microwave Irradiation Affects Radial-Arm Maze Performance in the Rat, *Bioelectromagnetics* 15, pp. 95-104, 1994.

[110] Kemerov, S., M. Marinkev, and D. Getova, Effects of Low-Intensity Electromagnetic Fields on Behavioral Activity of Rats, *Folia Med (Plovdiv)* 41, pp. 75-80, 1999.

[111] Bornhausen, M., and H. Scheingraber, Prenatal Exposure to 900 MHz, Cell-Phone Electromagnetic Fields had No Effect on Operant-Behavior Performances of Adult Rats, *Bioelectromagnetics* 21, pp. 566-574, 2000.

[112] Cameron, I. R., H. Davson, and M. Segal, The Effect of Hypercapnia on the Blood-Brain Barrier to Sucrose in the Rabit, *Yale Journal of Biology and Medicine* 42, pp. 241-247, 1970.

[113] Oscar, K. J., and T. D. Hawkins, Microwave Alteration of the Blood-Brain Barrier System of Rats, *Brain Research* 126, pp. 381-393, 1977.

[114] Shrivastav, S., W. G. Kaelin, W. T. Joins, and R. L. Jirtle, Microwave Hyperthermia and its Effects on Tumour Blood Flow in Rats, *Cancer Research* 43, pp. 4665-4669, 1983.

[115] Neilly, J. P., and J. C. Lin, Interaction of Microwaves on the Blood-Brain Barrier of Rats, *Bioelectromagnetics* 7, pp. 405-414, 1986.

[116] Winkler, T., H. S. Sharma, E. Stalberg, Y. Olsson, and P. K. Dey, Impairment of Blood-Brain Barrier Function by Serotonin Induces Desynchronization of Spontaneous Cerebral Cortical Activity: Experimental Observations in the Anaesthetized Rat, *Neuroscience* 68, pp. 1097-1104, 1995.

[117] Persson, B. R. R., L. G. Salford, and A. Brun, Blood-Brain Barrier Permeability in Rats Exposed to Electromagnetic Fields Used in Wireless Communication, *Wireless Network* 3, pp. 455-461, 1997.

[118] Ward, T. R., and J. Ali, Blood-Brain Barrier Permeation in the Rat During Exposure to Low-Power 1.7-GHz Microwave Radiation, *Bioelectromagnetics* 2, pp. 131-143, 1981.

[119] Ward, T. R., and J. S. Ali, Blood-Brain Barrier Permeation in the Rat During Exposure to Low Power 1.7 GHz Microwave Radiation, *Bioelectromagnetics* 6, pp. 131-143, 1985.

[120] Juutilainen, J., and R. de Seze, Biological Effects of Amplitude-Modulated Radiofrequency Radiation, *Scandinavian Journal of Environmental Health* 24, pp. 245-254, 1998.

9

Human and Epidemiological Studies

9.1 INTRODUCTION

Concerns regarding hazards of radio frequency radiation (RFR) from wireless equipment in general and cellular phones in particular are receiving heightened attention due to the hazards of energy absorption in the brain and other parts of the body. In Chapter 8, laboratory experimental investigations regarding the above effects were extensively discussed. However, human laboratory investigations as well as epidemiological studies are required to complement the above experimental-oriented research and clinical examinations.

Over the years, many studies have been performed with healthy volunteers recruited from different age groups. Various objective, performance, and subjective endpoints have been considered. However, there are several shortcomings of human studies related to the risk of intentionally keeping human beings under RF exposure for a long time.

There also exist a few epidemiological studies, probably incomplete, that are comparable to the ones discussed in Part I of this book for ELF fields, in which cancer incidences and other kinds of health risks in RF-exposed subjects were investigated. The value of epidemiology is that it can identify associations between diseases and RF exposure in humans. In the field of RFR, where the epidemiological evidence is weak at best, complementary research at the cellular and animal level is required to establish a cause and effect relationship of the interaction mechanisms involved.

In addition, there have been a few lawsuits, especially in the United States, alleging that a person's brain tumor was a result of cellular phone use, but none of these cases brought forward any evidence other than the anecdotal history of the subject's cellular phone usage.

9.2 HUMAN STUDIES

Human studies carefully utilize screened volunteers who participate in double-blind studies, where appropriate, utilizing a well-designed test performed in certified exposure facility. These studies investigate effects on various senses, hormones, and organs, such as hearing, the brain, the cardiovascular system, the immune system, melatonin, the eyes, etc.

9.2.1 Auditory Perception (RF Hearing)

It is believed when people are exposed to very low-level RF energy with certain frequency and modulation characteristics, they report hearing sounds [1-3]. This has been called auditory phenomena or RF hearing. These sounds, e.g., buzzes, clicks, tones, etc., vary as a function of the modulation. Pulsed microwaves have been heard as sound by radar operators (who used to stand close to an antenna) since radar was invented during World War II. This was reported in one of the earliest reports about the auditory perception of pulsed microwaves in 1956 as an advertisement of the Airborne Instruments Laboratory. The advertisement described observations made in 1947 on the hearing of sounds that occurred at the repetition rate of radar while the listener stood close to a horn antenna [4]. The incident average power density at the head needed to induce the effect is quite low, in $\mu W/cm^2$.

Many studies have been published over the years, especially those conducted by Dr. Chou and his colleagues investigating RF hearing [5-13]. They originally presented the RF-induced auditory phenomena as an example of RF interaction that has been widely accepted as a weak field effect. Although the hypothesis of direct nervous system stimulation was proposed, the alternative is that RF auditory or hearing effect does not occur from an interaction of RFR with the auditory nerves or neurons. Instead, the RF pulse, upon absorption by soft tissues in the head, launches a thermoelastic wave of acoustic pressure that travels by bone conduction to the inner ear and activates the cochlear receptors via the same mechanism for normal hearing

In 1999, Kellenyi et al. [14] found that a 15-minute exposure to GSM phone radiation caused an increase in auditory brainstem response in the exposed side of human subjects. The subjects also showed a hearing deficiency in the high frequency range (20 dB hearing deficiency from 2 kHz to 10 kHz).

9.2.2 Brain Activities

The close placement of RF sources such as cellular phones to the user's head has elevated possibilities of interference with brain activities. Eulitz et al. [15] reported that RF fields emitted by cellular phones alter distinct aspects of the brain's electrical response to acoustic stimuli. Their results demonstrate those aspects of the induced but not the evoked brain activity in higher frequency bands of the RFR, which can be different from those not influenced by the exposure. As the induced brain activity in higher frequency bands is proposed to be a correlate of coherent high-frequency neuronal activity, RFR provides a mean to systematically change the pattern fluctuations in neural mass activity.

Freude et al. [16] studied the influence of cellular phones on preparatory slow brain potentials (SP). As a result, RF exposure caused a significant decrease of SPs at central and temporo-parieto-occipital brain regions, but not at the frontal one. Similar findings were observed by Freude et al. [17].

Preece et al. [18, 19] reported that exposure of human volunteers (36 subjects in two groups) to RFR from simulated cellular phones at 915 MHz (about 1 W mean power) may affect cognitive function in humans, particularly, by decreasing reaction times (a decrease in reaction time of 15 ms). They used a quarter-wave antenna mounted on a physical copy of an analog phone, as a sine wave, or a wave modulated at 217 Hz with 12.5 percent duty cycle, or no power, was applied to the left squamous temple region of the subjects while they undertook a series of cognitive function tests lasting approximately 25-30 minutes. There was evidence of an increase in responsiveness, strongly in the analog and less in the digital simulation, in choice reaction time. They associated the finding with an effect on the angular gyrus that acts as an interface between the visual and speech centers and which lies directly under and on the same side as the antenna. Such an effect could be consistent with mild localized heating, or possibly a nonthermal response, which is power dependent. These studies were largely behind the report on mobile phone safety issued by a special committee in the U.K. called the Independent Expert Group on Mobile Phones [20].

A Finnish group led by Dr. Koivisto [21] has repeated the above work. The researchers found that exposure to RFR emitted by cellular telephones may have a facilitatory effect on brain functioning, especially in tasks requiring attention and manipulation of information in working memory. These findings were reported while investigating cognitive functioning in 48 healthy human volunteers who were exposed to 902-MHz RFR from a cellular phone. Although the two studies are similar there were a number of differences between them, especially the range of tests carried out.

Krause et al. [22] investigated patterns of brain waves of people using mobile phones on the ERD/ERS of the 4-6-Hz, 6-8-Hz, 8-10-Hz, and 10-12-Hz EEG frequency bands in 16 normal subjects performing an auditory memory task. All subjects performed the memory task both with and without exposure to a digital 902 MHz in counterbalanced order. The RF exposure significantly increased EEG power in the 8-10-Hz frequency band only. The presence of RFR altered the ERD/ERS responses in all frequency bands as a function of time and memory task. The results suggest that RF exposure alters the brain responses significantly during a memory task.

Hladky et al. [23] indicated that RF fields from the mobile phone Motorola GSM 8700 did not affect the visual evoked potentials. The researchers reached their conclusion through two experiments on twenty volunteers who participated to explore the acute effect of using the above phone.

Hietanen et al. [24] quantitatively analyzed the EEG activity of 19 volunteers. Ten of the subjects were men (28-48 years of age) and 9 were women (32-57 years of age). The sources of exposure were 5 different cellular phones (analog and digital) operating at a frequency of 900 MHz or 1800 MHz. The EEG activity was recorded in an awake, eyes-closed situation. Six 30-minute experiments, including 1 sham exposure, were made for each subject. The duration of a real exposure phase was 20 minutes. As a result, no abnormal effects on human EEG activity have been found.

There have been reports of headaches occurring in association with the use of cellular phones, especially the digital type [25]. More evidence goes back to the 1960s and 1970s, well before the use of cellular phones. This evidence came from the former Soviet and Eastern European literature describing a collection of symptoms, called microwave sickness, in personnel exposed to RFR, based on subjective complaints such as headache, sleep disturbances, weakness, impotence, chest pain, cardiovascular changes, stress, etc.

9.2.3 Cardiovascular System

Jauchem [26] reviewed cardiovascular changes in humans exposed to ELF fields and RFR. Both acute and long-term effects were investigated. He reported that most studies showed no acute effect of static or time-varying ELF fields on blood pressure, heart rate, or ECG waveform; others reported subtle effects on the heart rate. He noticed that if heating does not occur during exposure, current flow appears necessary for major cardiovascular effects to follow, such as those due to electric shock.

Braune et al. [27] conducted a study on seven healthy male and three female volunteers aged between 26 and 36 years who underwent a single-blind placebo-controlled protocol to investigate the influence of RFR of cellular phones (GSM 900-MHz, 2-W, 217-Hz frame repetition rate) on blood pressure, heart rate, capillary perfusion, and subjective well being. The cellular phone was fixed in a typical position on the right-hand side of the head and operated by remote control, so that the volunteer did not know whether or not the phone emitted RFR. The investigators noticed an increase in sympathetic efferent activity with increases in the resting blood pressure between 5-10 mm Hg.

However, Mann et al. [28] did not find any effect on the autonomic control of heart rate by applying weak-pulsed RFR emitted by digital mobile telephones during sleep in healthy humans.

9.2.4   Effects on Immune System

Tuschl et al. [29] investigated the influence of chronic exposure on the immune system of operators. Blood was sampled from physiotherapists working at the above-mentioned devices. Eighteen exposed and thirteen control persons, matched by sex and age, were examined. Total leucocyte and lymphocyte counts were performed and leucocytic subpopulations determined by flow cytometry and monoclonal antibodies against surface antigens. To quantify subpopulations of immunocompetent cells, the activity of lymphocytes was measured. No statistically significant differences between the control and exposed persons were found. In both groups, all immune parameters were within normal ranges.

9.2.5   Melatonin

According to Burch et al. [30], users that reported frequent to occasional cellular phone use had significantly lower mean urinary melatonin metabolite levels compared to those who reported infrequent (less than one per week) or no cell phone use. Results suggest that occupational cellular telephone use may be associated with reduced daytime melatonin production.

de Seze et al. [31] studied the effect of RFR from GSM/DCS cellular phones on the rhythmic secretion of the hormone melatonin in two healthy groups of male volunteers of 38 men, 20-32 years old. Exposures were for 2 hours/day, 5 days/week, for 4 weeks, at their maximum power. Analysis of blood samples taken before, during, and after the test period found no evidence of RF-related effects on melatonin secretion.

9.2.6   Cataract Induction

Cataract induction has been one of the most inculpated hazards of human exposure to RFR. The cornea and lens are the parts of the eye most exposed to RFR at high levels by their surface location and because heat produced by the RFR is more effectively removed from other eye regions by blood circulation.

The first microwave-induced human cataract was reported by Hirsch and Parker [32]. However, in 1966, Cleary and Pasternack [33] found no difference in cataract formation among U.S. Army and Air Force veterans. The exact conditions under which these changes may occur in humans are a subject of argument [34, 35].

9.3 EPIDEMIOLOGICAL STUDIES

In this section, occupational and public environments are considered separately, a classification that did not appear in Chapter 4 while considering epidemiological studies of ELF fields.

9.3.1 Occupational Exposure Studies

Occupational or controlled environments represent areas in which people are exposed as a result of their employment, and by personnel passing through such areas, provided that these people are fully aware of the impact of exposure and may exercise control over the level of exposure. There have been many epidemiological studies conducted among occupational groups concerned with the effect of RFR. In summarizing such studies, it is convenient to consider these situations separately according to the type of occupation.

Radar and Military Personnel

The American Armed Forces have been involved with the problem of radiation safety of radar personnel since 1940s in order to dispel fears of possible ill effects of microwaves upon personnel connected with radar work. The Department of Defense (DOD), through the U.S. Navy Force and the Tri-Service Committee, undertook a comprehensive analysis of the biological effects and associated hazards of RF exposure.

Most of the early work in the 1940s indicated that the major effect of RFR in biological tissues were due either to localized or to general elevation of temperature in the tissues, producing greatest danger to areas with poor blood circulation [36, 37].

Barron et al. [38] conducted a study to evaluate changes in various characteristics of 226 radar personnel of an airframe manufacturer grouped according to various duration of exposure. The exposure included two frequencies: 2.88 GHz and 9.375 GHz. Three ranges of power densities according to the distance from the radar were chosen: >131; 39-131 and <39 mW/m^2. Ocular anomalies were found in twelve of the exposed groups compared with only one of the controls. No serious health problems were observed.

Robinette and Silverman [39] conducted a study of mortality results on males who had served in the U.S. Navy during the Korean War. They selected 19,965 equipment-repair men who had occupational exposure to RFR. They also chose 20,726 Naval equipment-operation men who, by their titles, had lower occupational exposure to RFR as a control group. The researchers studied mortality records for 1955-1974, in-service morbidity for 1950-1959, and morbidity for 1963-1976 in veterans administration hospitals. As a result, there were 619 deaths (3.1%) from all causes in the exposed group versus 579 deaths (2.8%) in the age-specific general white male population. The death rate from trauma was higher in the exposed than the control group, 295 (1.5%) versus 247 (1.2%). No difference on cancer mortality or morbidity was seen among the high exposure and low-exposure groups. The information of this study was also presented in Robinette et al. [40].

A nested case-control study [41] was used to investigate the relation between a range of RF exposures and brain tumor risk in the U.S. Air Force (USAF). Men who were exposed to RF fields had a small excess risk for developing brain tumors, with the ELF fields and RFR age-race-senior military rank-adjusted odds ratios (OR) being 1.28. Military rank was consistently associated with brain tumor risk. Officers were more likely than enlisted men to develop brain tumors (age-race-adjusted OR=2.11), and senior officers were at increased risk compared with all other USAF members (age-race-adjusted OR=3.30).

A collaborative study [42] between the U.S. Army Biomedical Research and Development Laboratory (USABRDL) and the National Institute for Occupational Safety and Health (NIOSH) was designed to assess fecundity of male artillery soldiers with potential exposures to airborne lead aerosols. It became apparent from the extensive questionnaire data that many soldiers in the initial control population had potentially experienced RF exposure as radar equipment operators. A third group of soldiers without potential for lead or RF exposure, but with similar environmental conditions, was selected as a comparison population. Blood hormone levels and semen analyses were conducted. Concern about fertility problems motivated participation of some soldiers with potential artillery or RF exposure. Artillerymen with fertility concern demonstrated lower sperm counts/ejaculate and lower sperm than the comparison group. Men with potential RF exposure showed lower sperm counts and sperm/ejaculate than the comparison group.

In 2000, the medical records of 34 patients seen at the Aerospace Medicine Directorate, USAF Research Laboratory, for confirmed exposure to RFR exceeding the permitted exposure limits were reviewed by Reeves [43]. The author intended to see if RF overexposure created any detectable clinical or laboratory alterations that could be correlated with power density or the product of power density and time exposed. A sensation of warmth was positively associated with the increased power density. A negative correlation was observed between an abnormal tissue destruction screen and power density.

In a study of Polish military workers [44], cancer morbidity was registered in a cohort of about 127,800 military personnel during a period of 15 years (1971-1985). Subjects exposed occupationally to RFR were selected from the population on the basis of their service records and documented exposures at service posts. The cancer morbidity rate for RF-exposed personnel for all age groups (20-59 years) reached 119.1 per 100,000 annually (57.6 in nonexposed) with an observed/expected ratio (OER) of 2.07. The difference between observed and expected values resulted from higher morbidity rates due to neoplasms of the alimentary tract (OER = 3.19-3.24), brain tumors (OER = 1.91) and malignancies of the haemopoietic system and lymphatic organs (OER = 6.31). Overall, a strong association between RF exposure and several types of cancer was reported.

Traffic Radar Devices

Davis and Mostofi [45], in a brief communication, reported six cases of testicular cancer in police who used handheld radars between 1979 and 1991 among a cohort of 340 police officers employed at two police departments within contiguous counties in the north-central United States. The six cases had been employed as police officers as their primary lifetime occupation, and all had been exposed to traffic radar on a routine basis. The mean length of service prior to testicular-cancer diagnosis was 14.7 years, the mean age at diagnosis was 39 years, and all had used radar at least 4½ years before the diagnosis.

Finkelstein [46] presented the results of a retrospective cohort cancer study among 22,197 officers employed by 83 Ontario police departments. The standardized incidence ratio (SIR) for all tumor sites was 0.90. There was an increased incidence of testicular cancer (SIR=1.3) and melanoma skin cancer (SIR=1.45). No information about individual exposures to radar was provided.

Broadcast and Telecommunications Personnel

Milham [47] suggested a possibility of greater than normal leukemia risk in amateur radio operators. His finding was published in a study of mortality in male members of the American Radio Relay League (ARRL), a group of amateur radio operators likely exposed to RFR while they were operating their transmitters. For the years 1971-1983, 296 male-member deaths in Washington state and 1642 in California were listed in the monthly ARRL publication. Death certificates were obtained for 280 (95%) of the Washington decedents. Information on the age, date, and cause of death was obtained for 1411 (86%) of the California decedents, a total of 1691 deaths. The mortality rate of 281 was found for acute, chronic, and unspecified myelogenous leukemia (16 deaths found versus 5.7 deaths expected). The mortality for all leukemias was 191 (24 deaths versus 12.6 deaths expected). The author noted that many of the ARRL members are employed in occupations involving exposure to RF fields, but that occupational exposure alone does not explain the excess deaths. Likewise, Millham established his investigations with another two similar studies [48, 49].

An analysis [50] covering more than 93,000 Motorola employees found no increase in overall mortality and significantly fewer deaths from brain cancer by a factor of about one-third than would be expected based on national averages for people of similar age and sex in the United States.

In 1997, Bortkiewicz et al. [51] conducted a study to evaluate the function of the circulatory system in workers occupationally exposed to medium-frequency radiation. The subjects were 71 workers at four AM broadcast stations (0.738-1.503 MHz) aged 20-68 years and 22 workers at radio link stations aged 23-67 years. Workers at AM broadcast stations experienced between 2-40 years of exposure to RFR, while workers at radio link stations had no history of regular RF exposure. The ECG abnormalities detected in the resting and/or 24 hours ECG were more frequent in workers exposed to RFR than in nonexposed subjects (75% versus 25%). A notable tendency for a higher number of rhythms was observed in AM broadcast station workers.

In Norway, Tynes et al. [52] studied breast cancer incidence in female radio and telegraph operators with potential exposure to light at night, RFR (405 kHz-25 MHz), and ELF fields (50 Hz). The researchers linked the Norwegian Telecom cohort of female radio and telegraph operators working at sea to the Cancer Registry of Norway to conduct their study. The cohort consisted of 2619 women who were certified to work as radio and telegraph operators. The incidences of all cancers were not significant, but an excess risk was seen for breast cancer. They noted that these women were exposed to light at night, which is known to decrease melatonin levels, an expected risk factor for breast cancer.

Exposure in Industrial Settings

A few epidemiological studies have been performed with operators in industrial settings in order to assess specific problems that may arise: RF burns and/or burns from contact with thermally hot surfaces; numbness in hands and fingers, disturbed or altered tactile sensitivity; eye irritation; and warming and discomfort of legs of operators (perhaps due to current flow through legs to ground).

Kolmodin-Hedman et al. [53] investigated health problems from occupational exposure of men and women to RFR from plastic welding machines of various types in Sweden. The findings were based on interviews regarding general health and history, and on tests of eye coordination and neurological state. Operators of sewing machines composed the control group for female welders; an adequate control group for male welders could not be found. The fertility outcome of the female welders did not differ significantly from the averages of Swedish birth and malformation registers. About 83% of the control women reported being healthy, compared with about 75% of the welders of both genders. Data presented were insufficient in kind or number to assess the result.

In Florence, Italy, Bini et al. [54] investigated the exposure of 63 female workers to RFR levels in a room that contained 67 sealers used to make thermal seams in different plastic sheet articles, such as inflatable boats. Most of the sealers operated at 27.12 MHz and 13.56 MHz. The authors found that the electric field near most of the units exceeded the levels permitted in Italian exposure guidelines. They also noted that the stray fields were basically limited to the immediate proximity of the sealers, so the hands of the operators received the highest exposures, followed by the head and the abdomen. The authors interviewed the workers for possible health effects; of those, 30 had been exposed, 11 had been partially exposed, and 22 had been unexposed controls. The exposed group reported subjective complaints of eye irritation and upper-limb paresthesia (abnormal sensations such as burning, and prickling. Clinical examinations of specific organs and systems of the exposed group did not yield evidence that the paresthesias were of neurogenic origin. However vitreous body disorganization in different degrees was noticed.

Lagorio et al. [55] investigated the mortality experience of a cohort of Italian plastic ware workers exposed to RFR generated by dielectric heat sealers for the period 1962-1992. The standardized mortality ratio (SMR) analysis was applied to 481 women workers, representing 78% of the total person-years at risk. Mortality from malignant neoplasms was slightly elevated, and increased risks of leukemia and accidents were detected. The all-cancer SMR was higher among women employed in the sealing department than in the whole cohort.

Szmigielski et al. [56] selected 61 healthy workers (aged 30-50 years) who had been exposed to RFR at 0.738-1.503 MHz and 42 healthy workers at radio-line stations (aged 28-49 years) who had not been exposed to RFR occupationally. For workers exposed to RFR, they observed a significant lowering of the amplitudes of rhythms of blood pressure and heart rate and a shift of the acrophase to an earlier time. These changes were more pronounced among workers exposed to high intensities of RFR.

9.3.2 Public Exposure Studies

Much concern in the public eye is the claim that RF exposure increases the incidence of some cancers (particularly leukemia and brain tumors) or other health problems. This largely depends on a few studies with a tendency toward developing cancer or other illnesses due to RF exposure.

Radio and Television Transmitters

An association between proximity of residences to TV towers and an increased incidence of childhood leukemia was found in an Australian study conducted by Hocking et al. [57]. The researchers studied the leukemia incidence among people living close to television towers (exposed group) and compared this to the incidence among those living further out from the towers (unexposed or control group). People were assigned to one of the two groups based on data from the New South Wales Cancer Registry and their accompanying address. The Hocking study concluded that there was a 95% increase in childhood leukemia associated with proximity to TV towers. No such association was found between RFR and adult leukemia. The authors specified a number of environmental agents that might explain the association found in the study. One such agent was the RFR emitted by the TV towers. Since these radiation levels were not measured (but calculated), the authors stated no firm conclusion to be drawn until further detailed studies have been completed.

Dolk et al. [58, 59] conducted two studies on the same subject. The first study [58] was conducted around a television tower at Sutton Coldfield in United Kingdom using national cancer incidence rates as the control group. They reported increased risk of adult leukemia within a 2-km radius of the transmitter with a significant decline in risk with distance from the transmitter. The second study [59] was conducted on 20 different TV or FM transmitting towers in order to test the conclusions obtained from Sutton Coldfield. They found no significant excess of adult leukemia within a 2-km radius of the transmitters. However, there was some decline in risk with distance from the transmitters, but this did not replicate the data obtained from Sutton Coldfield and was small in comparison. The researchers concluded that the results give no more than very weak support to the Sutton Coldfield finding. No correlation was seen between the rates of childhood leukemia or brain cancer with distance from the transmitters. Also, the study did not support the findings in Hocking's study.

The study by Hocking et al. [57] was followed by a more detailed replication study by McKenzie et al. [60]. The researchers looked at the same area and at the same time period, but with more accurate estimates of the RF exposure that people received in various areas. They found increased childhood leukemia in one area near the TV antennas, but not in other similar areas near the same TV antennas. They found no significant correlation between RF exposure and the rate of childhood leukemia. They also found that much of the "excess childhood leukemia" reported by the Hocking study occurred before high-power 24-hour

TV broadcasting had started. This study plus the failure to find any effect in the larger U.K. studies [58, 59] dismiss the correlation reported by Hocking.

In Italy, Michelozzi [61] conducted a small area study to investigate a cluster of leukemia near a high-power radio transmitter in a peripheral area of Rome. The leukemia mortality within 3.5 km (5863 inhabitants) was higher than expected. The excess was due to a significant higher mortality among men (7 cases were observed). Also, the results showed a significant decline in risk with distance from the transmitter, only among men.

A Lativian study [62] presented the results of experiments on school children living in the area of the Skrunda Radio Location Station (RLS) in Latvia. Motor function, memory, and attention significantly differed between the exposed and control groups. Children living in front of the RLS had less-developed memory and attention span, their reaction time was slower, and their neuromuscular apparatus endurance was decreased.

Cellular Phones

The presence of an antenna in close vicinity to the user's body, especially the head, subjects the exposed parts to RFR several times more than the average background fields. This exposure has prompted concerns about adverse health outcomes. Epidemiologists are now evaluating the assumption that RF exposure from cellular phones causes brain cancer and other illnesses. Surveys and surveillance programs to monitor the effects of RF exposure to the human head, such as those emitted from mobile phones, have been conducted during the past few years [63-66]. Such surveys are important in classifying phones according to their frequency, power, nature of the signal, and user's holding patterns.

In 1998, Haugsdal et al. [67] carried out a joint Swedish-Norwegian study of cases using both GSM digital and analog mobile phones. A statistically significant association between calling time/number of calls per day and the prevalence of warmth behind/around the ear, headaches, and fatigue was reported. The GSM digital phones were less associated with these symptoms than analog phones. Warmth sensations were also reported lower among GSM users.

A case-control study on brain tumors and use of cellular phones was conducted by Hardell [68]. All cases, both male and female, with histopathologically verified brain tumors living in the Uppsala-Orebro region (1994-1996) and the Stockholm region (1995-1996) aged 20-80 at the time of diagnosis and alive at start of the study were included, 233 in total. Two controls to each case were selected from the Swedish Population Register matched for sex, age, and study region. Exposure was assessed by questionnaires supplemented over the phone. Use of cellular phone gave OR=0.97 for the digital GSM system and OR= 0.94 for the analog NMT system. Nonsignificantly increased risk was found for tumor in the temporal or occipital lobe on the same side as a cellular phone had been used, right side OR=2.45, left side OR=2.40. Increased risk was found only for use of the NMT system. For GSM use, the observation time was too short for definite conclusions.

Muscat [69] conducted a hospital-based case-control study of cellular phone use among 466 brain cancer patients and 422 control subjects. He found no increased risk of brain cancer among phone users and no increased risk related to the self-reported frequency or duration of phone use. There was an elevated risk of a rare nonmalignant tumor among phone users, but no correlation between that increased risk (35 cases) and the time length of phone use.

Regarding exposure from cellular base stations, there have been no significant epidemiological studies of cancer so far.

9.4   INDIVIDUAL CASES

There are many stories that tell of the harmful effects of RFR. One is the case of the U.S. embassy in Moscow. In March 1976, it became public that the embassy was being irradiated with microwaves by the Soviets. U.S. Navy Intelligence technicians during a routine electronic sweep at the embassy first detected irradiation in 1935. By 1963, the State Department concluded that the irradiation was advised and not accidental. Measurement between 1963 and 1975 detected radiation of maximum 0.05 W/m^2 for 9 hours per day at frequencies between 0.5 and 10 GHz. The Department started a classified project to assess the effects of the radiation. Experiments were carried out on laboratory animals using the duplicated low-level embassy signals (around 1 W/cm^2). In November 1975, the U.S. ambassador to Moscow was diagnosed with leukemia. A team of technical consultants was sent to Moscow to assess the situation. They reported that the low-power levels at the embassy had no health effects. The State Department contracted with the Department of Epidemiology at John Hopkins University in June 1976 to examine 1827 staff and their dependants who worked at the embassy for the period 1953-1976. Another group of staff comprising 2561 employees who had worked at other embassies during the same period along with their dependants was taken as controls. The study revealed that the embassy staff suffered no illnesses due the radiation [70].

Isa and Noor [71] presented three cases of exposure to RFR treated in a Malaysian outpatient clinic. The first person had maintained 1-kW TV transmitters during 2-hour sessions in the transmitter room for 11 years, with the transmitter off; during the 12th year, another transmitter was on while he was doing maintenance. The other two cases worked as aerial riggers, installing and maintaining antennas on 400-foot towers for about 10 years with the transmitters off, but did the work during the 11th year with the transmitters on. The three patients displayed symptoms of neck strain, headache, irritability, appetite loss, fatigue, memory difficulties, numbness of extremities, and loss of hair at specific areas of head. Blood and other laboratory tests yielded results within normal ranges, but scalp biopsies confirmed alopecia areata. Steroid injections into the bald areas produced complete hair regrowth. The authors noted that the subjective symptoms were reversible.

There also have been a handful of lawsuits regarding some kind of connection between mobile phone use and adverse health effects. In early 1991, woman named Norma Levitt in Oklahoma had hip surgery and died by a simple blood transfusion when a nurse warmed the blood in a microwave oven! Common sense suggests it does not matter what mode of heating one uses. Blood for transfusions is routinely warmed-but not in microwave ovens. In the case of Mrs. Levitt, the exposure altered the blood, and it killed her.

A case of actual injury was reported from Sandia Corporation. A technician used to hold his hand in front of a microwave beam to feel the heating effect, in order to make sure that the microwave set up was operational. He often looked directly into the beam of around 100 W/cm^2. After one year, he noticed a sudden loss of vision and found he had developed a cataract.

Another lawsuit involved the death of a woman in Florida from a brain tumor. The tumor was located on the area of brain above her ear. The cause was related to her extensive use of a cellular phone. Her husband David Reynard filed a lawsuit in mid-1992. He alleged that the use of a cellular phone had caused his wife's fatal brain cancer. A Federal court dismissed the suit in 1995 due to the lack of evidence [72].

Recently, a Maryland neurologist filed an $800 million lawsuit against Motorola as well as eight other telecommunications companies and organizations, claiming that his use of cell phones caused a malignant brain tumor. Dr. Christopher Newman, 41, said in the lawsuit filed in Baltimore City Circuit Court that his years of using handheld phones led to his brain cancer. The lawsuit accuses the companies of failing to inform consumers that cell phones produce high levels of RFR, which can cause cancer and other illnesses.

REFERENCES

[1] Frey, A. H., Auditory System Response to Radio Frequency Energy, *Aerospace Medicine* 32, pp. 1140-1142, 1961.

[2] Frey, A. H., Human Auditory System Response to Modulated Electromagnetic Energy, *Journal of Applied Physiology* 17, pp. 689-692, 1962.

[3] Frey, A. H., Headaches from Cellular Telephones: Are They Real and What Are the Implications? *Environmental Health Perspectives*, March 1998.

[4] An Observation on the Detection by the Ear of Microwave Signals, *Proceedings of the IRE* 44, 1956.

[5]   Chou, C. K., Effects of Electromagnetic Fields on the Nervous System, Ph.D Dissertation, University of Washington, Seattle, WA, 1975.

[6]   Chou, C. K., R. Galambos, A. W. Guy, and R. H. Lovely, Cochlear Microphonics Generated by Microwave Pulses, *Journal of Microwave Power* 10, pp. 361-367, 1975.

[7]   Chou, C. K., A. W. Guy, and R. Galambos, Microwave-Induced Auditory Response: Cochlear Microphonics Biological Effects of Electromagnetic Waves I, HEW Publication No. FDA 77-8010, pp. 89-103, 1976.

[8]   Chou, C. K., A. W. Guy, and R. Galambos, Microwave-Induced Cochlear Microphonics in Cats, *Journal of Microwave Power* 11, pp. 171-173, 1976.

[9]   Chou, C. K., A. W. Guy, and R. Galambos, Characteristics of Microwave Induced Microphonics, *Radio Science* 12, pp. 221-227, 1977.

[10] Chou, C. K., and A. W. Guy, Carbon-Loaded Teflon Electrodes for Chronic EEG Recordings in Microwave Research, *Journal of Microwave Power* 14, pp. 399-404, 1979.

[11] Chou, C. K., and A. W. Guy, Microwave-Induced Auditory Responses in Guinea Pigs: Relationship of Threshold and Microwave-Pulse Duration, *Radio Science* 14, pp. 193-197, 1979.

[12] Chou, C. K., A. W. Guy, K. R. Foster, R. Galambos, and D. R. Justesen, Holographic Assessment of Microwave Hearing, *Science* 209, pp. 1143-1144, 1980.

[13] Chou, C. K., and A. W. Guy, Auditory Perception of Radio-Frequency Electromagnetic Fields, *Journal Acoustical Society of America*, pp. 1321-1334, 1982.

[14] Kellenyi, L., G. Thuroczy, B. Faludy, and L. Lenard, Effects of Mobile GSM Radiotelephone Exposure on the Auditory Brainstem Response (ABR), *Neurobiology* 7, pp. 79-81, 1999.

[15] Eulitz, C., P. Ullsperger, G. Freude, and T. Elbert, Mobile Phones Modulate Response Patterns of Human Brain Activity, *NeuroReport* 9, pp. 3229-3232, 1998.

[16] Freude, G., P. Ullsperger, S. Eggert, and I. Ruppe, Effects of Microwaves Emitted by Cellular Phones on Human Slow Brain Potentials, *Bioelectromagnetics* 19, pp. 384-387, 1998.

[17] Freude, G., P. Ullsperger, S. Eggert, and I. Ruppe, Microwaves Emitted by Cellular Telephones Affect Human Slow Brain Potentials, *European Journal of Applied Physiology* 81, pp. 18-27, 2000.

[18] Preece, A. W., G. Iwi, A. Davies-Smith, K. Wesnes, S. Butler, E. Lim, and A. Varey, Effect of a 915-MHz Simulated Mobile Phone Signal on Cognitive Function in Man, *International Journal of Radiation Biology* 75, pp. 447-456, 1999.

[19] Preece, A. W., and A. Davies-Smith, The Effect of a 915 MHz Simulated Mobile Phone Transmission on Cognitive Function and Cerebral Blood in Humans, *Annual Bioelectromagnetics Society Meeting*, Long Beach, CA, 1999.

[20] Report on Mobile Phones and Health, Independent Expert Group on Mobile Phones, National Radiation Protection Board, Press Release IEGMP/P11, 2000.

[21] Koivisto, M., A. Revonsuo, C. Krause, C. Haarala, L. Sillanmaki, M. Laine, and H. Hamalainen, Effects of 902 MHz Electromagnetic Field Emitted by Cellular Telephones on Response Times in Humans, *NeuroReport* 11, pp. 413-415, 2000.

[22] Krause, C. M., L. Sillanmaki, M. Koivisto, A. Haggqvist, C. Saarela, A. Revonsuo, M. Laine, and H. Hamalainen, Effects of Electromagnetic Field Emitted by Cellular Phones on the EEG During a Memory Task, *NeuroReport* 11, pp. 761-764, 2000.

[23] Hladky, A., J. Musil, Z. Roth, P. Urban, and V. Blazkova, Acute Effects of Using a Mobile Phone on CNS Functions, *Central European Journal of Public Health* 7, pp. 165-167, 1999.

[24] Hietanen, M., T. Kovala, and A. M. Hamalainen, Human Brain Activity During Exposure to Radiofrequency Fields Emitted by Cellular Phones, *Scandinavian Journal of Work, Environment and Health* 26, pp. 87-92, 2000.

[25] Reports of Headaches Emerge Among Cellular Phone Users, *Microwave News* XVI (6), 10, 1996.

[26] Jauchem, J. R., Exposure to Extremely Low Frequency Electromagnetic Fields and Radiofrequency Radiation: Cardiovascular Effects in Humans, *International Archives of Occupational and Environmental Health* 70, pp. 9-21, 1997.

[27] Braune, S., C. Wrocklage, J. Raczek, T. Gailus, and C. H. Lücking, Resting Blood Pressure Increase during Exposure to a Radiofrequency Electromagnetic Field, *Lancet* 351, pp. 1857-1858, 1998.

[28] Mann, K., J. Roschke, B. Connemann, and H. Beta, No Effects of Pulsed High-Frequency Electromagnetic fields on Heart Rate Variability During Human Sleep, *Neuropsychobiology* 38, pp. 251-256, 1998.

[29] Tuschl, H., G. Neubauer, H. Garn, K. Duftschmid, N. Winker, and H. Brusl, Occupational Exposure to High Frequency Electromagnetic Fields and Its Effect on Human Immune Parameters, *International Archives of Occupational and Environmental Health* 12, pp. 239-251, 1999.

[30] Burch, J. B., J. S. Reif, C. A. Pitrat, T. J. Keele, and M. G. Yost, Cellular Telephone Use and Excreton of a Urinary Melatonin Metabolite (Abs.), *Annual Review of Research on Biological Effects of Electric and Magnetic Fields from the Generation, Delivery and Use of Electricity*, San Diego, CA, 1997.

[31] de Seze, R, J. Ayoub, P. Peray, L. Miro, and Y. Touitou, The Effects of Radiocellular Telephones on the Circadian Patterns of Melatonin Secretion, a Chronobiological Rhythm Marker, *Journal of Pineal Research* 27, pp. 237-242, 1999.

[32] Hirsch, F. B., and J. T. Parker, Bilateral Opacities Occurring in a Technician Operating a Microwave Generator, *American Medical Association Archives of Industrial Hygiene* 6, pp. 512-517, 1952.

[33] Cleary, S. F., and B. S. Pasternack, Lenticular Changes in Microwave Workers: A Statistical Study, *Archives of Environmental Health* 12, pp. 23-29, 1966.

[34] Lin, J. C., Health Aspects of Radio and Microwave Radiation, *Journal of Environmental Pathology and Toxicology* 2, pp. 1413-1432, 1979.

[35] Michaelson, S. M., and J. C. Lin, *Biological Effects and Health Implications of Radio Frequency Radiation*, Plenum Press, New York, NY, 1987.

[36] Daily, L. E., A Clinical Study of the Results of Exposure of Laboratory Personnel to Radar and High Frequency Radio, *U. S. Navy Medical Bulletin* 41, pp. 1052-1056, 1943.

[37] Follis, R. D., Studies on the Biological Effects of High Frequency Radio Waves (Radar), *Journal of Physiology* 147, pp. 281-283, 1946.

[38] Barron, C. I., et al., Physical Evaluation of Personnel Exposed to Microwave Emanations, *Journal of Aviation Medicine* 26, pp. 442-452, 1955.

[39] Robinette, C. D., and C. Silverman, Causes of Health Following Occupational Exposure to Microwave Radiation (Radar) 1950-1974, *Symposium on Biological Effects and Measurement of Radiofrequency/Microwaves* (ed. Hazzard, D. G.), Dept. of Health, Education, and Welfare, HEW Publication No. (FDA) 77-8026, Washington, DC, 1977.

[40] Robinette, C. D., C. Silverman, and S. Jablon, Effects Upon Health of Occupational Exposure to Microwave Radiation, *American Journal of Epidemiology*, 112, pp. 39-53, 1980.

[41] Grayson, J. K., Radiation Exposure, Socioeconomic Status, and Brain Tumor Risk in the US Air Force: A Nested Case-Control Study, *American Journal of Epidemiology* 143, pp. 480-486, 1996.

[42] Weyandt, T. B., S. M. Schrader, T. W. Turner, and S. D. Simon, Semen Analysis of Military Personnel Associated with Military Duty Assignments, *Reproductive Toxicology* 10, pp. 521-528, 1996.

[43] Reeves, G. I., Review of Extensive Workups of 34 Patients Overexposed to Radiofrequency Radiation, *Aviation, Space, and Environmental Medicine* 71, pp. 206-215, 2000.

[44] Szmigielski, S., Cancer Morbidity in Subjects Occupationally Exposed to High Frequency (Radiofrequency and Microwave) Electromagnetic Radiation, *Science Total Environment* 180, pp. 9-17, 1996.

[45] Davis, R. L., and F. K. Mostofi, Cluster of Testicular Cancer in Police Officers Exposed to Hand-Held Radar, *American Journal Industrial Medicine* 24, pp. 231-233, 1993.

[46] Finkelstein, M. M., Cancer Incidence Among Ontario Police Officers, *American Journal of Industrial Medicine* 34, pp. 157-162, 1998.

[47] Milham, S., Jr., Silent Keys: Leukemia Mortality in Amateur Radio Operators, *Lancet* 8432, p. 812, 1985.

[48] Milham, S., Jr., Increased Mortality in Amateur Radio Operators Due to Lymphatic and Hematopoietic Malignnancies, *American Journal of Epidemiology* 127, pp. 50-54, 1988.

[49] Milham, S., Jr., Mortality by License Class in Amateur Radio Operators, *American Journal of Epidemiology* 128, pp. 1175-1176, 1988.

[50] Morgan, R. W., Epidemiologic Analysis of Mortality Among Motorola Employees, Chicago, Illinois, 1993.

[51] Bortkiewicz, A., M. Zmyslony, E. Gadzicka, C. Palczynski, and S. Szmigielski, Ambulatory ECG Monitoring in Workers Exposed to Electromagnetic Fields, *Journal of Medical Engineering and Technology* 21, pp. 41-46, 1997.

[52] Tynes, T., M. Hannevik, A. Andersen, A. I. Vistnes, and T. Haldorsen, Incidence of Breast Cancer in Norwegian Female Radio and Telegraph Operators, *Cancer Causes Control* 7, pp. 197-204, 1996.

[53] Kolmodin-Hedman, B., M. K. Hansson, E. Jonsson, M. C. Andersson, and A. Eriksson, Health Problems Among Operators of Plastic Welding Machines and Exposure to Radiofrequency Electromagnetic Fields, *International Archives of Occupational and Environmental Health* 60, pp. 243-247, 1988.

[54] Bini, M., A. Checcucci, A. Ignesti, L. Millanta, R. Olmi, N. Rubino, and R. Vanni, Exposure of Workers to Intense RF Electric Fields that Peak from Plastic Sealers, *Journal of Microwave Power* 21, pp. 33-40, 1986.

[55] Lagorio, S., S. Rossi, P. Vecchia, M. De Santis, L. Bastianini, M. Fusilli, E. Ferrucci, and P. Comba, Mortality of Plastic-Ware Workers Exposed to Radiofrequencies, *Bioelectromagnetics* 18, pp. 418-421, 1997.

[56] Szmigielski, S., A. Bortkiewicz, E. Gadzicka, M. Zmyslony, and R. Kubacki, Alteration of Diurnal Rhythms of Blood Pressure and Heart Rate to Workers Exposed to Radiofrequency Electromagnetic Fields, *Blood Pressure Monitoring* 3, pp. 323-330, 1998.

[57] Hocking, B., I. Gordon, H. Grain, and G. Hatfield, Cancer Incidence and Mortality and Proximity to TV Towers, *Medical Journal of Australia* 65, pp. 601-605, 1996.

[58] Dolk, H., G. Shaddick, P. Walls, B. Grundy, B. Thakrar, I. Kleinschmidt, and P. Elliot, Cancer Incidence Near Radio and Television Transmitters in Great Britain. Part I: Sutton Coldfield Transmitter, *American Journal of Epidemiology* 145, 1-9, 1997.

[59] Dolk, H., P. Elliot, G. Shaddick, P. Walls, and B. Thakrar, Cancer Incidence Near Radio and Television Transmitters in Great Britain. Part II: All High Power Transmitters, *American Journal of Epidemiology* 145, pp. 10-17, 1997.

[60] McKenzie, D. R., Y. Yin and S. Morrell, Childhood Incidence of Acute lymphoblastic Leukemia and Exposure to Broadcast Radiation in Sydney-A Second Look, *Australia and New Zealand Journal of Public Health* 22, pp. 360-367, 1998.

[61] Michelozzi, P., C. Ancona, D. Fusco, F. Forastiere, and C. A. Perucci, Risk of Leukemia and Residence Near a Radio Transmitter in Italy, *Epidemiology* 9 (Suppl), p. 354, 1998.

[62] Kolodynski, A. A., and V. V. Kolodynska, Motor and Psychological Functions of School Children Living in the Area of the Skrunda Radio Location Station in Latvia, *Science of The Total Environment* 180, pp. 87-93, 1996.

[63] Rothman, K. J., C. K. Chou, R. Morgan, Q. Balzano, A. W. Guy, D. P. Funch, S. Preston-Martin, J. Mandel, R. Steffens, and G. Carlo, Assessment of Cellular Telephone and Other Radio Frequency Exposure for Epidemiologic Research, *Epidemiology* 7, pp. 291-298, 1996.

[64] Rothman, K. J., J. E. Loughlin, D. P. Funch, and N. A. Dreyer, Overall Mortality of Cellular Telephone Customers, *Epidemiology* 7, pp.303-305, 1996.

[65] Funch, D. P., K. J. Rothman, J. Loughlin, and N. A. Dreyer, Utility of Telephone Company Records for Epidemiologic Studies of Cellular Telephones, *Epidemiology* 7, pp. 299-302, 1996.

[66] Dreyer, N. A., J. E. Loughlin, and K. J. Rothman, Epidemiologic Safety Surveillance of Cellular Telephones in the U.S., *Radiation Protection Dosimetry* 83, pp. 159-163, 1999.

[67] Haugsdal, B., E. Hauger, K. H. Mild, G. Oftedal, M. Sandstrom, J. Wilen, and T. Tynes, Comparison of Symptoms Experienced by Users of Analogue and Digital Mobile Phones: A Swedish-Norwegian Epidemiological Study, *Arbetslivsrapport* 23, 1998.

[68] Hardell, L., A. Nasman, A. Pahlson, A. Hallquist, and K. H. Mild, Use of Cellular Telephones and the Risk for Brain Tumours: A Case-Control Study, *International Journal of Oncology* 15, pp. 113-116, 1999.

[69] Muscat, J., Epidemiological Study of Cellular Telephone Use and Malignant Brain Tumors, *WTR Second State of the Science Colloquium*, Long Beach, CA, 1999.

[70] Lilienfield, A. M., J. Tonascia, and C. A. Libaur, Foreign Service Health Status Study: Evaluation of Health Status of Foreign Service and Other Employees from Selected Eastern European Posts, Final Report, U.S. Department of State, Washington D.C., 1978.

[71] Isa, A. R., and M. Noor, Non-Ionizing Radiation Exposure Causing Ill-Health and Alepecia Areata, *Medical Journal of Malaysia* 46, pp. 235-238, 1991.

[72] Foster, K. R., and J. E. Moulder, Are Mobile Phones Safe, *IEEE Spectrum* 37, pp. 23-28, 2000.

10

RF Regulations and Protection Guidelines

10.1 INTRODUCTION

Wireless communication is expanding worldwide. For example, in the last two decades we have witnessed a huge increase in cellular networks; and in the coming years, new personal communication services will become widespread. Wireless technology first started with high-power transmitting equipment during the 1940s and 1950s. Such transmitters were used for radar, the military, and telephony. In the following years, development and application of devices that emit RFR have significantly increased the quality of life throughout the world. Yet, the beneficial aspects have been somewhat overshadowed in recent years by the public's fear of harmful effects. This fear, in turn, has resulted in increased research and a better understanding of EM bioeffects, which ultimately lead to an awareness of safety.

As discussed in Chapter 5, the concept of safety or safety standard needs serious examination. Scientists and regulators have devoted efforts to decide upon safe RFR limits. This is indeed a very complex issue, involving public health, life sciences, engineering, and economic considerations. Currently, there are various safety standards, limits, and protection guidelines established for RF exposure in most of the industrial world, but a comprehensive set of safety standards for all kinds of exposure to all frequency bands of RFR is not practical or probable. Sensible agreement may exist from time to time, which ultimately leads to guidelines as the only realistic answer regarding the health effects associated with RF exposure. However, there are still too many questions related to main parameters such as field strength, duration of exposure, pulse effects, exposure geometry, modulation technique, etc., that require answers in order to define levels at which harmful effects can occur. Therefore, it is not possible to state conclusively that health safety has been established according to the current protection guidelines.

To efficiently protect against risk of harmful effects of RFR, regulatory agencies, in addition to setting safety limits, need to incorporate a "safety margin" to allow for uncertainty. This is contrary to the requirements of a simple technical standard that has to be based on measurable quantities. The question that now faces various standard-setting bodies is how to deal with the uncertainty and weakness of the available knowledge on risk of RFR, and how big the safety margin should be to sufficiently cover possible risks.

Another critical issue refers to an international effort to secure various standard-setting bodies, health agencies, governments, and international organizations to cooperate on safety standard development. It does not certainly mean that the world will have only one accepted standard, but it does mean that the ground for the differences should be known.

The United States, Canada, European Union, Russia, Asia Pacific as well as a few international organizations have all established RF protection guidelines. The reason for the large number of guidelines is the manner in which they are defined, e.g., by frequency, duration of exposure, body mass, and periodicity of exposure. Many guidelines have also been revised downward several times in recent years, but not all scientific bodies agree on this matter.

10.2   REGULATIONS IN THE UNITED STATES

In the United States, various nongovernmental organizations such as the American National Standards Institute (ANSI), the Institute of Electrical and Electronic Engineers (IEEE), and the National Council on Radiation Protection and Measurement (NCRP) have developed RF protection guidelines. Other federal agencies, which have been actively involved in standardization, monitoring, and investigating matters, are the Occupational Safety and Health Administration (OSHA), the National Institute of Occupational Safety and Health (NIOSH), the American Conference of Governmental Industrial Hygienists (ACGIH), the Food and Drug Administration (FDA), the Environmental Protection Agency (EPA), the Federal Communications Commission (FCC), the Department of Defense (DOD), and the National Telecommunications and Information Administration (NTIA) of the Commerce Department.

10.2.1   ANSI/IEEE C95.1

The safety standards most widely used in the Unites States are the ANSI C95.1 guidelines. ANSI is a voluntary standard body, which has served in its capacity as administrator and coordinator of the U.S. private sector voluntary standardization system for more than 80 years. Founded in 1918 by five engineering societies and three government agencies as the American Standard Association (ASA), ASA became the United States of America Standard Institute (USASI) in 1966. By 1974, USASI had become the American National Standards Institute (ANSI). The Institute remains a private, nonprofit membership organization supported by a diverse constituency of private and public sector organizations.

The history of the C95.1 standards goes back to the 1940s and the fear of the safety of military personnel working close to radars during World War II. In 1942, the U.S. Navy directed the Naval Research Laboratory to investigate the possible health effects of RFR. Other military agencies in the United States were also involved within a short period. Early results showed no reason to fear, but proposed that procedures should be put in place to avoid extensive exposure. No guidelines were endorsed. Immediately after the war, very little research was conducted on the bioeffects of RFR. In 1948 and the following years, a few researchers reported the formation of cataracts in dogs and other animals. During the 1950s, researchers reported concerns over other adverse health effects such as leukemia, brain tumors, heart problems, and headaches.

According to the available empirical data, scientists could set a safety factor of 10, basing on an exposure of 0.1 W/cm^2. The above figure took into account an average male weighting 70 kg and having a surface area of 3000 cm^2. Sometime later, Professor Herman Schwan, a pioneer researcher in the field at the University of Pennsylvania, noticed that the absorbing surface of the body is closer to 20,000 cm^2 rather than 3000 cm^2. He figured out that the pure effect of absorbed radiation was twenty times greater than the body could resolve. Therefore, the standard was lowered to 10 mW/cm^2, and this was the base for the C95.1 recommendations of 1966.

The industry was more interested in setting up guidelines for its employees. For example, in 1953, the Central Safety Committee of Bell Telephone Laboratories issued a bulletin that recommended reduction of the power density 100 W/cm^2 to a 30-dB safety margin. This led to a recommendation of 0.1 mW/cm^2. This figure was the first safety standard decided for a human being under RF exposure. In 1954, General Electric recommended a stricter standard by a factor of 100, at 1 mW/cm^2. In 1957, Bell Telephone developed a standard at 1 W/cm^2 for continuous exposure. However, the Bell Telephone standard allows for the higher exposure levels for shorter periods of time. The Bell standard limits were based on certain biological effects (especially cataracts), which may occur at this level. In 1958, General Electric adopted a 10-mW/cm^2 limit. However, the U.S. Air Force (USAF) adopted an upper limit of 10 mW/cm^2 through its first Tri-Service Conference [1] held in 1957.

All of the above safety limits were not intended to be final guidelines, but only the beginning of long-term research and investigation. The intention was to provide some kind of protection until enough data were available to set up solid safety guidelines.

C95.1-1966

The USASI C95.1-1966 Standard [2], "An American National Standard-Safety Levels of Electromagnetic Radiation with Respect to Personnel" was a joint project between the U.S. Department of Navy, IEEE, and ASA (in 1966, ASA became USASI). The applicable frequency range was 10 MHz to 100 GHz, and it fixed a power density limit of 10 mW/cm^2 for the protection of public health and safety. The time-averaging exposure level was allowed only for 6 minutes.

C95.1-1974

The C95.1-1966 was updated in 1974 with only minor changes. The time-average exposure for continuous radiation was removed, admitting time-average exposure only for modulated fields. This was meant, perhaps, to apply to radar, with its known difference in peak and average power levels. The electric and magnetic field limits for the C95.1-1974 standard in the 10-300 MHz frequency range are 200 V/m and 0.5 A/m (both RMS). In the far-field zone, the limits are 300 V/m and 0.8 A/m. This means a power density of 250 W/m^2. The C95.1-1974 recommended a limit of 10 mW/cm^2 for frequencies lower than 10 MHz. Just like the previous standard, C95.1-1974 allowed exposure above the RF exposure limits, provided the average level did not exceed these limits for longer than 6 minutes.

C95.1-1982

Research and investigation continued through the 1970s and resulted in a substantial amendment to the standards in 1982, considering the fact that RF energy absorption in human is frequency dependent. This frequency dependency concept established a defensible metric for exposure, that is the SAR as a common indicator for biological effects.

These standards state that for normal environmental conditions and for incident EM energy from 10 MHz to 100 GHz, the radiation projection guide for both short- and long-term exposure is 10 mW/cm^2 for exposures in excess of 6 minutes, and 100 mW/cm^2 for exposures less than 6 minutes. The C95.1-1982 standard was based entirely on thermal effects.

Table 10-1 The ANSI C95.1-1982 RF Protection Guidelines [3]

Frequency (MHz)	Electric Field (V^2/m^2)	Magnetic Field (A^2/m^2)	Power Density (mW/cm^2)
0.3-3.0	400,000	2.5	100
3.0-30	$4,000 \times (900/f^2)$	$0.025 \times (900/f^2)$	$900/f^2$
30-300	4,000	0.025	1.0
300-1,500	$4,000 \times (f/300)$	$0.025 \times (f/300)$	$f/300$
1,500-100,000	20,000	0.125	5.0

f is the frequency in MHz.

The limit of 10 mW/cm^2 was lowered in 1981 from 10 to 1 mW/cm^2 over the frequency range 30-300 MHz, but still solely on the basis of thermal effects. The peak SAR should not exceed 8 W/kg, and the whole-body average SAR of power deposition should not exceed 0.42 W/kg. This is based on power densities in the frequency range 3 MHz-100 GHz as given in Table 10-1.

In terms of incident power density, the permissible levels are 1 mW/cm^2 at 150 MHz, 1.5 mW/cm^2 at 450 MHz, and 2.75-2.83 mW/cm^2 for frequencies between 824 and 850 MHz (the transmitting frequency band used for mobile cellular transceivers). It is also understood that in most cases of exposure, the field is far from being plane waves. Significant leakage fields are encountered in close proximity of EM sources, which may pose a health risk to equipment operators. Hence, plane wave exposure gives an upper limit of the whole-body SAR as compared to partial body near-field exposure of similar power density.

In 1985, the FCC adopted the ANSI C95.1-1982 protection guidelines for use as the standard that all FCC licensees would need to meet. This was to guarantee all regulated transmitters not expose members of the public and workers to radiation levels in excess of the ANSI C95.1-1982 limits.

C95.1-1992

IEEE, the largest professional institution in the world, published a standard that is used to determine the safety of exposure to RFR [4, 5]. This is also recognized as an ANSI document. It was developed after reviewing a large number of studies on the bioeffects of RF energy. The ANSI/IEEE-C95.1-1992 (originally issued as IEEE-C95.1-1991) maximum permissible exposure (MPE) limits are frequency dependent and time dependent in controlled and uncontrolled environments as shown in Table 10-2.

Table 10-2   ANSI/IEEE C95.1-1992 Maximum Permissible Exposures [4, 5]

Frequency Range (MHz)	Electric Field (E) (V/m)	Magnetic Field (H) (A/m)	Power Density (P) (mW/cm^2)	Averaging Time ($|E|^2$), S (min)
Controlled Environments				
0.003-0.1	614	163	100;1,000,000*	6
0.1-3.0	614	16.3/f	100;10,000/f^2*	6
3-30	1824/f	16.3/f	900/f^2;10,000/f^2	6
30-100	61.4	16.3/f	1.0;10,000/f^2	6
100-300	61.4	0.163	1.0	6
300-3,000	-	-	f/300	6
3,000-15,000	-	-	10	6
15,000-300,000	-	-	10	616,000/$f^{1.2}$
Uncontrolled Environments				
0.003-0.1	614	163	100;1,000,000*	6
0.1-1.34	614	16.3/f	100;10,000/f^2*	6
1.34-3.0	823.8/f	16.3/f	180/f^2;10,000/f^2	f^2/3
3-30	823.8/f	16.3/f	180/f^2;10,000/f^2	30
30-100	27.5	158.3/$f^{1.668}$	0.2;940,000/$f^{3.336}$	30
100-300	27.5	0.0729	0.2	30
300-3,000	-	-	f/1,500	30
3,000-15,000	-	-	f/1,500	90,000/f^2
15,000-300,000	-	-	10	616,000/$f^{1.2}$

f is the frequency in MHz.
* Plane wave equivalent power density, not suitable for near-field region, but useful for comparing them with the power density limits for the higher frequency ranges.

One hundred and twenty-five scientists, engineers, and physicians developed the ANSI/IEEE C95.1-1992 guidelines over a period of nine years with extensive expertise in the area of EM biological effects. These guidelines were approved by IEEE in 1991, and were subsequently adopted by ANSI in 1992 as a replacement for the previous ANSI C95.1-1982. In April 1993, the FCC proposed using the ANSI/IEEE C95.1-1992 for evaluating environmental RF fields created by transmitters it licenses and authorizes.

Table 10-3 ANSI/IEEE C95.1-1992 Maximum Permissible Exposure Limits on Induced and Contact RF Current [4]

Frequency (MHz)	Maximum Current Both Feet (mA)	Maximum Current Each Foot (mA)	Contact
	Controlled Environments		
0.003-0.1	2000 f	1000 f	1000 f
0.1-100	200	100	100
	Uncontrolled Environments		
0.003-0.1	900 f	450 f	450 f
0.1-100	90	45	45

f is the frequency in MHz.

Table 10-2 shows a complex mixture of MPE limits differ not only for controlled and uncontrolled environments but also for electric fields and magnetic fields. In both environments, the exposure values in terms of electric and magnetic field strengths are obtained by spatially averaging values over a plane area equivalent to a vertical cross section of a human body facing a RF source.

The lowest electric field exposure limit occurs at frequencies between 30 and 300 MHz. The lowest magnetic field limit occurs at the range 100-300 MHz. The maximum electric field limit occurs between 30 and 300 MHz at a power density of 1 mW/cm^2 (61.4 V/m) in controlled environments, but at lower level (0.2 mW/cm^2 or 27.5 V/m) in uncontrolled environments. The magnetic field limit drops to 0.163 A/m at 100-300 MHz in controlled environments and 0.0728 A/m in uncontrolled environments. Higher power densities are permitted at frequencies below 30 MHz (below 100 MHz for magnetic fields) and above 300 MHz, assuming that the human body will not be resonant at those frequencies and will therefore absorb less RF energy.

The maximum time-averaged SAR is 8 W/kg for six or more minutes for controlled environments and a corresponding value at 1.6 W/kg for exposure in uncontrolled environments for 30 or more minutes. Higher local SARs are permitted for shorter exposure periods.

The ANSI/IEEE C95.1-1992 guidelines require averaging the power level over time periods ranging from 6 to 30 minutes for power density calculations, depending on the frequency. The exposure limits for uncontrolled environments are lower than those for controlled environments. To compensate for that, the guidelines allow exposure levels in those environments to be averaged over much longer time periods (30 minutes). Time averaging is based on the concept that the human body may bear a greater rate of body heating (that is a higher level of RF energy) for a shorter time than for a longer period. However, time averaging may not be appropriate in considerations of nonthermal effects of RF energy.

Table 10-3 shows the ANSI/IEEE C95.1-1992 guidelines for maximum allowable values of RF current induced within the feet of a person immersed in a RF field, or by physical contact of a person with an electrically charged object, such as a vehicle or fence. The valid range of frequency is 3 kHz to 100 MHz. The guidelines also specify 100 kV/m as the MPE limits on pulsed RFR for controlled environments at the frequency range 0.1 to 300 GHz. For a single pulse of duration less than 100 ms in the above range, the peak MPE is defined as

$$\text{Peak MPE} = \text{MPE} \times \frac{\text{Averaging time (seconds)}}{5 \times \text{Pulse duration}} \qquad (10.1)$$

A maximum of 5 pulses, with a pulse repetition period of at least 100 ms, is allowed during a period of time equivalent to the averaging time. For series of pulses more than 5 or for pulse duration higher than 100 ms, Equation (10.1) will be defined as

$$\sum \text{peak MPE} \times \text{Pulse duration (seconds)} = \text{MPE} \times \frac{\text{Averaging time (seconds)}}{5} \qquad (10.2)$$

Importantly, the subcommittee revising the ANSI/IEEE RF protection guidelines is thinking of a single-tier standard that would apply to all members of the population, whether they are public or workers [6].

10.2.2 The National Council on Radiation Protection and Measurements

The National Council on Radiation Protection and Measurements (NCRP) is a group chartered by the U.S. Congress to develop documentation and recommendations pertaining to the safety of both ionizing and nonionizing radiation. The Council's mission is also to facilitate and stimulate cooperation among organizations concerned with scientific and related aspects of radiation protection and measurements. The standards developed by the NCRP are based on the evaluation of thousands of scientific and medical reports. These reports summarize laboratory and epidemiological studies and serve as the basis for defining the limits of safe exposure to EM radiation for equipment ranging from cellular phones and amateur radio transmitters to radio and TV stations. Because the U.S. Congress created the NCRP, it has been the body to which the EPA has deferred for guidance in this field. The main body of work by the NCRP comprises a series of publications. Three of its reports are related to RFR.

Report No. 67 (1981)

The NCRP Report No. 67 [7], "Radio Frequency Electromagnetic Fields Properties, Quantities and Units, Biophysical Interaction, and Measurements," represents the first result of the NCRP Council's decision to enter the area of nonionizing radiation. The initial objective stemming from that decision was the development of a report on quantities, units, and measurement techniques. Report No. 67 is concerned with the first objective, although the report represents an expansion of efforts to include the material properties and biophysical interactions of RF fields. Inclusion of these subjects permits a unified treatment of background material, which is expected to be useful in the preparation of a subsequent report treating biological bioeffects. Report No. 67 was intended to be an extensive discussion of fundamentals, especially those related to radiation protection. Also, it developed a perspective for those quantities and units that are needed to relate, quantitatively, certain biological effects to particular exposures.

Report No. 86 (1986)

The NCRP Report No. 86 [8], "Biological Effects and Exposure Criteria for Radio Frequency Electromagnetic Fields," is considered the NCRP standard to which a reference is sometimes made. The report presents the results of an extensive evaluation of the available literature on the biological effects of RF fields. This report starts with a discussion of studies at the molecular level and continues to a larger scale of interaction, covering macromolecular and cellular effects, chromosomal and mutagenic effects, and carcinogenic effects.

Report No. 86 treats effects such as those related to reproduction, growth and development, hematopoesis and immunology, endocrinology and autonomic nerve function, cardiovascular and cerebrovascular effects, and interaction of EM fields with the CNS. Table 10-4 shows the limits recommended by the Report No. 86. The NCRP recommendations are also based on a maximum, time-averaged, localized SAR of 8 W/kg for occupational exposure and one-fifth of the occupational level, i.e., 1.6 W/kg, for the general public. The fivefold safety factor was based on the assumption that the general public is exposed continuously (168 hours per week) compared with 40 hours in the week for occupational environments. The ratio is approximately 5.

Table 10-4 NCRP Report No. 86 (1986) RF Protection Guidelines

Frequency Range (MHz)	Electric Field (V/m)	Magnetic Field (A/m)	Power Density (mW/cm^2)	Contact Current (mA)
Occupational Exposure				
0.3-1.34	614	1.63	100	200
1.34-3.0	614	1.63	100	200
3.0-30	1824/f	4.89/f	900/f^2	200
100-300	61.4	0.163	1.0	-
300-1,500	3.54$\sqrt{f}$	$\sqrt{f}$/106	f/300	-
1,500-100,000	194	0.515	5.0	-
General Population				
0.3-1.34	614	1.63	100	200
1.34-3.0	823.8/f	2.19/f	180/f^2	200
3.0-30	823.8/f	2.19/f	180/f^2	200
100-300	27.5	0.0729	0.2	-
300-1,500	2.59$\sqrt{f}$	$\sqrt{f}$/238	f/1500	-
1,500-100,000	106	0.23	1.0	-

Report No. 119 (1993)

The NCRP Report No. 119 [9], "A Practical Guide to the Determination of Human Exposure to Radiofrequency Fields," was designed as a guide to people who are responsible for the assessment of RF exposure with less knowledge of principles and practices of the subject. This report provides broad information on various RF sources and guidelines for estimating the associated exposures. Major sections of Report No. 119 include: concepts and definitions of terms and units, procedures for evaluation of RF exposures, instruments and measurement techniques, and recommended areas for further research and development.

Comparing the ANSI/IEEE and NCRP power density limits, one of the few differences is that the NCRP limits are more restrictive at higher frequencies (above the 1.5 GHz, for example). Accordingly, the industry generally supports the ANSI/IEEE limits, while the public generally favors the NCRP limits.

Table 10-5 ACGIH Threshold Limit Values

Frequency	Electric Field (V^2/m^2)	Magnetic Field (A^2/m^2)	Power Density (mW/cm^2)
10 kHz-3 MHz	377,000	2.65	100
3 -30 MHz	$3,770 \times 900/f^2$	$900/37.7\,f^2$	$900/f^2$
30-100 MHz	3,770	0.027	1
100-1 GHz	$3,770 \times f/300$	$f/37.7 \times 100$	$f/100$
1-300 GHz	37,700	0.265	10

10.2.3 The American Conference of Governmental Industrial Hygienists

In 1983, the American Conference of Governmental Industrial Hygienists (ACGIH) published new threshold limit values (TLVs) for RF exposure [10]. The TLVs confine human absorption to SAR of 0.4 W/kg or less averaged over any 6-minute period. The TLVs cover the frequency range from 10 kHz to 300 GHz. The ACGIH limits are established as safety guidelines for the workplace. They are intended for use in the practice of industrial hygiene and should be applied only by a person trained in this practice. Table 10-5 shows the ACGIH TVLs.

Because the TLVs are applied in occupational environments, they are based on the assumption that no children (or small humans) should be in the workplace. This hypothesis allows an average incident power density of 10 mW/cm² at frequencies higher than 1 GHz, while maintaining the same 0.4-W/kg whole-body absorption limits. The arbitrary 100-mW/cm² cap applied in the frequency range from 10 kHz to 3 MHz appears to be safe on the basis of whole-body SAR. But RFR intensities of 100 mW/cm² may result in shocks or burns under certain conditions. The 100-mW/cm² limit should not restrict many operations but serves as a reminder that at this level potentially significant shock and burn problems may occur. The ACGIH TLVs provide procedures to minimize operational constraints while maintaining personnel safety.

10.2.4 The Department of Defense

The Department of Defense (DOD), as the world's largest user of RFR, is concerned about the safety aspects of a large number of emitters and devices ranging from cellular phones to more complicated apparatuses. The DOD wants to be sure that there are no harmful effects on either its own personnel or the general public at large.

Over the past few decades, the DOD has conducted research and investigation on the areas of human exposure to RFR. The guidelines are promulgated by those agencies based on the DOD instruction DODI 6055.11 [11]. Among the standards is the Air Force Occupational Safety and Health (AFOSH) Standard 48-9, Radio Frequency Radiation (RFR) Safety Program, 1997 [12]. In fact, the AFOSH guidelines are similar to the ANSI/IEEE C95.1-1992 guidelines.

10.2.5 The Environmental Protection Agency

The Environmental Protection Agency (EPA) is an independent federal agency established in 1970. The mission of the EPA is to protect human health and to safeguard the natural environment. The EPA's Office of Radiation Program (ORP) has studied the subject of EM bioeffects since 1972. A number of reviews, including studies on both ELF fields and RFR, have been conducted. In addition, the EPA has reviewed various clinical, epidemiological, and toxicological studies of *in vivo* and *in vitro* systems exposed in the near- and far-field regions. In 1984, the EPA was poised to fix a limit that would have been 10 times tighter than the ANSI C95.1-1982 in the body resonance range (0.1 mW/cm^2 instead of 1 mW/cm^2). But the EPA's Office of Policy, Planning, and Evaluation (OPPE) expressed concern regarding the failure of ORP to enumerate any adverse health effect in humans. As a result, the EPA decided not to adopt that limit at all.

Instead, the EPA developed a list of options published as a report by Elder and Cahill [13] in 1984. The EPA report was conducted to offer guidelines for protection of the public. The review of RFR bioeffects concluded that maximum heating occurs at resonant frequencies. It was reported that SARs in the range of 1 to 4 W/kg for short periods of exposure (1 hour) produce a significant increase in body temperature at an ambient temperature of 25 to 30°C. No biological effects at the molecular or subcellular level other than those associated with temperature increase were observed. Laboratory animals were found affected by SARs in the range of 10 to 30 W/kg, even for short period of exposures.

In June 1990, the EPA drafted the report entitled, "An Evaluation of the Potential Carcinogenicity of Electromagnetic Fields." The report reviewed research work published through mid-1989, covering the frequency range from 3 Hz to 30 GHz (including ELF fields and RFR). The evaluation of the findings ranged from neutral to negative, with indication for a need to assess the information from ongoing studies and to further evaluate the mechanisms of carcinogenic action and the characteristics of exposure that lead to these effects. This report was released only in draft form and then was withdrawn under some kind of controversy. A rewrite of the 1990 EPA report was completed, and progressed through several steps of scientific and administrative review, but has not been released to the public to date.

In 1995, the EPA fixed its purpose to issue guidelines for RF exposure, based entirely on thermal effects, for the general public. However, the EPA abandoned the idea due to lack of information about the long-term effects of RF exposure.

Finally, the EPA supported the FCC RF exposure guidelines issued in August 1996 as providing sufficient protection of public health. This recent view of the EPA finds that the current FCC guidelines sufficiently protect the public from all scientifically established effects that may result from RFR. This is despite the fact that the FCC guidelines categorically take into account thermal effects of RF energy, but do not directly address postulated nonthermal effects.

10.2.6   The Food and Drug Administration

The Food and Drug Administration (FDA) was founded in 1927. In 1968, the Radiation Control for Health and Safety Act authorized the FDA to develop standards for emission of radiation from electronic products. Accordingly, the Center for Devices and Radiological Health (CDRH) of the FDA had established a performance standard for microwave ovens that limits the amount of radiation leaking from the oven. Separate standards for maximum leakage from microwave ovens went into effect on October 6, 1971. Under these standards, radiation leakage from microwave ovens cannot exceed 1 mW/cm^2 measured 5 cm away from the oven prior to factory release, and 5 mW/cm^2 thereafter. This FDA limit is far below the level known to harm people and it provides a large margin of safety. The measuring equipment to be used is also specified in the standard. Before the standard for microwave ovens went into effect, the industry had operated with voluntary standard of 10 mW/cm^2 [14].

The FDA belongs to an interagency working group of the federal agencies that have responsibility for different aspects of mobile phone safety to ensure a coordinated effort at the federal level. These agencies are NIOSH, EPA, FCC, OHSA, and NTIA. Accordingly, the FDA participated in establishing standards for devices such as cellular phones. The FDA's particular engagement with cellular phones began in early 1993 through the CDRH. That was when the issue of brain cancer and its possible association with cellular phone use was raised via a nationally televised interview with a man who attributed his wife's death from brain cancer to her frequent use of a cellular phone [see Section 9.4 for details]. In early 1993, the CDRH requested several meetings with industry to discuss the inadequacy of the data that exists with which to evaluate claims of health risks such as cancer. At the meetings, the CDRH presented the need for reliable research, proper labeling, and possible redesigns to address issues related to potential effects from RF energy emitted by handheld cellular phones. Industry groups represented at the meeting were manufacturers and distributors of cellular phones, communications firms, and related trade associations. In response to the industry request for federal agencies playing a role in directing essential research, the CDRH offered to explore the possibility of working under a cooperative research and development agreement. But the Cellular Telecommunications Industry Association (CTIA) finally rejected this agreement and the role of the CDRH in the industry program became advisory only [15].

10.2.7 The National Institute for Occupational Safety and Health

The Occupational Safety and Health Act of 1970 established the National Institute for Occupational Safety and Health (NIOSH). NIOSH is part of the Centers for Disease Control and Prevention (CDC) and is the only federal institute responsible for conducting research and making recommendations for the prevention of work-related illnesses and injuries. NIOSH was established to conduct research and support education of occupational health professionals. It is involved in issues related to occupational exposure to both chemical and physical agents. Also, NIOSH conducts research and health-hazard assessment related to occupational RF exposure. NIOSH conducted an extensive review and evaluation of the biological effects of RFR covering the period up to 1982. The document was not released to the public. The aim was to develop occupational RF exposure guidelines, but those guidelines have never been issued.

10.2.8 The Occupational Safety and Health Administration

The Occupational Safety and Health Administration (OSHA) is part of the U.S. Department of Labor. The mission of OSHA is to save lives, prevent injuries, and protect the health of America's workers. Sometimes, OSHA staff inspects RF transmitting facilities, such as broadcast stations, for failure to conform to OSHA regulations related to access to areas where high RF fields exist.

In 1971, OSHA issued a federal protection guide for workers (29 CFR 1910.97) limiting occupational exposures to RFR. The guide covers the frequency range 10 MHz to 100 GHz was based on the C95.1-1966 protection guideline. It was established as a limit for occupational environments with a maximum power density of 10 mW/cm^2, as averaged over any possible 6-minute period [16]. In the far fields, a power density of 10 mW/cm^2 is equivalent to mean squared electric field strength of 40,000 V^2/m^2 or a mean squared magnetic field strength of 0.25 A^2/m^2.

In 1976, OSHA's regulation was ruled to be advisory and not mandatory. In

1982, OSHA proposed to repeal the regulation, but after deliberating the issue, it decided in 1984 to retain it. Currently, actions related to exposure of workers are carried out using OSHA's "general duty clause," which depends largely on the use of voluntary consensus standards [17]. Personnel of OSHA usually use the ANSI/IEEE C95.1-1992 guidelines as criteria for safe exposure levels [18].

10.2.9 The Federal Communications Commission

In the United States, the Communications Act of 1934 established the Federal Communications Commission (FCC) as a regulatory agency, which regulates the radio and all wire communications. Since the FCC is responsible for licensing and regulating most of the communication systems in the United States, it has been directly involved in ensuring safety of communication technology use.

Since 1985, the FCC has determined the potential for human exposure to RF energy from FCC-regulated transmitters as a potential environmental effect that needs evaluation [19]. In its original order, the FCC specified that it would use the ANSI C95.1-1982 guidelines as a rule for RFR analysis [20].

The FCC practiced its rule to indicate which transmitters are of great concerns. High-powered radio and TV transmitters and satellite uplink equipment were categorized as utilities, which require environmental evaluation. Meanwhile, low-powered transmitters such as mobile and cellular radio were excluded from undergoing environmental evaluation [21]. This policy was justified due to the lack of evidence that such transmitters are in excess of the ANSI C95.1-1982 guidelines because of their low operating power.

In 1993, the FCC responded to developments in the area of RF standards by proposing to rewrite its safety rules in Docket 93-62. The FCC issued a proposal to adopt the ANSI/IEEE C95.1-1992 guidelines [22].

In 1996, the FCC was set to enforce RF safety levels. Although it has acknowledged that it is not a public health agency, the FCC adopted a set of RF guidelines that regulates cellular radiation levels, FCC 96-326.

The FCC's action also fulfilled requirements of the Telecommunication Act of 1996 for adopting new guidelines. The FCC examined comments submitted by NIOSH, OSHA, the FDA, and the EPA. In addition, the FCC considered comments received from the government, the industry, and the public.

In August 1996, the FCC adopted the NCRP's recommended limits for transmitters operating at frequency range of 300 kHz to 100 GHz. Also, the commission adopted SAR limits for devices operating within close proximity to the body as specified in the ANSI/IEEE C95.1-1992 guidelines. Both the ANSI/IEEE and NCRP guidelines are based on a determination that potentially harmful bioeffects can occur at a SAR level of 4 W/kg as averaged over the entire

Table 10-6 FCC Limits for Maximum Permissible Exposure Limits [23]

Frequency Range (MHz)	Electric Field (E) (V/m)	Magnetic Field (H) (A/m)	Power Density (P) (mW/cm²)	Averaging Time ($|E|^2$), P, ($|E|^2$) (min)
Occupational/Controlled Environment				
0.3-3.0	614	1.63/f	100*	6
3-30	1824/f	4.89/f	(900/f^2)*	6
30-300	61.4	0.163	1.0	6
300-1,500	-	-	f/300	6
1,500-100,000	-	-	5.0	6
General Population/Uncontrolled Environment				
0.3-1.34	614	1.63	100*	30
1.34-30	824/f	2.19/f	(180/f^2)*	30
30-300	27.5	0.073	0.2	30
300-1,500	-	-	f/1500	30
1,500-100,000	-	-	1.0	30

f is frequency in MHz
* Plane wave equivalent power density.

body. Safety factors of 10 and 50 respectively, were applied to arrive at limits for whole-body exposure (0.4 W/kg for controlled or occupational exposure and 0.08 W/kg for uncontrolled or general population exposure, respectively), and localized exposure SAR limits (8 W/kg for controlled environments and 1.6 W/kg for uncontrolled environments) [23].

Table 10-6 shows the FCC whole-body limits, while Table 10-7 shows the FCC SAR limits for localized (partial-body) exposure in the frequency range 100 kHz to 6 GHz. The FCC guidelines are specified in terms of MPE limits. They are given in terms of electric field, magnetic field, and power density. For multiple-frequency exposure, the fraction of MPE limits produced by each frequency is determined and these fractions must not exceed unity (100 percent).

The most notable change in the FCC order from the previous standards is that cellular phones must now comply with SAR exposure limits of 1.6 W/kg. Previously, cellular phones could exceed MPE limits if their radiated power was less than $1.4 \times 450/f$, where f is the operating frequency in MHz. For most of the cellular phones, this is approximately 0.6 W of radiated power.

Table 10-7 FCC SAR Limits for Localized Exposure in the Range 100 kHz-6 GHz [23]

Occupational/Controlled Exposure	General/Uncontrolled Exposure
< 0.4 W/kg whole body ≤ 8 W/kg partial body	< 0.08 W/kg whole body ≤ 1.6 W/kg partial body

The deadline for compliance to the MPE limits was September 1, 2000, for all FCC-regulated transmitters and licensed sites. Compliance can be required even earlier for any site where a license is to be renewed. If a license at an existing site needs to be renewed, then all of the transmitters and licenses at that site need to come into compliance at the same time. Compliance to the FCC MPE limits is legally enforceable. Noncompliance can lead to FCC license suspension and possible penalties. FCC's enforcement authority is limited only to licensed sites and operators and does not apply to nonlicensed operators, such as site owners, roofers, tower painters, or air conditioning repairmen.

10.3 REGULATIONS IN CANADA

The Canadian Ministry of Health has taken up various safety codes for protection of Canadian citizens. These codes specify the requirements of a safe use of RF devices that operate in the frequency range 3 kHz to 300 GHz. In 1979, the Bureau of Radiation and Medical Devices of the Ministry adopted the first Safety Code 6, setting limits for human RF exposure. Safety Code 6 (EHD-TR-160) was also published in 1991 and reprinted in 1994 as 93-EHD-160.

In 1999, a new version of Safety Code 6 was published (99-EHD-237) [24]. The RF limits specified in the code are based on a review of the scientific research conducted over the past 30 years on EM bioeffects. Table 10-8 shows Safety Code 6 exposure limits for occupationally exposed persons and the general public. According to the code, a worker or member of the public shall not be exposed to EM levels exceeding the values listed in Table 10-8.

Table 10-9 shows Safety Code 6 SAR limits for occupationally exposed persons and the general public. SAR limits should be determined for cases where exposure takes place at 0.2 meters or less. For conditions where SAR determination is impractical, field strength or power density shall be carried out.

Safety Code 6 also, fixed the limits for induced and contact currents in order to reduce the potential for RF shocks or burns. The limits for both occupationally exposed persons and general public are given in Table 10-10.

Table 10-8   Exposure Limits for Safety Code 6 [24]

Frequency Range (MHz)	Electric Field (RMS) (V/m)	Magnetic Field (RMS) (A/m)	Power Density (W/m²)	Averaging Time (min)
		Exposed Workers		
0.003-1	600	4.9	-	6
1-10	600/f	4.9/f	-	6
10-30	60	4.9/f	-	6
30-300	60	0.163	10*	6
300-1,500	3.54 $f^{0.5}$	0.0094 $f^{0.5}$	f/30	6
1,500-15,000	137	0.364	50	6
15,000-150,000	137	0.364	50	616,000/$f^{1.2}$
15,000-300,000	0.354$f^{0.5}$	9.4×10⁻⁴ $f^{0.5}$	3.33×10⁻⁴ $f^{0.5}$	616,000/$f^{1.2}$
		General Public		
0.003-1	280	2.19	-	6
1-10	280/f	2.19/f	-	6
10-30	28	2.19/f	-	6
30-300	28	0.037	2*	6
300-1,500	1.585 $f^{0.5}$	0.0042 $f^{0.5}$	f/150	6
1,500-15,000	61.4	0.163	10	6
15,000-150,000	61.4	0.163	10	616,000/$f^{1.2}$
15,000-300,000	0.1584 $f^{0.5}$	4.21×10⁻⁴ $f^{0.5}$	6.67×10⁻⁵ f	616,000/$f^{1.2}$

f is the frequency in MHz.
A magnetic field strength of 1 A/m corresponds to 1.257 μT or 12.57 mG.
* Power density level is applicable at frequencies greater than 100 MHz.

The RF exposure guidelines for public in Safety Code 6 are based on the thermal effects. They are based on studies that have demonstrated tolerance of power densities at various radio frequencies before the body's temperature is increased by 1°C within 30 minutes of exposure. A protection factor of 10 has been applied to these power densities to arrive at the levels fixed for occupational environments. This protection factor compensates for the variation in physical activity such as temperature and humidity. For the safety of public, a safety factor of 5 has been implemented (for a total of 50) to extrapolate from occupational to

Table 10-9   SAR Limits for Safety Code 6 [24]

Condition	SAR (W/kg)
Occupationally Exposed Persons	
SAR averaged over the whole body mass	0.4
Local SAR for head, neck and trunk, averaged over one gram of tissue	8
SAR in limbs, as averaged over 10 g of tissue	20
General Public	
SAR averaged over whole body mass	0.08
Local SAR for head, neck and trunk, averaged over one gram of tissue	1.6
SAR in the limbs, as averaged over 10 g of tissue	4

The tissue is defined in the shape of cube.

Table 10-10   Induced and Contact Current Limits for Safety Code 6 [24]

Frequency (MHz)	Induced Current (RMS) (mA) Through Both Feet	Each Foot	Contact Current (RMS) (mA) Hand Grip and Through Each Foot	Averaging Time
Occupationally Exposed Persons				
0.003-0.1	$2000\,f$	$1000\,f$	$1000\,f$	1 s
0.1-110	200	100	100	6 min
General Public				
0.003-0.1	$900\,f$	$450\,f$	$450\,f$	1 s
0.1-110	90	45	45	6 min

f is the frequency in MHz.

public exposure levels. However, it is common practice to apply two factors, 4.2, and 10. The protection factor of 4.2 is applied to extrapolate from occupational to public environments to account for the longer exposure that can be experienced by the public. The protection factor of 10 is applied to members of society, such as children, pregnant women, and the aged, who may be more sensitive to health effects associated with chemical and physical agents.

Basically, Safety Code 6 is based on the assumption that there are no nonthermal effects even though a number of studies suggest that a few biological effects do occur at lower levels of exposure. It is also based on short-term health effects even though several long-term animal studies at lower levels of exposure have demonstrated adverse health effects such as behavioral changes and increased cancer rates. Moreover, Safety Code 6 is based on a threshold for irreversible effects rather than on a "no adverse effect level" that is normally given preference when developing environmental health standards.

10.4 REGULATIONS IN EUROPE

There is a large number of RF guidelines, limits, and ranges of tolerance established in most of Europe. An underlying reason for this is due to differences in philosophy in standard-setting approach of various countries in the continent.

10.4.1 The European Union

On 8th June 1999, the European Union (EU) Health Council agreed on a recommendation, with the support of the U.K. government, for limiting EM exposure, thereby establishing, for the first time, EU-wide EM safety standards, especially for mobile phone emissions. The recommendation was based on exposure limits recommended by the ICNIRP [25]. The recommendation proposes limiting public exposure to a SAR of 0.2 W per 10 g of tissue for the head, and 0.08 W/kg for the whole body (one-fifth of the exposure permitted by the NRPB), but permissible occupational exposure would remain at the level defined by the NRPB [26].

10.4.2 The Commission of the European Communities

The Commission of the European Communities has proposed limits of exposure in the workplace for nonionizing radiation through its Directorate General (DG) V (Health and Safety). The proposed limits for electric and magnetic fields are intended as a European Council directive on the minimum safety and health requirements regarding exposure of workers to the risk arising from physical agents. DG XIII of the European Communities (Directorate General Telecommunications Information Industry Innovation) has mandated the 18-country European Committee for Electromechanical Standardization (CENELEC), to prepare an exposure standard for the protection of people against EM fields. CENELEC Technical Committee TC111, "Human Exposure to Electromagnetic Fields" and its subcommittees are carrying out the work.

In 1994, CENELEC issued a draft standard (Prestandard No. 2). The standard uses specific reference levels for exposures of unlimited duration. The CENELEC TC211 working group WGMTE has submitted the document, "Considerations for Evaluation of Human Exposure to Electromagnetic Fields (EMFs) from Mobile Telecommunication Equipment (MTE) in the Frequency Range 30 MHz-6 GHz," as a European specification [27]. The CENELEC pre-standard places a SAR of 2 W/kg as a limit for the public.

10.4.3 Regulations in EU Member States

RF Exposure has become a subject of great interest, and even has developed into a national issue in many European countries. In these countries, critical incidents were reported, supported by few scientific reports, and backed by citizens' groups and nongovernmental organizations (NGOs). The focus of the controversy is on cellular base stations and handheld cellular phones.

Austria

In 1985, Austria released the standard ÖVE MW-ÖVE-HG 335, Teil 2 [2500] [28]. However, another standard ON-ÖNORM S1120, "Microwave and Radiofrequency Electromagnetic Fields-Permissible Limits of Exposure for the Protection of Persons in the Frequency Range 30 kHz to 3000 GHz," replaced the previous standard in 1992.

Belgium

Recently, the Belgium government has voted for exposure limits of 21 V/m for 900 MHz and 29 V/m for 1800 MHz.

Finland

The Finnish Centre for Radiation and Nuclear Safety is a public agency and expert organization committed to prevent and limit the harmful effects of radiation. It acts under the direction of the Ministry of Social Affairs and Health in respect of issues governed by the Health Protection Act. Research carried out by the Centre yields information related to the use and effects of ionizing and nonionizing radiation. In 1991, the Centre released the document entitled, "FIN SG 9.2-Radiation Safety of Pulsed Radar." In 1992, another document was released, "FIN SG 9.3-Radiation Safety on Mastworks at FM/TV Stations."

Germany

Until 1978, there was a prevailing 10-mW/cm^2 limit for RF protection adopted by the German Association of Radar and Navigation [29]. In 1978, the German Electrotechnical Commission (VDE) published the first draft of the standard, revising it in 1984 as VDE-DIN 57 848 VDE 0848 Part 2, "Hazards by Electromagnetic fields, Protection of Persons in the Frequency Range from 10 kHz to 300 GHz." In 1991, the draft was revised again, and designated DIN-VDE 0848 Part 2, "Safety in Electromagnetic Fields, Protection of Persons in the Frequency Range from 30 kHz to 300 GHz."

Italy

The Italian standard [30] was published in 1998, in which Italy introduced "cautionary" limits that are as low as one-hundredth of the international guidelines. At mobile phone frequencies the standard is 0.10 mW/cm^2. For situations where exposure is expected to exceed 4 hours/day, the limit is further reduced to 0.010 mW/cm^2. Local regional administrations to be more definite have the authority to further reduce these limits, and several regions appear to have limits 4 times lower (0.0025 mW/cm^2). For example, the limit for mobile phone towers and broadcast is 6 V/m or 10 µW/cm²; for other RF/MW exposures is 100 µW/cm² in the frequency range 3 MHz to 3 GHz; and it is 400 µW/cm² in the frequency range 3 GHz to 300 GHz.

The Netherlands

The electromagnetic health issue was not regarded as a major problem in The Netherlands. So far, no mandatory limits for nonionizing radiation exposure exist. Several different government ministries including Environment and Housing, Health Council, and Social Affairs and Employment are involved in this matter. The question of limiting exposure was dealt with under a framework act involving these ministries but with no specific limits for the general public. The Health Council of the Netherlands, which is a national advisory body, was addressing the EM health aspects. The Council issued a report on 50-Hz fields in 1992, which called for a reevaluation of research on health effects after five years. In 1995, a brochure (without a limit) was released. Recently, the Health Council again has issued a report concluding that only acute exposures to EM fields present a known health risk. The government will probably make either the Council's or ICNIRP's limits legally binding [31].

Sweden

In Sweden, RF protection regulations have been applicable since 1976. The current regulations are called ASF 1987:2, which are issued by the National Board of Occupational Safety and Health.

In 1995, the European Standard was established as the Swedish Standard SS-ENV 50 166-2. This standard includes recommendations about occupational and general public environments. The permitted power density level for the general public, at 900 MHz, is 4.5 W/m^2 or 41 V/m for the electric field strength. The permitted levels for occupational environments are five times higher than the general public environments [32].

Switzerland

The Swiss standard was published in 1999 [33]. Accordingly, Switzerland instituted similarly low RF exposure limits for "sensitive-use areas" (such as residential areas, schools, and hospital wards) and banned new construction in areas in which the precautionary limits are exceeded. For wireless transmitters above 6 W (ERP) the limit is 4 V/m (0.0042 mW/cm^2) at 900 MHz, and 6 V/m (0.0095 mW/cm^2) at 1800 MHz. For broadcast radio and TV transmitters, the exposure limit is between 3 to 8.5 V/m (0.0024 to 0.019 mW/cm^2). Higher values are for long and middle waves. The Swiss limits were based on the lowest levels that were economically expected and technically achievable. They do not apply to industrial and medical equipment, or even cellular phones.

United Kingdom

In 1960, the limit 10 mW/cm^2 was fixed for exposure of continuous radiation, regardless of frequency. This was a kind of first standard adopted by the U.K. Post Office and published as, "Safety Precautions Relating to Intense Radiofrequency Radiation."

In 1989, the National Radiological Protection Board (NRPB) released the guidelines NRPB-GS11. The guidelines were for electric shock and heating effects only, and did not attempt to address low-level (nonthermal) effects. The NRPB set 0.4 W/kg as its basic restriction and then established field investigation levels for electric fields, magnetic fields, and currents.

The most recent guidance was issued in 1993 [34] after an extensive consultation exercise. The NRPB advice has been accepted and supported by government departments as an effective basis for protection standard in the U.K. for EM fields. The NRPB enforced the current guideline, "Restrictions on Exposure to Static and Time-varying Electromagnetic Fields." This is a set of established guidelines within which the mobile phone operators are bound to operate. The levels set by the NRPB are not limits, as such, but investigation levels. In several cases, the NRPB levels are more restrictive than the ANSI/IEEE C95.1-1992 limits, although both are based on the SAR level of 0.4 W/kg.

Averaging times for NRPB-93 are 15 minutes for whole-body exposure and 6 minutes for partial-body exposure. Currently, the U.K. RFR limits are 112 V/m and 0.57 mW/cm^2 at 900 MHz, and 194 V/m and 1 mW/cm^2 at 1800 MHz.

In Scotland, new BTSs may be subject to tighter controls. The Scottish Environment Ministry is planning to publish proposals that recommend "common sense regulations." A consultation for new regulations is also underway in England, where tightening up of planning controls is expected, especially after the publication of the U.K.'s IEGMP (Stewart) report on mobile phone safety in May 2000 [see 13.7.3 for details].

10.4.4 Eastern Europe and Russia

The work done in Eastern Europe and Russia, however, indicated that effects on the CNS were taking place at nonthermal levels below 10 mW/cm^2. As a result of their work, Russians, in 1958, set their standard level for continuous exposure three orders of magnitude lower (10 W/cm^2) than that set later by the ANSI. Western researchers criticized the Soviet research on the grounds that they lacked adequate reporting of methodology and data.

The exposure guidelines of the Soviet Union before its transformation into a confederation of independent republics are shown in Table 10-11 and Table 10-12 [35]. For the frequencies range 300 MHz-300 GHz, a maximum power density limit of 1 mW/cm^2 was fixed for occupational environments. For the same frequency range, a power density limit of 0.01 mW/cm^2 was fixed for general population. No magnetic field limits were specified for the general population.

Sanitary Rules by the State Commission of Sanitary and Epidemiological Supervision of Russia became effective on May 8, 1996, as mandatory for all government and public enterprises [40]. For occupational exposure [Table 10-13], MPE levels are determined by a so-called "maximum exposure energy (MEE)." In the frequency range 30 kHz-300 MHz, MEE is defined as a product

Table 10-11   USSR Occupational Standard [35]

Frequency (MHz)	Electric Field (V/m)	Magnetic Field (A/m)
0.06-1.5	50	5
1.5-3	50	
3-30	20	
30-50	5	
300-300,000	0.125	

Table 10-12   USSR General Population Standard [35]

Frequency (MHz)	Electric Field (V/m)
0.03-0.3	25
0.3-3	15
3-30	10
30-300	3

Table 10-13   Russian MPE Limits for Occupational Environments [36]

Frequency (MHz)	Electric Field (V^2/m^2)	Magnetic Field (A^2/m^2)
0.03-3	20,000	200
3-30	7,000	
30-50	800	0.72
50-300	800	
300 MHz-300 GHz	200 µW/cm²	

Table 10-14 Russian MPE Limits for General Population Environments [36]

Frequency	Electric Field (V/m)
30 kHz-300 kHz	25
300 kHz-3 MHz	15
3 MHz-30 MHz	10
30 MHz-300 MHz	3
300 MHz-300 GHz 10 μW/cm^2	

of the square of the electric or magnetic field strength (in V/m or A/m), and the duration of exposure in hours per day. For the 300 MHz-300 GHz range, MEE is defined as a product of the incident power density (in μW/cm^2) and the duration of exposure in hours per day. The MPE limits are calculated by dividing the MEE in the frequency ranges by the number of exposure hours per day.

According to the above exposure limits in the frequency range 300 MHz-300 GHz, the MPE limit for 10 hours of exposure per day is 200/10=20 μW/cm^2. However for 0.2 hour exposure per day, it is 200/0.2=1000 μW/cm^2. If the exposure duration is less than 0.2 hour per day in the frequency range 300 MHz-300 GHz or less than 0.08 hour per day in the 30 kHz-300 MHz range, no further MPE limit increase is required.

For the general population, MPE limits, which are not dependent on the exposure duration, are shown in Table 10-14. In addition to above MPE limits, there are certain exceptions. For example, the MPE limits for the following TV broadcasting frequencies are:

48.4 MHz	5 V/m
88.4 MHz	4 V/m
192 MHz	3 V/m
300 MHz	2.5 V/m

The MPE limits for beam-scanning radar in the frequency range 150-300 MHz are 10 μW/cm^2 in the near-field region, and 100 μW/cm^2 in the far-field region. Also specified in the Russian limits are safety limits for various home appliances and for people living near cellular base stations or users of cellular phones. The Republic of Byelorussia as well as the Russian Federation adopted the limits.

10.5 REGULATIONS IN ASIA PACIFIC

There is increasing research on the bioeffects of RFR in Asia Pacific region. The various nations in the region address RF standard issues seriously. Japan, Australia, and New Zealand are the countries where major regulatory activities to limit human RF exposure have been carried out. Also, other countries like China and Korea have recently increased their activity in the area of EM bioeffects research. Committees have been formed to review research, compare international standards, and make recommendations.

10.5.1 Japan

The Japanese guidelines for EM fields were established under the auspices of Ministry of Posts and Telecommunications (MPT). In 1990, the MPT issued the guideline (TTC/MPT) for human RF exposure, which is similar to the ANSI/IEEE C95.1-1992 standard [37]. The guideline is divided into two parts: the *fundamental guide* and the *administrative guide*. The fundamental guide deals with biological-related quantities such as SAR and induced currents. SAR limits are 0.4 W/kg averaged over any 6 minutes with regard to the whole body and 8 W/kg with regard to the maximum local SAR within 1g tissues except extremities and skin, where SAR limit is 25 W/kg for any 1g tissues.

The two-tier administrative guide provides quantities related to EM environments such as electric and magnetic fields. It is constituted of condition P and condition G. Condition P is related to controlled environments and condition G to uncontrolled environments in the ANSI/IEEE standard. Primarily, there are no real differences between the exposure limits in the administrative guide and the ANSI/IEEE standard, except the exclusion clause for low-power devices. The administrative guide excludes low-power devices with nominal power 7 W or less at frequencies lower than or equal to 3 GHz for both P and G conditions [38].

10.5.2 China

With increasing use of RF devices such as cellular phones, China is increasingly interested in the issue of RF standards. However, there is limited information about the research and RF regulatory activities in China. The only available source of information is the few papers published by the Chinese researchers in conference proceedings and journals. However, the public exposure limits recognized currently in China are much stricter than those in the United States: 5.0 V/m or 6.6 $\mu W/cm^2$ at 900 MHz [33].

10.5.3   Australia/New Zealand

The Standards Association of Australia takes the responsibility of fixing RF exposure standards in Australia, while the responsibility in New Zealand goes to Standards New Zealand.

In 1985, Australia developed its first standard for limiting exposure to RF fields. This standard was reaffirmed in Australia in 1990 and adopted by New Zealand in the same year. In the following years, the Australian standard [39], "AS/NZS 2772.1 RF Fields Part 1: Maximum Exposure Levels-3 kHz to 300 GHz," has provided the basis for standards and practices to limit public and occupational exposure to RFR. Over this period, there were a number of attempts to update the standard taking into account the new scientific findings.

Amid argument and increasing public concern over the possibility of adverse health effects of RF sources, Standards Australia has published a joint revision with Standards New Zealand of the existing Standard (AS 2772.1). The revised Standard is "AS/NZS 2772.1 (Int): 1998 Radiofrequency Fields Part 1: Maximum Exposure Levels -3 kHz to 300 GHz." This standard specifies limits on public exposure to RFR. Due to the high level of public interest in the subject, the new edition has been released as an interim standard. This left the content open to public comment and debate for a period of 12 months.

The level at which these limits are set is much lower than the level at which any thermal (heating) effect can occur. The standard specifies limits of exposure of all or part of the human body to EM fields in the range 100 kHz-300 GHz. In this standard, the allowable general public exposure limit for the frequencies used by mobile phone services is 0.2 mW/cm^2; this is a factor of 2–6 lower than the ANSI/IEEE, ICNIRP, and NCRP standards. This standard is kept under revision, and the allowable general public exposure limits in the new draft appear to be 0.45 mW/cm^2 at 900 MHz and 0.90 mW/cm^2 at 1800 MHz.

The New Zealand standard NZS6609 [40] published as the Australian standard AS 2772.1-1990 divides exposure levels into occupational and nonoccupational. It further subdivides the occupational exposure limits into Condition A where the possibility for RF shock and burns exist and Condition B where the possibility for RF shock and burns has been eliminated [41, 42]. The cities of Auckland and Christchurch have adopted a 50 μW/cm^2 exposure limit, which is stricter than the 200 μW/cm^2 guideline New Zealand adopted in 1990.

Although the standard, AS/NZS 2772.1(Int): 1998, expired at the end of April 1999, it remains the basis of the Australian Communications Authority (ACA) for its proposed health exposure framework. Representatives of the telecommunications carriers, unions, and the community have agreed in principle to the proposal by the ACA to develop a dual approach for the regulation of RFR. However, implementation of this proposal may require participation by other standard-making bodies in the process.

After abandoning the joint Australian/NZ standards, New Zealand has adopted the ICNIRP standard but included a precautionary policy that was based on common practice. The final result was the standard, "NZS 2772.1:1999 Radiofrequency Fields Part 1: Maximum Exposure Levels-3 kHz to 300 GHz." It complies adequately with the ICNIRP limits [25] excluding the reduced exposure levels at higher frequencies that were part of the earlier standards.

The ministries of Health and Environment considered the limits to provide adequate protection but recommended minimizing, as appropriate, RF exposure which is insignificant or incidental to achievement of service objectives or process requirements, provided that this can be readily achieved at modest expense. They also asked the industry to reduce community concern through nonregulatory approaches. These two approaches contrast sharply; in one case, by setting compulsory exposure limits for precautionary reasons and, in the other, by supplementing international limits with precautionary policies aimed at improving the public acceptability of new RF transmitters. The latter is clearly more consistent with traditional approaches to setting exposure limits and is easier to apply in a consistent way to the diverse sources of RF energy in modern society. However, none of these precautionary approaches were based on any newly identified hazard from low-level exposures.

10.6 INTERNATIONAL REGULATORY ACTIVITIES

10.6.1 The International Radiation Protection Association

The International Radiation Protection Association (IRPA) is a worldwide organization, which was initiated in 1964. The primary purpose of IRPA is to provide a medium whereby those engaged in radiation protection activities in all countries may communicate more readily with each other.

The International Nonionizing Radiation Committee (INIRC) as an independent scientific commission established by IRPA approved interim guidelines on limits of RF exposure in the range 100 kHz-300 GHz. The INIRC worked with other bodies to promote safety and standardization in the field of RFR. They have suggested in 1981 that power densities not exceeding 10 mW/cm^2 could be allowed for occupational exposure continuously throughout a working day. The general population limits were lower.

In 1984, IRPA issued more specific recommendations, based on a threshold of 0.4 W/kg for continuous RF exposure. The recommendations were revised in 1988 [43] as shown in Table 10-15. The derived limits are extremely conservative in the frequency range 10-30 MHz. For occupational environments,

Table 10-15 IRPA Exposure Limits [43]

Frequency Range (MHz)	Electric Field (V/m)	Magnetic Field (A/m)	Power Density (mW/cm^2)
Occupational			
0.1-1	194	0.51	10
>1-10	$194/f^{1/2}$	$0.51/f\,f^{1/2}$	$10/f$
>10-30	61	0.16	1
>400-2,000	$3 \times f^{1/2}$	$0.008 \times f^{1/2}$	$f/400$
>2,000-300,000	137	0.36	5
General Public			
0.1-1	87	0.23	2
>1-10	$87/f^{1/2}$	$0.23/f^{1/2}$	$2/f$
>10-30	27.5	0.73	0.2
>400-2,000	$1.375 \times f^{1/2}$	$0.0037 \times f^{1/2}$	$f/2,000$
>2,000-300,000	61	0.16	1

the IRPA limits are frequencies greater than 10 MHz, 0.4 W/kg, when averaged over any 6 minutes and over the whole body, or 4 W/kg when averaged over any 6 minutes and any 1 g of tissue. For the general public, IRPA exposure limit is 5 times lower, i.e., 0.08 W/kg when averaged over any 6 minutes over the whole body or 0.8 W/kg when averaged over any 6 minutes and any 1 g of tissue.

10.6.2 The International Commission on Non-Ionizing Radiation Protection

In 1992, the International Commission on Non-ionizing Radiation Protection (ICNIRP) was chartered as the successor to IRPA/INIRC. The ICNIRP's mission is to coordinate knowledge of protection against various nonionizing exposures in order to develop internationally accepted recommendations.

In April 1998, the ICNIRP published guidelines [see Table 10-16] for limiting RF exposure in the frequency range up to 300 GHz. The development of the guidelines was based on reviews of a large body of studies.

Table 10-16 ICNIRP Protection Guidelines [25]

Frequency Range	E-field Strength (V/m)	H-field Strength (A/m)	B-field (µT)	Power Density (W/m²)
Occupational Exposure				
Up to 1		1.63×10^5	2×10^5	
1-8 Hz	20,000	$1.63 \times 10^5/f^2$	$2 \times 10^5 /f^2$	
8-25 Hz	20,000	$2 \times 10^4/f$	$2.5 \times 10^4/f$	
25-820 Hz	$500/f$	$20/f$	$25/f$	
820 Hz-65 kHz	610	24.4	30.7	
65 kHz-1 MHz	610	$1.6/f$	$2/f$	
1-10 MHz	610/f	$1.6/f$	$2/f$	
10-400 MHz	61	0.16	0.2	10
400 MHz-2 GHz	$3f^{0.5}$	$0.008f^{0.5}$	$0.01f^{0.5}$	$f/40$
2-300 GHz	137	0.36	0.45	50
General Public				
Up to 1		3.2×10^4	4×10^4	
1-8 Hz	10,000	$3.2 \times 10^4/f^2$	$4 \times 10^4/f^2$	
8-25 Hz	10,000	$4000/f$	$5000/f$	
25-800 Hz	$250/f$	$4/f$	$5/f$	
800 Hz-3 kHz	$250/f$	5	6.25	
3-150 kHz	87	5	6.25	
150 kHz-1MHz	87	$0.73/f$	$0.92/f$	
1-10 MHz	$87/f^{0.5}$	$0.73/f$	$0.92/f$	
10-400 MHz	28	0.073	0.092	2
400-2000 MHz	$1.375^{f0.5}$	$0.0037f^{0.5}$	$0.0046f^{0.5}$	$f/200$
2-300 GHz	61	0.16	0.2	10

The ICNIRP guidelines include a reduction factor of five in maximum SAR for the general public as opposed to occupational environments. The reason for this approach was the possibility that some members of the general public might be exceptionally sensitive to RFR. However, no detailed scientific evidence to justify this additional safety factor was provided. The basic restriction for occupational exposure to electric and magnetic fields with frequencies up to 1 kHz is 10 mA/m² and above that it is frequency dependent. The value of 10

mA/m^2 was chosen as less than one-tenth of the value of the current density above. This is the same value recommended by NRPB in the U.K.

For exposures received by general public, a reduction factor of five is applied, resulting in a basic restriction of 2 mA/m^2. In its clarification, the ICNIRP notes that compliance with this basic restriction may permit higher current densities in body tissues other than the CNS under the same exposure conditions.

The basic restriction for occupational exposure to EM fields with frequencies between 100 kHz and 10 GHz is 0.4 W/kg for whole-body SAR. Again, this is the same as the value recommended by the NRPB. For the general public, the reduction factor of five, results in a basic restriction on whole-body SAR of 0.08 W/kg. The factor of five reductions also applies to the basic restriction on localized SAR (head and trunk). The values for those occupationally exposed and for the general public being 10 W/kg and 2 W/kg respectively averaged over any 10-g tissue. However localized SAR values at limbs for those occupationally exposed and for the general public are 20 W/kg and 4 W/kg, respectively.

In 1999, the ICNIRP guidelines for the public have been incorporated in a European Council Recommendation, which has been agreed in principle by all countries in the EU, including the U.K.

REFERENCES

[1] Pattishal, E. G., (ed.), *Proceedings of the 1st Annual Tri-Service Conference on Biological Hazards of Microwave Radiation*, 1957.
[2] American National Standard-Safety Levels of Electromagnetic Radiation with Respect to Personnel, ANSI C95.1-1966, Institute of Electrical and Electronics Engineers, New York, NY, 1966.
[3] American National Standard Safety Levels with Respect to Human Exposure to Radio Frequency Electromagnetic Fields, 300 kHz to 100 GHz, ANSI C95.1-1982, American National Standards Institute, New York, NY, 1982.
[4] IEEE Standard for Safety Levels with Respect to Human Exposure to Radio Frequency Electromagnetic Fields, 3 kHz to 300 GHz, ANSI/IEEE C95.1-1992 (Revision of ANSI C95.1-1982), Institute of Electrical and Electronics Engineers, Piscataway, NJ, 1992.
[5] IEEE Standard for Safety Levels with Respect to Human Exposure to Radio Frequency Electromagnetic Fields, 3 kHz to 300 GHz, ANSI/IEEE C95.1-1999 Edition (Incorporating IEEE Std C95.1-1991 and IEEE Std C95.1a-1998), Institute of Electrical and Electronics Engineers, Piscataway, NJ, 1999.
[6] ANSI/IEEE Group Favors a Single RF/MW Safety Standard, *Microwaves News* XX No. 3, pp. 6-7, 2000.
[7] Radio frequency Electromagnetic Fields Properties, Quantities and Units, Biophysical Interaction, and Measurements, NCRP Report No. 67, NCRP, Bethesda, MD, 1967.
[8] Biological Effects and Exposure Criteria for Radio Frequency Electromagnetic

Fields-Recommendations of the National Council on Radiation Protection and Measurements, National Council on Radiation Protection and Measurements, NCRP Report No. 86, NCRP, Bethesda, MD, 1986.

[9] A Practical Guide to the Determination of Human Exposure to Radiofrequency Fields, National Council on Radiation Protection and Measurements, NCRP Report No. 119, pp. 171-174 & 186-188, Bethesda, MD, 1993.

[10] Threshold Limit Values for Chemical Substances and Physical Agents in the Work Environment with Intended Changes for 1983-1984, American Conference of Governmental Industrial Hygienists (ACGIH), Cincinnati, Ohio, 1983.

[11] DODI 6055.11-Protection of DOD Personnel from Exposure to Radiofrequency Radiation and Military Exempt Lasers, DOD, 1995.

[12] Radio Frequency Radiation (RFR) Safety Program, *Air Force Occupational Safety and Health Standard* 48-9, 1997.

[13] Elder, J. A., and D. F. Cahill, (eds.), Biological Effects of Radiofrequency Radiation, EPA Report No. EPA-600/8-83-026F, U.S. Environmental Protection Agency, Research Triangle Park, NC, 1984.

[14] Microwave Oven Radiation, Publication No. 79-8058, FDA, Reissued 1982.

[15] Letter to Congress from the Food and Drug Administration in Response to Questions Regarding Alleged Health Hazards Associated with the Use of Cellular Phones, FDA, 1997.

[16] Occupational Safety and Health Administration: OSHA Safety and Health Standards, 29 CFR 1910.97, OSHA 2206, Revised, U.S. Department of Labor, Washington, D.C., 1978.

[17] Cleveland, R. F, and J. L. Ulcek, Questions and Answers About Biological Effects and Potential Hazards of Radiofrequency Electromagnetic Fields, FCC OET Bulletin 56, Fourth Edition, 1999.

[18] Curtis, R. A., Elements of a Comprehensive RF Protection Program: Role of RF Measurements, OSHA Health Response Team, *National Association of Broadcasters Engineering Conference*, Las Vegas, Nevada, 1995.

[19] Report and Order, Gen. Docket 79-144, 100 FCC 2d 543, and Memorandum Opinion and Order, FCC, 50 Federal Register 38653, 1985.

[20] Cleveland, R. F., Regulatory Activities in the U.S.A., In *Mobile Communications Safety* (eds. Kuster, N., Q. Balzano, and J. C. Lin), Chapman & Hall, London, UK, 1997.

[21] Second Report and Order, Gen. Docket 79-144, FCC Record 2064 and FCC Record 2526, FCC, 1987.

[22] Guidelines for Evaluating the Environmental Effects of Radiofrequency Radiation, Notice of Proposed Rule Making, ET Docket 93-62, 8 FCC Record 2849, 58 Federal Register 1993.

[23] Cleveland, R. F., D. M. Sylvar, and J. L. Ulcek, Evaluating Compliance with FCC Guidelines for Human Exposure to Radiofrequency Electromagnetic Fields, *OET Bulletin* 65, Edition 97-01, August 1997.

[24] Limits of Human Exposure to Radiofrequency Electromagnetic Fields in the Frequency Range from 3 kHz to 300 GHz, Safety Code 6, Environmental Health Directorate, Health Protection Branch, Health Canada, Canada, 1999.

[25] ICNIRP Guidelines for Limiting Exposure to Time Varying Electric, Magnetic and

Electromagnetic Fields (Up to 300GHz), *Health Physics* 74 (4), pp. 494-522, 1998.

[26] Board Statement: Advice on the 1998 ICNIRP Guidelines for Limiting Exposure to Time-Varying Electric, Magnetic and Electromagnetic Fields (Up to 300 GHz), Documents of the NRPB 10(2), NRPB, 1999.

[27] Proposal for Council Directive on the Minimum Health and Safety Requirements Regarding the Exposure of Workers to the Risks Arising from Physical Agents, COM (92) 560 Final (Luxembourg: Office for Official Publications of the European Communities), CB-CO-92-626-EN-C, CEC, 1992.

[28] Bogers, M., Regulatory Environment in the E.U., In *Mobile Communications Safety* (eds. Kuster, N., Q. Balzano, and J. C. Lin), Chapman & Hall, London, UK, 1997.

[29] Hammett, W. F., *Radio Frequency Radiation: Issues and Standards*, McGraw Hill, New York, NY, 1997.

[30] Regulations for Determination of the Threshold of Radio Frequency Compatibility with Human Health, p. 381, Ministry of Environmental Health, Italy, 1998.

[31] Dutch Advisory Panel Limits Still in Line with ICNIRP, *Microwave News* XX No. 3, p. 3, 2000.

[32] Regulation About Protection Against Nonionizing Radiation, Swiss Federal Council, Switzerland, 1999.

[33] The Swedish Association for the ElectroSensitive, FEB, Internet Document at http://www.feb.se/, 2000.

[34] Board Statement on Restrictions on Human Exposure to Static and Time Varying Electromagnetic Fields and Radiation, Documents of the NPRB 4(5), NRPB, Chilton, Didcot, Oxon, UK, 1993.

[35] Czerski, P., Radiofrequency Radiation Exposure Limits in Eastern Europe, *Journal of Microwave Power and EM Energy* 20, pp. 233-239, 1985.

[36] Heynick, L. N., Radiofrequency Electromagnetic Fields (RFEMF) and Cancer: A Comprehensive Review of the Literature Pertinent to Air Force Operations, Air Force Research Laboratory, 1998.

[37] Amemiya, Y., Researches on Biological and Electromagnetic Environment in RF and Microwave Regions in Japan, *IEICE Transactions* E77-B, pp. 693-698, 1994.

[38] Massao, T., and M. H. Repacholi, Regulatory Environment in the EU, In *Mobile Communications Safety* (eds. Kuster, N., Q. Balzano, and J. C. Lin), Chapman & Hall, London, UK, 1997.

[39] Radiofrequency Radiation-Part 1: Maximum Exposure Levels-100 kHz to 300 GHz, Standards Australia AS2772.1-1990, 1990.

[40] New Zealand Standard NZS6609: Part 1: Maximum Exposure Levels-100 kHz to 300 GHz, Australian Standard AS 2772.1, 1990.

[41] New Zealand Standard NZS6609-NZS 9901.1:1990: Part 1: Radiofrequency Radiation-Part 1: Maximum Exposure Levels-100 kHz to 300 GHz, Australian Standard AS 2772.1, 1990.

[42] New Zealand's History of Public Participation on Environment Issues Extends to Siting of Phone Towers, *Electromagnetics Forum* 1, 1996.

[43] IRPA Guidelines on Limits of Exposure to Radio Frequency Electromagnetic Fields in the Frequency Range from 100 kHz to 300 GHz, *Health Physics* 54, pp. 115-123, 1988.

11

Incident Field Dosimetry

11.1 INTRODUCTION

Dosimetry consists of two parts [1]. The first part involves the evaluation of *incident* fields, which are produced by certain source(s). These fields are either measured (with no object present) or calculated from the information of the source. Second is the evaluation of *internal* fields inside an object, which are also either measured or calculated. The first part of dosimetry is the one considered in this chapter.

Engineering contributions in the field of EM bioeffects have made it possible to evaluate the field strength or power density due to exposure from an EM source and check its compliance with protection guidelines. It should be noted that it is not always possible to evaluate the levels of RFR in and around areas of concern. This is due to the fact that RF fields are absorbed, reflected, or refracted by the surrounding objects in a random way. Theoretical calculations are adequate in some situations; but measurements often prove more conclusive and less expensive, particularly at multiple-source sites. Therefore, theoretical calculations are not enough to assess the exposure in certain region. For this reason, RF measurements are usually performed to assure compliance with relevant standards in order to prevent overexposure conditions that may pose short- and long-term health problems. Measurements also are needed when the calculated fields are close to the threshold for overexposure or when fields are likely to be distorted by reflection from various objects.

11.2   RFR MODELING

Modeling means theoretical calculation of RF fields at various points from a source. With basic data, the field strength can be estimated before the start of actual measurement. In order to apply modeling, it is necessary to understand the characteristics of the radiating antenna. In general, it is possible to calculate the probable power density near the antenna using simple equations. But such calculations have many drawbacks. Most of the situations in which the power density would be high enough to be of concern are in the near-field region of the antenna, where the average power density varies inversely with the distance from the antenna. This is an area approximately bounded by several wavelengths of the antenna in which the spatial characteristics of RF fields are very complex. The average power density within the near-field region varies inversely with the distance from the antenna.

Further away from the antenna we reach the far-field region, where the beam has developed and propagates in a behaved manner. The power density decreases inversely with the square of distance from the antenna. Far field calculation of signal strength is the normal approach for estimating signal strength at the RF receiver. The power density decreases much faster in the far field than the near field. There is a distance from the antenna were the field strength of near field and far field is equal or intersects. The point of intersection, which is the boundary for the two regions, is called the *crossover point*. The near- and far-field regions are shown in Figure 11-1.

Calculation methods discussed in this chapter are helpful in evaluating certain exposure situations. Equations given may be used for predicting field strength and power density in the vicinity of most sources.

11.2.1   Power Density

Power density calculation could be the best exercise for RF predictions. Primarily, the formula to calculate the power density is generated from the following simple form [2-10]:

$$\text{Power density} = \frac{\text{Radiated power}}{\text{Area impacted by the source}}$$

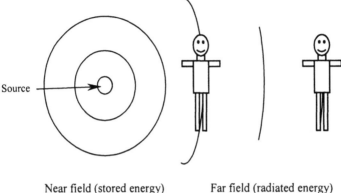

Near field (stored energy)   Far field (radiated energy)

Figure 11-1 Near- and far-field regions.

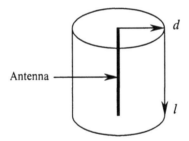

Figure 11-2 Near-field region of a vertical antenna.

Near-Field Region

The power density in the near field of a vertical antenna [Figure 11-2] is calculated using the cylinder shape (circular radiation pattern and the height of the antenna). The area of a cylinder placed around this antenna is assumed to be uniformly filled by the power radiated from the antenna. No RF power is emanated from the top or bottom. This power density is almost the same as the average power density a person of a certain height would be exposed to when standing very close to the antenna. The following formula is referred to as the *cylindrical model* since it utilizes a cylinder appearance for the modeling:

$$P_d = \frac{P_t}{2\pi dl} \qquad\qquad (11.1)$$

Where P_d is the power density on the surface in watts per square meter (W/m^2), P_t

is the power input to the antenna in watts (W), d is the distance to the center of radiation of the antenna in meters (m), and l is the length of the antenna in meters (m).

Far-Field Region

In the far-field region, the radiation pattern does not change with distance from the antenna. The maximum radiating power density becomes related to the gain of the antenna. For an isotropic point source, the power density is the distribution of power over a sphere having a radius equal to the distance from the antenna. It is defined as

$$P_d = \frac{P_t}{4\pi d^2} \tag{11.2}$$

For a directional antenna, the power density of Equation (11.2) will be defined as

$$P_d = \frac{P_t G_t}{4\pi d^2} \tag{11.3}$$

where G_t is the gain ratio of the transmitting antenna based on an isotropic radiator. Figure 11-3 shows the relation between transmitted and received power in a wireless communication system.

Usually, the term EIRP (equivalent isotropic radiated power) can be used in the nominator of Equation (11.3). EIRP can also be expressed in antilogarithm (watts) and decibel expressions (dBW), respectively

$$EIRP = P_t G_t \tag{11.4}$$

$$[EIRP] = [P_t] + [G_t] \tag{11.5}$$

EIRP is an important concept to show the capabilities of RF transmission. It is significant to note that G_t is usually numeric gain. Therefore, when the gain is expressed in logarithmic term (dB), a conversion is needed according to the following relation

$$G = 10^{dB/10} \tag{11.6}$$

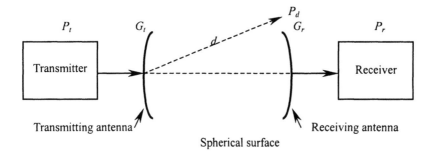

Figure 11-3 Transmitted and received power in a wireless communication system.

The power, sometimes, is expressed in terms of effective radiated power (ERP) instead of EIRP. ERP is power referred to a half-wave dipole antenna instead of to an isotropic radiator. It is needed, therefore, to convert ERP into EIRP in order to be able to use it in Equation (11.3). EIRP can be obtained by multiplying ERP by the factor 1.64, which is the gain of a half-wave dipole relative to the isotropic radiator. Equation (11.3) can then be rewritten as

$$P_d = \frac{\text{EIRP}}{4\pi d^2} = \frac{1.64\text{ERP}}{4\pi d^2} \tag{11.7}$$

While predicting the field near a surface, such as at the ground level or on the rooftop, double reflection of incoming radiation may be assumed, resulting in a fourfold increase in far-field equivalent power density. In such case, Equation (11.3) and Equation (11.7) are modified to

$$P_d = \frac{4P_tG_t}{4\pi d^2} = \frac{P_tG_t}{\pi d^2} = \frac{\text{EIRP}}{\pi d^2} \tag{11.8}$$

In the case of FM radio and television broadcast antennas, the U.S. Environmental Protection Agency (EPA) has developed models for predicting ground level field strength and power density [11]. An approximation for ground reflection is made by assuming a maximum 1.6- fold increases in field strength resulting in an increase of power density of 2.56 (1.6 × 1.6). Equation (11.7) may then be modified to:

$$P_d = 2.56\frac{\text{EIRP}}{4\pi d^2} = 1.05\frac{\text{ERP}}{\pi d^2} \tag{11.9}$$

If the power density P_d is given in units of $\mu W/cm^2$ instead of mW/cm^2, then Equation (11.9) can be written as

$$P_d = 33.4 \frac{\text{ERP}}{d^2}$$
(11.10)

While considering the received power P_r by a receiving antenna, which has a gain G_r, additional parameters should be considered. This is defined as

$$P_r = P_t G_t G_r \left(\frac{\lambda}{4\pi r}\right)^2$$
(11.11)

where λ is the wavelength of the signal in meters (m). Equation (11.11) includes power loss from the spreading of the transmitted wave but does not include other losses such as atmospheric absorption or ohmic losses of the coaxial or waveguide leading the energy to the antenna.

Considering all ohmic losses (L) and expressing Equation (11.11) in terms of decibels, we get

$$P_r = 20\log\left(\frac{\lambda}{4\pi r}\right) + P_t + G_t + G_r - L$$
(11.12)

The term $20\log\left(\frac{\lambda}{4\pi r}\right)$ refers to free-space loss in dB.

11.2.2 Field Strength

The field strength at the receiving antenna is related to the received power P_r by considering the fact that the received power is the antenna effective aperture area multiplied by the power density. In receiver sensitivity measurements, the field strength E as RMS quantity is considered rather than the peak amplitude, which is common in EM analysis. The electric field strength E, in volts per meter (V/m), is defined as

$$E = \sqrt{\frac{P_r \eta_0}{A_e}}$$
(11.13)

where η_0 is the intrinsic impedance of free space (377 Ω), and A_e is the antenna effective aperture area in square meters (m²).

In the far-field region, the electric and magnetic fields are interrelated with each other as

$$\frac{E}{H} = \eta_o \qquad (11.14)$$

where H is the magnetic field strength, in amperes per meter (A/m). The RMS electric field E at a distance d from a source with EIRP on the main beam axis is defined as

$$E = \frac{(30\text{EIRP})^{0.5}}{d} \qquad (11.15)$$

11.2.3 Computer Modeling

Various modeling software packages are available that allow a theoretical study of site situations. The software creates maps of the area showing the RF levels. Calculations may use different methods, standards, and antenna heights for evaluation.

Computer modeling programs are suitable for estimating RF electric and magnetic fields around antenna systems, and yet, these too have limitations. Ground interactions must be considered in estimating near-field power densities. Computer modeling is not sophisticated enough to predict hot spots in the near-field region where the field intensity is far higher than would be expected. These hot spots are often found near wiring in the shack and metal objects such as antenna masts or equipment cabinets. Professional measuring instruments often can detect intensely elevated but localized fields. However, even with the best instrumentation, these measurements may also be misleading in the near fields. Taking precise measurements or modeling the exact antenna system is not needed but there is a need for some data to develop an idea of the relative fields around the source. Computer modeling using approximations of the geometry and power input of the antenna will generally suffice.

11.3 MEASUREMENT TECHNIQUES

The first step in the process of measurement is to classify the area under investigation either as occupational/controlled or public/uncontrolled. Such distinction is necessary before measurements are carried out, so that, exposure levels are used for evaluation and comparison.

11.3.1 Instrumentation

There are a few necessary steps for the accurate assessment of RFR. First, the source and exposure situation must be characterized so that the most accurate measurement technique and instrumentation can be selected. Second, the correct use of this instrumentation requires knowledge of the quantity to be measured and the limitations of the instrument used. Third, knowledge of a relevant exposure standard is needed.

Unlike ELF fields, determining the power density of RFR is not a simple task. Although sophisticated instruments are used to measure RF power densities quite accurately, they are costly and require frequent recalibration. The public does not have access to such equipment, and the inexpensive field strength meters that we do have are not suitable for measuring RF power density. Therefore, the best way to estimate RF power density is to depend on the results of computer modeling techniques.

Still, it is not possible to rely on a single measurement technique or instrumentation setting to obtain reliable measurements over the entire RF frequency range. Suitable meters should also be made available with variety of probes for electric and magnetic field measurements. Commercially available meters give indications of RFR in several possible units like mW/cm^2 (power density), V^2/m^2 or A^2/m^2 (field strength square) and V/m or A/m (field strength). In this case, ability to convert from unit to unit according to suitability of the standard is necessary. Also, a spectrum analyzer may make a number of measurements almost simultaneously and may display the individual signals at the same time. Narrowband meters may also be used to some extent to measure the field strength across a wide range of frequencies. Such measurements can be cumbersome, requiring frequent readjustment of the receiving antenna and frequent recalibration.

A broadband meter can be used to assess a large site. Broadband meters used in RF measurements respond to either the electric or magnetic field component of the EM field. When making near-field measurements, it is necessary to consider both the electric and magnetic components. While it is possible to calculate the power density in mW/cm^2 or W/m^2, the calculation is based on assumptions that do not hold true in the near-field region. However, most safety measurements performed at frequencies less than 300 MHz are made in the near-field region.

At low frequencies (below approximately 30 MHz), measurement of only one field component could lead to conclusions as to compliance with the RF protection guidelines. Accordingly, below 30 MHz, both electric and magnetic fields shall be determined to evaluate compliance of exposure fields with the guidelines. Between 30 and 300 MHz, it may be possible through analyses to show that measurement of only one of the two fields is sufficient to determine compliance with the guidelines.

In general, all instruments used for RF measurement have basic components [5, 6]: a probe or antenna, a detector, a cable, electronic conditioning circuitry, a display device, and an external data collection device. Figure 11-4 shows basic components of a RF measurement system.

Probe

The simplest types of antenna are the probes (rods) and loops (coils), which are used to measure electric and magnetic fields, respectively. It is necessary to align the probe/loop with the field direction. More than a dipole or loop may be used to perform the measurement more accurately, for example, a three-dipole or loop probe, which is an orthogonal array providing isotropic response. In both cases, there are three elements arranged at right angles to each other in three dimensions as shown in Figure 11-5. This enables the probe to measure the field, regardless of the probe's orientation, and makes the probe similar to an ideal antenna. There are also probes, which have both rod and loop, making them fit to measure both electric and magnetic fields.

Several factors control the response of probes to the field. These factors include:

1. Variation of probe impedance with proximity to nearby reflective surfaces.
2. Capacitive coupling between the probe and the field source.
3. Nonuniform illumination of the sensing elements that make up the probe (for example, the three orthogonal elements that comprise an isotropic, broadband electric field probe).

Maintaining enough separation distance between the probe elements and the field source can exclude the influence of each of these factors, which may result in faulty measurement of fields. Experts recommend that measurement should be made at a distance equal to the three-probe dimensions between the surface of the nearest probe element and any object.

Currently, there are various types of probes and any one is suitable for use at a site with knowledge of frequency range. Care should be taken to provide separate probes to measure both electric and magnetic fields. At frequencies above 100 MHz, measurement of only electric field could be sufficient to make sure that a site complies with the safety standards. At lower frequencies, like AM broadcast stations, separate electric, and magnetic field measurements are necessary. For example, while measuring low RF levels in areas around a cellular base station, a sensitive probe is necessary; however, a broadcast antenna would need less sensitive probes for measurement.

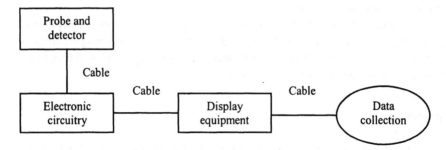

Figure 11-4 Basic components of a RF measurement survey system.

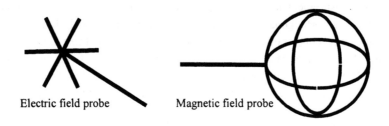

Figure 11-5 Electric and magnetic fields probes.

Detectors

There are two main types of detectors, a *diode* detector, and a *thermocouple* detector. Both types respond to the square of the voltage induced in the probe, and the outputs can be converted to equivalent power density depending on the far-field relationship between electric and magnetic fields.

Diode detector probes are suitable for low-field levels. They have a linear and square law combination of response. It is useful to divide diode detector operation into three regions: linear (above 20 dBm), transition (-20 dBm to 20 dBm) and square law (below −20 dBm). The square law simply means that the DC component of the diode output is proportional to the square of the AC input voltage. So, if RF input voltage is reduced by half, the DC output will be one quarter. If the applied RF is ten times as much RF input, the DC output will be 100 times higher.

Thermocouple detector responds to average power. A disadvantage of the thermocouple type of instrument is the possibility of getting fired. The thermocouple cannot sustain a power of more than twice of its upper power density. Thermocouple-based probes are also too sensitive to temperature and their accuracy is usually in the range of 2-3 dB.

Cable

The DC signal from the probe is transferred to the electronic circuitry via a cable. It is necessary that the cable does not interact with the field or conduct RF current from the field to the sensor.

Electronic Circuitry and Display

Such circuit provides signal conditioning, which may include filtering, amplification, digitizing, etc. Usually the conditioning circuit is connected with the display unit by either coaxial or optical cables. Also, the display unit could be connected via coaxial or fiber optic cable to a remote data collection device.

11.3.2   Calibration Techniques

There are various methods to calibrate RF instruments for exposure assessment under conditions simulating free space with an overall uncertainty of less than about 1 dB. One technique, which is suitable at frequencies above 500 MHz, involves the use of *anechoic chamber* and a waveguide horn antenna whose gain is accurately calibrated. The use of *transverse electromagnetic cell* is preferred below 500 MHz [12]. Using this technique for calibration requires a moderate amount of RF power to generate fields of sufficient strength to calibrate probes over the range of their operation. Probe sensitivity varies with frequency. For high frequency probe, variation of about 1 dB is typical, while the variation for lower frequency probes is 2 dB. In general, an accuracy of about 0.5 dB should be achievable.

11.3.3   Special Considerations

Exposure to RFR below 3 MHz and particularly below 200 kHz requires special consideration. Practical experience has shown that avoidance of shock because of voltages induced by RFR in ungrounded conductive objects, such as vehicles, fencing, metal roofing, and guy wires, can have a significant safety effect. The major concern arises from the induction of RF currents in conductive objects that are immersed in ambient RF fields [Figure 11-6]. These induced currents may flow through the body of an individual who contacts them. RF currents can be induced in the individual's body even without touching the object. The amount of current that will flow through the human body depends on the object (size and shape), the frequency, the impedance between the object and the person, and how well the individual is electrically grounded. The impedance between the object

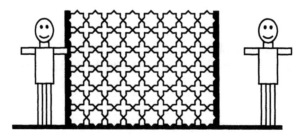

Figure 11-6 Induction of current into the human body.

and person depends on the person's weight, height, body composition, and type of contact (surface area of contact, i.e., finger or grasp, skin wet or dry), and the type of footwear. The current flowing through the person's body is perceived at certain level, but it becomes disturbing at higher levels and may lead to injury. Below a frequency of about 100 kHz, the perception is of a tingling or prickling feeling in the finger [9].

RF exposures at low frequencies, even at very low field strengths, may cause high values of electrically induced current to flow from large conducting objects to a grounded individual. In conditions where the potential for RF burns exist, mitigation measures should be taken in order to reduce the induced currents through each foot to below 100 mA for $f > 0.1$ MHz and below 1000 mA for $0.003 < f \leq 0.1$ MHz. Possible methods for reducing currents include restricting area access, reduction in source power, shielding, and other procedures of safety.

11.3.4 Time Averaging

Averaging time is the appropriate time period over which exposure is averaged, for the purpose of complying with safety standards [10]. Most of the safety standards discussed in Chapter 10 include averaging time because the effects of exposure are the result of signal level and exposure time. In general, the signal level is changing in which case the time-averaged values should be calculated from multiple measurements. A single measurement is sufficient in case the signal level is constant or changing within small level (less than 20%).

Time average is defined as the sum of the product (or products) of the actual exposure level(s) times the actual times(s) of exposure. The time-averaging capability is available in some modern RF measurement equipment. However, if this capability is not available, then the following set of equations can be followed to calculate the time-averaged RMS electric (E) or magnetic (H) field strength [9]:

$$E = \left[\frac{1}{\text{Averaging time (min)}} \sum_{i=1}^{n} E_i^2 . \Delta t_i \right]^{1/2} \qquad (11.16)$$

or

$$H = \left[\frac{1}{\text{Averaging time (min)}} \sum_{i=1}^{n} H_i^2 . \Delta t_i \right]^{1/2} \qquad (11.17)$$

where E_i and H_i are the sampled RMS electric and magnetic field strengths, respectively, which are considered to be constant in the i-th time period, Δt_i is the duration in minutes of the i-th time period, and n is the number of time periods within the averaging time.

The time-averaged power density P, is defined as

$$P = \frac{1}{\text{Averaging time (min)}} \sum_{i=1}^{n} P_i \Delta t_i \qquad (11.18)$$

where P_i is the sampled power density in the i-th time period.

The time-averaged SAR is defined as

$$SAR = \frac{1}{\text{Averaging time (min)}} \sum_{i=1}^{n} (SAR)_i \Delta t_i$$

$$(11.19)$$

where $(SAR)_i$ is the sampled SAR in the i-th time period. For equations (11.16-11.19), the following equation shall be satisfied

$$\sum_{i=1}^{n} \Delta t_i = \text{Time averaging (min)} \qquad (11.20)$$

For pulsed fields, E_i and H_i are RMS values, and P_i is the value averaged over the time interval Δt_i. If peak values are measured, the RMS or average values shall be calculated.

The particular applicable time averaging depends on the adopted protection guideline. These average times are either fixed or vary with the frequency range in order to regulate the RF exposure so that the total energy delivered over the average time does not exceed the exposure limits. This means it is permissible to exceed the recommended limits for certain duration as long as the average along the period of exposure remains within the limits, so no harmful effects occur.

Example 1

Consider that at 3 GHz, exposure of workers at 10 mW/cm^2 would be permitted for 3 minutes in any 6-minute period as long as during the remaining 3 minutes of the 6-minute period the exposure was at or near zero level of exposure. This is defined as

$$20 \text{ mW/cm}^2 \times 3 \text{ minutes} + 0 \text{ mW/cm}^2 \times 3 \text{ minutes} = 10 \text{ mW/cm}^2 \times 6 \text{ minutes}$$

Similarly, during any 6-minute period, exposure at 15 mW/cm^2 would be allowed for 4 minutes if the remaining 2 minutes were at or near zero.

$$15 \text{ mW/cm}^2 \times 4 \text{ minutes} + 0 \text{ mW/cm}^2 \times 3 \text{ minutes} = 10 \text{ mW/cm}^2 \times 6 \text{ minutes}$$

Also, 15 mW/cm^2 would be allowed for 3 minutes and 5 mW/cm^2 would be allowed for the remaining 3 minutes of a 6-minute period.

$$15 \text{ mW/cm}^2 \times 3 \text{ minutes} + 5 \text{ mW/cm}^2 \times 3 \text{ minutes} = 10 \text{ mW/cm}^2 \times 6 \text{ minutes}$$

Example 2

Also consider that exposure of the public at 2 mW/cm^2 would be permitted for 15 minutes only as long as during the previous and following 15 minutes the exposure was at or near zero level. This is defined as

$$4 \text{ mW/cm}^2 \times 15 \text{ minutes} + 0 \text{ mW/cm}^2 \times 15 \text{ minutes} = 2 \text{ mW/cm}^2 \times 30 \text{ minutes}$$

Likewise, during any 30-minute period, exposure at 3 mW/cm^2 would be allowed for 20 minutes if exposure during the remaining 10 minutes was at or near zero.

$$3 \text{ mW/cm}^2 \times 20 \text{ minutes} + 0 \text{ mW/cm}^2 \times 3 \text{ minutes} = 2 \text{ mW/cm}^2 \times 30 \text{ minutes}$$

Also, 3 mW/cm^2 would be allowed for 15 minutes and 1 mW/cm^2 would be allowed for the remaining 15 minutes of a 30-minute period

$$3 \text{ mW/cm}^2 \times 15 \text{ minutes} + 1 \text{ mW/cm}^2 \times 15 \text{ minutes} = 2 \text{ mW/cm}^2 \times 30 \text{ minutes}$$

In general, if the time of exposure is very short, the body can still safely process a proportionately higher-level exposure as long as the average based on the protection guidelines is not exceeded.

Time averaging is an important RF mitigation measure in occupational environments since the exposure can be controlled or monitored. In public environments, it is difficult to conclude how long an individual would stay in the exposed area. This process may provide solutions for accessing or traversing areas where fields exceed the exposure limits. For correct time averaging of exposure, the time both before and after the period of high exposure should be considered [6].

11.3.5 Spatial Peak

The whole body peak (WBP) is the maximum RF energy across the area of human body (about 2 meters high) that an individual can be exposed to RFR [6]. This level should be considered as the highest level that is found in the area of interest. If there are no WBP exposures above the safety limits, the area is considered below the limits and requires no additional evaluation.

11.3.6 Spatial Averaging

Spatial averaging is a means of measuring RF field by taking the total body average. Both, the ANSI/IEEE C95.3-1992 standard and NCRP Report No. 119 provide information on spatial averaging. The NCRP states [13], "the concept of spatial may be appropriate from a thermal standpoint due to the dynamics of the body's thermal regulation characteristics." The assumption of spatial averaging means the human body can regulate the thermal load caused by high-localized RFR as long as the total exposure does not exceed the whole-body average limit.

If peak levels exceed the exposure limits during evaluation of a site, then spatial-averaging is required. Spatial-averaging considers the whole area of the human body in the evaluation of exposure. If there is an area that has RF fields above the applicable exposure limit, additional vertical measurements should be taken to understand the levels between ground level and 2 meters high. The average of these vertical measurements is the spatial-averaged exposure, which is used to evaluate compliance with the exposure limit. The spatially averaged values are defined as [9]:

$$E = \left[\frac{1}{n} \sum_{i=1}^{n} E_i^{\,2} \right]^{1/2} \tag{11.21}$$

$$H = \left[\frac{1}{n} \sum_{i=1}^{n} H_i^2 \right]^{1/2} \qquad (11.22)$$

$$P = \frac{1}{n} \sum_{i=1}^{n} P_i \qquad (11.23)$$

where n is the number of locations, E_i, H_i, and P_i are the electric field strength, the magnetic field strength, and the power density, respectively, measured in the i-th location.

11.3.7 Multiple Frequency Environment

When the radiation consists of a number of frequencies, the ratio of the measured value at each frequency to the limit at that given frequency should be determined and the sum of all ratios obtained for all frequencies must not exceed unity (100 percent) when averaged spatially along the time. For electric and magnetic fields, the measured values and the limits should be squared before determining the ratios. The limit is defined as [9]

$$\sum_{f_1}^{f_n} R_f \leq 1 \qquad (11.24)$$

where f_1 is the lowest frequency band, f_n is the highest frequency band, R_f is the relative value with respect to exposure limit. For electric or magnetic field, the relative value is defined as

$$R_f = \left(\frac{\text{Measured value of field strength at } f}{\text{Exposure limit of field strength at } f} \right)^2 \qquad (11.25)$$

Where f is the frequency for which measurements were taken. However, the relative value for the power density is defined as

$$R_f = \frac{\text{Measured value of power density at } f}{\text{Exposure limit of power density at } f} \qquad (11.26)$$

Example

Suppose a worker is exposed to RFR at three different frequencies. Timely- and spatially-averaged measurements were carried out, producing the following conditions:

Magnetic field of 0.2 A/m at 13 MHz.
Electric field of 20 V/m at 250 MHz.
Power density of 1 mW/cm^2 at 2.45 GHz.

Let us consider the three relative values with respect to a specific RF protection guideline (for example, ANSI/IEEE C95.1-1992) in the above frequency bands. By using Equation (11.25) for electric and magnetic fields, and Equation (11.26) for power density, we obtain

$R_1 = (0.2/1.25)^2 = 0.02656$ for 13 MHz (in the frequency band 3-30 MHz)
$R_2 = (20/27.5)^2 = 0.528$ for 250 MHz (in the frequency band 100-300 MHz)
$R_3 = 1/1.63 = 0.613$ for 2.45 GHz (in the frequency band 300-3000 MHz)
$R = R_1 + R_2 + R_3 = 1.168.$

Since the resultant R is higher than unity, the exposure environment of the worker does not comply with the ANSI/IEEE C95.1-1992 safety limit.

11.4 MITIGATION IN PUBLIC ENVIRONMENTS

In general, regulations define two main RF exposure environments: occupational/controlled and public/uncontrolled. Public environments are those open to the general public access, where individuals would normally be unaware of RF exposure. This applies to all areas near transmitters and their associated antennas where the public is not restricted from access such as sidewalks, roads, and neighboring homes.

It is evident from Chapter 10 that exposure limits in public environments are lower than those for occupational environments. This is justified by the fact that exposure to the public is potentially 24 hours a day for 7 days a week, while exposure to workers is for 8 hours a day for 5 days a week.

11.4.1 Classification

An evaluation and classification should be performed after RFR levels are determined. Classifying the RFR allows site supervisors to realize the entire

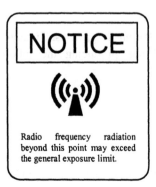
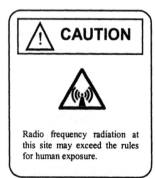

Figure 11-7   (a) Example of RF notice signs. (b) Example of RF caution sign.

situation and develop procedures to ensure exposure to public is kept below the safety limits. This is accomplished by comparing the levels found against the exposure limits for public environment. To further classify areas, a standard color-coding can be adopted to precisely show RFR levels. On a site where transmitters and their associated antennas are situated, it is substantive to restrict the access of general population. Walls, fences, and other natural or man-made structures frequently bound such areas.

11.4.2   Notice and Caution Signs

Notice or caution signs or appropriate substitutes, indicating the presence of RF fields, should be posted in areas where an overexposure could occur. Such signs are available from a variety of sources. Notice signs are usually used to distinguish between the public and the occupational areas. Boundaries are usually fences, gates, or roof doors to equipment rooms.   Caution signs represent additional precautions on fenced areas. They identify RF areas where exposure levels exceed exposure limits. Signs should be clearly visible and identifiable at all viewing distances. Figure 11-7 shows standard RF caution signs.

11.5   MITIGATION IN OCCUPATIONAL ENVIRONMENTS

In occupational/controlled environments people know that RFR is present and can take steps to control their exposure. This applies to sites where access can be controlled. The limits for occupational environments are evaluated differently (less stringent) than those for public environments.

11.5.1   Zoning Regulations

The purpose of zoning is to identify exposure levels in order to protect individual safety on sites where RF transmitters, antennas, and their cables are situated. Within these areas distinctive coloration is used (usually three colors: green, yellow, and red) to determine the warning for compliance to the RF protection guidelines [7].

The green zone is an area where the time (as appropriate) and spatial average is below 20% of the occupational safety limits. Areas so classified afford the highest level of protection for individuals working in RF fields. Time limit and special safety practices are not required for these areas. Workers in these areas need only basic exposure awareness. This may be conveyed with signs to provide necessary information.

The yellow zone is any area where the spatial average is between 20%-100% of the occupational safety limits. While fields in this area are within acceptable limits, caution must be exercised because nearby locations may exceed the limits. Workers in these areas should be aware of their potential for exposure. Usually, there will never be a yellow zone without another zone of higher level in the neighborhood. Only personnel with proper understanding of protection procedures should be allowed to work in such areas. Caution signs should be posted to inform workers of the situation.

The red zone is an area where the spatial-averaged levels fall above 100% of the occupational safety limits. When locations are found to require red zoning, special procedures, engineering, or restricted access must be implemented to secure compliance.

11.5.2   Site Characterization

Understanding the characteristics of site aids the surveyor in predicting the possible levels of RFR and subsequently helps in the prevention of levels that exceed the limits, which may cause health risks.

Building-Mounted Antennas

Building-mounted antennas means any antenna, other than an antenna with its supports resting on the ground, directly attached or affixed to a building, tank, tower, a mounted mast less than 3 meters tall, or structure other than a telecommunication tower. Building-mounted antenna sites are usually in metropolitan cities. The buildings used are generally the highest structures in the city and offer unique opportunity of height without a need for long feeding cables. The facility that houses the radio transmitters is also close to the antenna, which reduces the loss between the antenna and transmitter, permitting maximum power to the antenna. While this maximum power provides an extended range, it also increases the exposure levels around the antennas. The main determinants of exposure are frequency, power into the antenna, and aperture height. The greater the power, the higher the EM fields. The shorter the aperture, the higher the EM fields for a given power.

The mounting arrangement is normally laid out on a single plane and distributed in a grid arrangement, within the confines of the roof. The mounting is normally on a pipe structure and the separation can be as close as one meter in some cases. This arrangement provides for maximum mounting density, but it may leave little space for workers performing maintenance.

When the antenna is placed on the roof of a building in such a way those maintenance personnel could be exposed when working in the roof, appropriate engineering design and applicable safety precautions should be applied to avoid such condition. For the maintenance personnel, additional measures, e.g. instructions, test equipment, power switch-off rules, protective clothing and other measures are extremely necessary. Since close approaches or even direct contact with antennas is involved in such situations, it is necessary to reduce the radiated power, or sometimes even suspend the operation. Also, it is possible that certain RF levels could be present on the rooftop when antennas are mounted at rooftop locations. This might be harmful to maintenance personnel or others. On the other hand, the roof of a building introduces significant signal attenuation. This minimizes chances for harmful exposure of personnel living or working within the building itself. By reducing the level of fields on a building the potential for high exposure is eliminated, in addition to better compliance resolution.

Tower-Mounted Antennas

Throughout the world, there is a proliferation of new structures on the landscape, designed especially to serve the expanding market of mobile communications. Thousands of telecommunication towers have been already installed and more are required to meet the expected need.

A telecommunications tower means a mast, pole, monopole, guyed tower, lattice tower, freestanding tower, or another structure designed and principally used to support antennas. A ground- or building-mounted mast greater than 3 meters tall and 15 centimeters in diameter supporting one or more antenna, dish, or array is also considered a telecommunications tower.

Normally, towers are designed to elevate antennas in accordance with the intended coverage area. Some broadcast towers are hundreds of meters high, but these services have a very low frequency and a very high power function.

Cellular communication facilities have no need for such heights. However, if cellular antennas are found on a broadcast tower as a collocation (a single telecommunication tower or building supporting one or more antennas, dishes, or similar devices owned or used by more than one public or private entity), they are usually much lower in position, regardless of the height of the supporting structure. Cellular towers usually have directional antennas mounted on a single face to define a sector. There may be several faces and several directional antennas per face. Towers may have several antennas mounted in a star configuration to maximize the density of antennas at a position on the tower.

There is a significant power difference between the front and the backside of the antenna. This difference is called *front-to-back ratio*. While the front-to-back ratio can be as great as 25 dB in the far-field region, it is less well developed in the near-field region. There is still reduction of the exposure of workers in the near field behind, as compared to the front of the antenna, but the amount may be considerably less than the advertised far field front-to-back ratio.

The situation on towers is significantly different. As workers climb up a tower they may encounter several antenna mounts at various locations on the tower. These mounting areas might hold different types of transmitters ranging from high-power paging transmitters to large antennas for transmitters in other frequency ranges. While the antennas and the resulting mounting arrangement can be notably different, in some conditions the exposure levels may advance or exceed the RF protection guidelines.

In the case of paging transmitter, the antenna will normally be an omnidirectional with an aperture length of one meter to five meters. The antenna will be mounted from one meter to two meters from the tower. Fields immediate to the aperture present the highest levels. Therefore, workers must be cautious while working or standing instantly in front of these antennas unless the transmitters are deactivated. If the antenna is grouped with other antennas at the same level more than one transmitter may need to be deactivated.

11.5.3 RF Mitigation Measures

To guarantee compliance at some sites, it is necessary to apply certain changes of a technical, engineering or physical nature. Such changes are intended to provide the necessary assurance that neither workers nor the public would be exposed to RF fields in excess of the adopted exposure limits. Examples of such changes may include:

1. Place antennas at a height above head level (above 2 meters). This may decrease the power densities at nearby areas on the rooftop. Elevating antennas to heights of considerably less than 2 meters may, on a spatially

averaged basis, significantly reduce the power densities in areas very close to the antenna. This procedure is especially effective for rooftops where multiple antennas are located.

2. Antennas should be mounted on long side arms (1 to 2 meters length) rather than mounted directly to the tower in order to reduce the high level of exposure to tower climbers.

3. Decrease power fed to the antenna; therefore, cumulative RF fields at the site, as well as in publicly accessible areas will be reduced.

4. Consideration should be given to individuals working on antenna sites during maintenance. Coordination ahead of time should be performed to reduce the transmitted power if a person is working on the antenna site. Extra attention should be paid when a person is passing through fields of strong radiation.

5. Combination of fields from several antennas may produce exposure levels exceeding the exposure limits. This may be resolved by relocating individual antennas and arrays that affect the power densities at various locations at and around the site. Special attention should be given to traffic passageways that workers or employees would use while on the site.

6. Increase spacing between antennas in order to reduce prevailing RF fields in some controlled location areas. The spacing between antennas affects the power densities at the site. Where the antenna density in the grid is higher (less distance between antennas), the power density at any point on the site is likely to be higher.

7. Precautions should be taken to make sure that maintenance workers are not exposed to hazardous RFR. A clearance distance of at least 1 meter should be kept if their presence is required. Such distance is needed in order to assure exposure level remains within the limits.

8. Workers may use RF personal monitors while being very close to sources of radiation. A personal monitor is a RF threshold detector that sounds an alarm when RF energy exceeds the threshold of the device.

9. After considering all the safety measures and if the situation is not under the control of work practice, realization of personal protective equipment (PPE), such as protective clothes, is the final solution for reducing RF exposure. Such clothes may provide up to 10-dB reduction in RF energy absorption within the body. These clothes are necessary when exposure levels are many times higher than the exposure limits.

10. All workers must have a basic understanding of EM exposure safety. This is achieved through regular training. They should understand the potential exposure and steps they can take to reduce the exposure levels.

REFERENCES

[1] Durney, C. H., and D. A. Christensen, *Basic Introduction to Bioelectromagnetics*, CRC Press, Boca Raton, FL, 1999.

[2] Lee, W. C. Y., Mobile Radio Performance for a Two-Branch Equal-Gain Combining Receiver with Correlated Signals at the Land Site, *IEEE Transactions on Vehicular Technology* 27, pp. 239-243, 1978.

[3] Lee, W. C. Y., *Mobile Communication Engineering*, McGraw Hill, New York, NY, 1982.

[4] Garg, V. K., and J. E. Wikes, *Wireless and Personal Communications Systems*, Prentice Hall, Upper Saddle River, NJ, 1996.

[5] Cleveland, R. F., D. M. Sylvar, and J. L. Ulcek, Evaluating Compliance with FCC Guidelines for Human Exposure to Radiofrequency Electromagnetic Fields, *OET Bulletin* 65, Edition 97-01, August 1997.

[6] Hammett, W. F., *Radio Frequency Radiation: Issues and Standards*, McGraw Hill, New York, NY, 1997.

[7] Release of EME Evaluation and Management for Antenna Sites, Motorola Network Service Division, October 1997.

[8] Ohmori, S., W. Hiromitsu, and K. Seiichiro, *Mobile Satellite Communications*, Artech House, Norwood, MA, 1998.

[9] Limits of Human Exposure to Radiofrequency Electromagnetic Fields in the Frequency Range from 3 kHz to 300 GHz, Safety Code 6, Environmental Health Directorate, Health Canada, Canada, 1999.

[10] IEEE Standard for Safety Levels with Respect to Human Exposure to Radio Frequency Electromagnetic Fields, 3 kHz to 300 GHz, ANSI/IEEE C95.1-1999 Edition (Incorporating IEEE Std C95.1-1991 and IEEE Std C95.1a-1998), Institute of Electrical and Electronics Engineers, Piscataway, NJ, 1999.

[11] Gaily, P. C., and R. A. Tell, An Engineering Assessment of the Potential Impact of Federal Radiation Protection Guidance on the AM, FM, and TV Broadcast Services, U.S. Environmental Protection Agency, Report No. EPA 520/6-85-011, April 1985.

[12] Crawford, M., Generation of Standard EM Fields Using TEM Transmitted Cells, *IEEE Transactions on Electromagnetic Compatibility* 16, p. 189, 1974.

[13] A Practical Guide to the Determination of Human Exposure to Radiofrequency Fields, National Council on Radiation Protection and Measurements, NCRP Report No. 119, Bethesda, MD, pp. 171-174 & 186-188, 1993.

12

RF Site Surveys

12.1 INTRODUCTION

There are certain steps in formulating programs that will protect workers or the public from being exposed to RF energy above the allowable limits, as well as protect utilities from litigation or possible penalties. The first and foremost is to survey any utility owned or leased sites that have transmitters, or for that matter, heat sealers, induction units or any other devices that emit RF to determine if RF hazards are present. Taking an inventory of all site hazards is the necessary first step in choosing the correct course of compliance action.

Throughout surveying, it is not possible to specify whether a site under investigation is safe or not. The only expected result is to show whether the site is complying with the adopted protection guideline. The aim through evaluation is to find the highest fields and upon such finding the safety relief program may be developed. In addition, periodic site surveys are identical when RF sources are replaced or changed in order to identify the effects that these changes have on RF coverage. Once identified, remedial action can be recommended to return to a state of optimal performance and a safer environment.

12.2 SURVEY OF MOBILE SYSTEMS

The attainable data through research work show concentrations of electric field energy or hot spots located in and around vehicles with RF transmitters operating at VHF and lower bands. The hot spots are practically absent in vehicles with center-of-the-roof-mounted antennas operating at 450 MHz and higher bands. The same phenomenon was detected with center-of-the-trunk mounted antennas. The hot spots may cause some harmful effects because of the possibility of sharp, localized high values of SAR.

In principle, the vehicle passengers are significantly shielded by the metal surfaces of the car body, if the antenna is located on the roof or on the vehicle. Measured radiation patterns of antennas mounted on cars show little dependence on the number of passengers in the car or their location in the cabin. At high frequencies (450 MHz and higher bands), the occupancy or lack of passengers makes no difference in the radiated level from mobile antennas.

The main factors in determining the RF emission from a mobile antenna is its location on the vehicle and the size and shape of the vehicle. The dimensions of the vehicle roof are essential factors for the antenna efficiency and general radiation pattern shape. The characteristics of the antenna and its height above the ground determine the details of the radiation pattern. At low frequencies (150 MHz and lower bands), with wavelengths comparable to a vehicle size, the entire metal body of the car participates in the radiation process by supporting the RF currents emanating from the antenna feed point. These currents terminate in electric charges where the conducting external surfaces of the vehicle come to a steep end.

In general, high-power (5 watts and above) mobile radio equipment emits strong fields. Roof gutter and fender mounts are not recommended for high-power mobile radios because of the possibility for overexposure of a bystander.

Importantly, for vehicles with plastic bodies, enormous care should be placed to position the mobile radio antenna and its grounding surfaces, if any, at a sufficient distance from the passengers so as to avoid potential overexposure.

12.3   SURVEY OF CELLULAR BASE STATIONS

The fast growth of the cellular communication industry has resulted in the installation of large number of base transceiver stations (BTSs), which are mounted on freestanding towers, on rooftops, or on the sides of buildings. Such transmitters represent the core of cells in the cellular system. They usually transmit between 20 and 50 watts depending on the type of the BTS.

As discussed in 6.9.1, large cells can be split into smaller cells, which can be split further into even smaller cells by decreasing the power of the transmitter. These may be of three types: macrocells, microcells, and picocells, depending upon their size and the power output of the antenna.

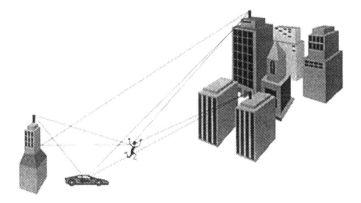

Figure 12-1 RF exposure from various BTS antennas.

Macrocells provide the main structure for the base station network. The BTS for macrocells have power outputs of tens of watts and communicate with phones up to about 30 km. Microcells are used to improve the main network, especially when the network is congested. They are located in different places such as airports, railway stations, markets, etc. BTSs for picocells have lower power output than those of microcells (a few watts) and are almost always situated inside buildings.

BTSs are different from each other in terms of radiated power. For example, BTSs for AMPS radiate up to 50 watts per channel and many sites have six or seven channels per sector, using three-sectored antennas, which concentrate the signals into 120 degrees of arc. Meanwhile, GSM digitals BTSs require less power per channel than analog because there are eight digital users time-sharing a single carrier. Since GSM emphasizes capacity rather than geographic coverage of AMPS, the inclination is to confine both the power and the cell size, rather than boost them. Usually, smaller cells produce excellent capacity.

12.3.1 Implementation of Safety Standards

It is known that power density from the antenna decreases as the inverse square of the distance, and therefore, the exposure at ground level in the vicinity of the antenna tower is relatively low compared with the exposure very close to the antenna. Also, exposures of people from BTSs are to the whole body but at levels of power many times less than levels radiated by cellular handsets.

The installation of BTS antennas frequently raises concerns about their human health impacts and safety, mostly for people who live in the vicinity of these sites. There might be circumstances where people could be exposed

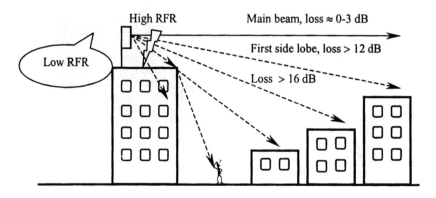

Figure 12-2   Conditions of RFR around a BTS.

to fields greater than the exposure limits. Figure 12-1 shows the scenario of human exposed to various BTS antennas.
Because of building attenuation, levels of power density inside buildings at corresponding distances from the BTS antenna would be from 10 to 20 times smaller than the outside. It is only in specific areas on the rooftop, depending on the proximity to the antenna, that the exposure levels are higher than those allowed by the RF protection guidelines. Also, access to such locations should be restricted. Therefore, measurements in rooms exactly below roof-mounted antennas show the power density levels lower than that of the roof top locations. This depends on the construction material. The level of power densities behind sector antennas is hundreds of times less than in front. Therefore, levels are too low in rooms located behind sector antennas. Figure 12-2 illustrates the conditions of RFR around a BTS.

The exposure situation around a typical BTS can be computed easily. The field strength data can then be analyzed with respect to possible conflicts with the available guidelines for limiting RF exposure. In general, the maximum exposure levels near the base of a typical BTS antenna are, really, lower than all national and international recommended safety limits. These maximum exposure levels may occur only at limited distances close to the base of the BTS antenna. Typical safety distances for BTS range from 1 to 5 meters for one RF carrier in the direction of the main beam of the antenna. However, it is difficult to specify a typical BTS since the configuration (i.e., service, power output, frequencies, antenna configuration, etc.) may vary considerably. Therefore, operators need to check the compliance of a given BTS with the protection guidelines or applicable regulations according to their needs. In addition, the residual radiation (side lobes) from the antenna must also be considered.

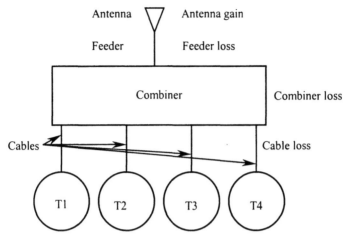

Transmitting power from N numbers of transmitters

Figure 12-3 Components of a BTS.

Consider the BTS components illustrated in Figure 12-2. The power density transmitted in the main lobe direction is defined according to Equation 11.3. Combining Equation 11.3 and 11.6, we obtain

$$P_d = \frac{P_t 10^{G_t/10}}{4\pi d^2}$$ (12.1)

where G_t is the gain of the antenna in dB. However, with several transmitters connected to the same antenna, Equation (12.1) can be written as if we consider the ohmic losses shown in Figure 12-3 between the transmitter and the antenna (cable loss + combiner loss + feeder loss = L), then the power density can be defined as

$$P_d = N\frac{P_t 10^{G_t/10}}{4\pi d^2}$$ (12.2)

$$P_d = N\frac{P_t 10^{(G_t-L)/10}}{4\pi d^2}$$ (12.3)

The safety distance d_{min} from an antenna is derived from Equation (12.3) as

$$d_{min} = \sqrt{NP_t 10^{(G_t-L)/10} / 4\pi P_d}$$
(12.4)

where P_d represents the maximum allowed power density in air (W/m^2) due to the adopted safety standard at the relevant frequency band.

Example

Calculate the minimum safety distance d_{min} according to the FCC protection guidelines for a worker at a BTS with the following specifications:

Operating frequency:	900 MHz
Maximum transmitting power:	50 watts
Losess (L):	4 dB
Gain (G_t):	16 dB
Number of transmitters (N):	4

According to the FCC guidelines [see Table 10-6], P_d at 900 MHz should be 30 W/m^2 for occupational environments. Using Equation (12.4), we obtain

$$d_{min} = \sqrt{4 \times 50 \times 10^{(16-4)/10} / 4\pi \times 30} = 2.9 \text{ meters}$$

This means that the worker is safe (according to the FCC guidelines) as long as the distance separating the worker and the antenna is either 2.9 meters or more.

12.3.2 RF Survey Studies

Measurements near typical BTSs have shown those exposure levels encountered by the public to be well below the recommended protection guidelines. However, there may be circumstances where workers could be exposed to RF fields higher than the safety limits, generally on rooftops and close to antennas.

An example of data submitted to the FCC [1] showed a maximum measured ground-level power density at the base of a 45 meters tower in the order of 0.00002 mW/cm^2 per radio channel, corresponding to 0.002 mW/cm^2 for a 96 channel, 100 watts ERP per channel, fully implemented system. The maximum was found to occur typically at distances between 18 and 25 meters from the base of the tower. At other points within 90 meters the levels were considerably lower than 0.0001 mW/cm^2.

Similar measurements made by Bonte and Habash [2] in the vicinity of BTS in Finland yielded accordingly lower values. The power densities at distances greater than 50 meters from all commonly used BTS antennas were less than 0.010 mW/cm^2 including points in the main beam. But measurements made directly in the beam of a GSM directional antenna with 12 radio channels indicated that the power density was less than 1 mW/cm^2 at a distance of 10 meters away from the antenna and less than 0.010 mW/cm^2 beyond 30 meters. Therefore, in certain areas on the rooftop, depending on the proximity to the antenna, the exposure levels might be higher than those allowed by the guidelines. Access to these areas should be restricted. It is also possible that in rooms directly below roof-mounted installations, the power density levels are considerably lower than roof locations, depending on the construction.

Thansandote et al. [3] conducted a RF survey in and around 5 schools selected in consultation with the concerned parents regarding the health of their children due to the installation of a BTS in a church cross located across the street from an elementary school in Vancouver, Canada. Three of these schools were selected because they had a BTS on or near the school property. The others, which were not located near a BTS, were selected as controls. Although the purpose of the survey was to determine the actual levels of RFR in the analog and PCS cellular BTS frequency bands, measurements also covered AM, FM, and TV broadcast frequencies where possible. The researchers presented a brief report of the survey findings and compared the results with the exposure limits outlined in Health Canada's Safety Code 6. The power density, expressed as μW/m^2, was taken as a practical indicator of exposure. More than 160 measurements were carried out at the selected schools at indoor and outdoor sites frequented by both staff and students. The measured power densities did not exceed the Safety Code limits. For example, the maximum power densities from the PCS BTS across the street, the analog BTS on the roof, the analog BTS across the street, no BTS nearby were 0.00016 mW/cm^2, 0.0026 mW/cm^2, 0.00022 mW/cm^2, and less than 0.00001 mW/cm^2, respectively. The researchers concluded that the levels measured during their study posed no health risk to the students, school staff, or the general public in or around the five Vancouver schools involved.

In the United Kingdom, Mann et al. [4] of the NRPB measured RFR levels at 118 sites around 17 BTSs. The maximum exposure at any location was 0.00083 mW/cm^2 (on a playing field 60 meters away from a school building with an antenna on its roof). Typical power densities were less than 0.0001 mW/cm^2. Levels of power densities indoors were substantially less than levels of power densities outdoors.

12.4   SURVEY OF BROADCAST STATIONS

Broadcast stations are usually located near densely populated areas so that large audiences can receive the signals. The radiation patterns from broadcast antennas are not as highly collimated as those from other RF sources, such as dish antennas used for satellite earth stations. Therefore, exposure of persons to main-beam radiation intensities near the broadcast antenna is possible, especially if individuals are at eye level with the antenna bays, as may be the case for residents of high-rise buildings.

Public access to broadcast antennas is normally restricted, either through fencing, placement on a communication tower, or installation in rugged terrain. However, there are some instances where overexposure of the general public may occur. In certain cases, simple measures can be taken to prevent this overexposure, such as the installation of fencing or the posting of warning signs. In cities, broadcast antennas may be located on the roofs of buildings and thus building maintenance personnel may unknowingly be exposed to RFR.

The intensity and location of the radiation fields from broadcast antennas depend on several factors, including type of station, characteristics of the antenna being used, power transmitted to the antenna, and distance from the antenna. Usually, calculations and/or measurements are performed to predict what levels of field intensities would exist at various distances from the antenna.

In general, standard AM radio broadcast stations can produce power densities exceeding 0.0004 mW/cm^2 at all points within a radius of one kilometer of the antenna and above 0.04 mW/cm^2 at ranges of a quarter kilometer.

In Sydney, Australia, McKenzie et al. [5] repeated the Hocking et al. [6] study [see 9.3.2 for details]. McKenzie and colleagues looked at the same area at the same time period and surveyed RF exposure from the North Sydney TV towers. They took readings at roof level, street level, and inside houses. At a particular house there were three different readings: 3.0, 0.066, and 0.017 mW/cm^2, respectively. A significant difference in readings between indoor/ outdoor and home/away was observed.

12.5   SURVEY OF TRAFFIC RADAR DEVICES

Large estimations of exposure to RFR emitted from traffic radar devices were conducted under a variety of operating conditions. A number of studies have been conducted concerning potential operator exposures to radiation emitted by traffic radars. Most of these studies measured some feature of the emitted radiation intensity, and some of them measured levels of exposure at other locations away from the aperture of the antenna.

Baird et al. [7] of the National Bureau of Standards (NBS), now known as the National Institute of Standards and Technology (NIST), published the most widely referenced of these studies. The emissions of 22 (seven K-Band and 15 X-Band) radar devices from six different manufacturers were measured. Radar units were mounted at different positions inside a patrol car, as in typical operation. The maximum level measured at any passenger position within the vehicle was $0.36\ \text{mW/cm}^2$, while typical levels were less than $0.01\ \text{mW/cm}^2$. From those measurements, they formulated a simple model for predicting average power densities from measured aperture power densities for both fixed-mounted and handheld X-band and K-band antennas at specific distances within the near- and far-field regions of radars used for measuring speed. The study was important in that it fixed a NBS protocol for measuring exposures in the vehicle in which traffic radar is used.

In 1991, the Institute of Police Technology and Management (IPTM) conducted a similar study [8] of 310 randomly selected radar units from four manufacturers. At two inches from the face of the antenna, IPTM found a maximum level of $0.55\ \text{mW/cm}^2$, and an average level of $0.17\ \text{mW/cm}^2$.

Fisher [9, 10] conducted the largest study of exposure from traffic radar units for measuring the levels of radiation using various radars at various locations inside and outside a police vehicle. He measured the X-band and K-band RFR levels emitted by 30 models of police traffic radars from six manufacturers (about 95% of the radar units tested had fixed-mounted antennas, and the remaining 5% were handheld devices). The data were collected during 1982-1991. The total number of antennas evaluated was 5000 (1075 for X-band and 3925 for K-band). The average aperture power densities ranged from a low of $0.69\ \text{mW/cm}^2$ for K-band handheld units to a high of $2.66\ \text{mW/cm}^2$ for X-band handheld units. The minimum and maximum power densities measured for any unit were $0.1\ \text{mW/cm}^2$ for X-band fixed mounted unit and $6.4\ \text{mW/cm}^2$ also for an X-band fixed mounted unit. As a result, Dr. Fisher concluded that there is no evidence to support the allegation that police traffic radar operators are at risk due to prolonged exposure to microwave emission from their radar guns.

Lotz et al. [11] of NIOSH measured and evaluated microwave emissions from ten models of radar guns. Specific measurements included both fixed-mounted and handheld radar units operated both inside and outside the police vehicle. The measurement procedures were based, in part, upon the IEEE recommended practice for the measurement of potentially hazardous RFR [12], the technical report by Dr. P. David Fisher [9], and the technical report from the NBS [8]. For potential personnel exposures, they indicated that only in cases where the person would actually be in the main beam path in close proximity to the radar would the exposure be above 20 $\mu W/cm^2$, the lowest limit of detectability on the exposure survey meter they used. This meant that only if the radar antenna was mounted inside the car and directed toward an occupant was the exposure strong enough to be measured by their measurement techniques.

Balzano et al. [13], in response to claims of a link between testicular cancer and exposure to the RFR from handheld traffic radar devices, presented measurements of equivalent power density at the antenna aperture of 24-GHz handheld traffic radar. The authors also measured depth of penetration and energy absorption in a material that had similar electrical characteristics to that of human tissue. As a result, the authors indicated that for the 12-mW radar unit, the maximum power density incident on the skin when the antenna was in close proximity is less than 0.5 mW/cm^2. Also more than 95% of the energy was absorbed in the first millimeter of depth when the antenna was placed in contact with tissue.

Fink et al. [14] evaluated police officers' exposures to RFR emitted by 54 traffic radar units; 17 different models, encompassing 4 frequency bands and 3 antenna configurations. Exposure measurements were taken at approximated ocular and testicular levels of officers seated in patrol vehicles. Comparisons were made of the radar manufacturers' published maximum power density specifications and actual measured power densities taken at the antenna faces of those units. Four of the 986 measurements taken exceeded the 5-mW/cm^2 limit accepted by IRPA and the NCRP, though none exceeded the ACGIH, ANSI, IEEE, or OSHA standard of 10 mW/cm^2. The four high measurements were maximum power density readings taken directly in front of the radar. Of the 812 measurements taken at the officers' seated ocular and testicular positions, none exceeded 0.04 mW/cm^2; the highest of these (0.034 mW/cm^2) was less than 1% of the most conservative current safety standards.

12.6 SURVEY OF RF HEATING EQUIPMENT

RF ovens and RF dryers, along with RF sealers and heaters, and microwave ovens provide the flexibility and speed to heat, dry, and cure a vast spectrum of products with demonstrated increase in productivity as well as less cost. Such devices have been among the major sources of employee RF overexposure.

12.6.1 RF Heaters and Sealers

The exposure of operators occurs from fringing EM fields emerging outward and away from the electrodes. Strong magnetic fields can exist due to the RF current flow within the material being sealed or heated between the electrodes. A matter of concern is the leakage of EM fields in excess of all existing RF protection guidelines, which may be hazardous to the workers around. The leakage field is often extensive, resulting in whole-body exposure of operators in these occupational situations.

Many studies [15-21] show that safe limits for EM fields from such devices and induced electric currents in the human body are often exceeded for heater operators. In the frequency range of such equipment, fields may penetrate the human body and cause heating of internal tissues. Workers nearby may be unaware of their exposure to RF fields, because the fields can penetrate deeply into the human body without activating the heat sensors located in the skin.

Precautional steps should be followed in order to keep the level of power densities below the protection guidelines. Control of the emission of RF energy from sealers and heaters depends on the use of efficiently designed and installed shielding material. Shielding of heaters is an effective way to reduce operator exposures [22-24]. All shielding material must be properly grounded.

Other emission controls are proper grounding; use of thick stand-on insulating pads to reduce body-to-ground currents; locating RF sealers away from reflecting surfaces; placing a wooden or plastic table between the operator and the heater; and proper maintenance of equipment. Also, when these machines are used, employees should use mechanical or electrical devices that allow them to stay as far away form the source of radiation as possible.

12.6.2 Microwave Ovens

The use of microwave ovens provides a big deal of usefulness to our lives, however, care must be taken to avoid human exposure to the microwaves that heat and cook food. The main concern is about microwave leakage from around the oven door. Currently, oven doors have at least two independent interlocks to ensure that the door cannot be opened until the microwave power generator has been turned off and that the power generator cannot be turned on while the door is open. Some doors of earlier models were relatively loose fitting, particularly after being in use for a while, although leakage is not a function of age. Leakage is possible if the door is bumped, dropped, or misaligned, or if the hinges are loose. However, with the current technological advances in door seal design and with appropriate maintenance, microwave oven leakage has been exceedingly minimized. The design of a microwave oven is such that the microwaves are contained within the cavity of the oven, but it is likely for some leakage to occur around the door, just like light can be seen under a door to a lighted room. The only difference is that RFR is not seen. In such circumstances, a neon lamp (not connected to any electrical source) will light up when held close to a leaky microwave oven door. A very simple and safe test is to run your finger around the edge of the door while the oven is operating; if slight warmth is felt at any point, the oven is probably leaking in excess of 5 mW/cm². When carrying out these checks, it is necessary to be sure to have at least a cup of cold water in the oven. It is also useful to check if the door flange and faceplate are free of food spatters. Spills and spatters can build up in these areas and affect the door seal enough to cause leakage.

Surveys were carried out in order to evaluate radiation leakage levels from used microwave ovens [25-29]. Thansandote et al. [29] conducted a survey for the Radiation Protection Bureau of Health Canada in order to determine the compliance of these ovens to the leakage radiation, labeling requirements, and design and construction of the Canadian radiation emitting devices regulations. A total of 60 microwave ovens from 14 different national and international manufacturers (including the most popular brands) were inspected and measured to confirm their compliance with the Canadian regulations. The average levels of radiation leakage with and without water test load were 0.1 and 0.3 mW/cm², respectively. Accordingly, none of the oven models evaluated was found to emit microwave radiation in excess of the maximum allowed leakage. The levels of leakage did not only meet but were well below the requirements of the regulations.

12.7 SURVEY OF RF ENVIRONMENTAL LEVELS

The U.S. Environmental Protection Agency (EPA) has measured the environmental field intensities at chosen locations in 15 U.S. cities. Although those measurements are from the 1970s, the data stay important in the lack of extensive succeeding measurement [30].

Janes et al. [31] and Tell and Mantiply [32] presented the results for those cities (a total of 486 sites). Those results were also summarized in Hankin [33] and in EPA [34]. Janes et al. [31] conducted a survey measurement of field intensity at 6.4 meters above ground at each site in the following frequency ranges: 0.5-1.6 MHz (the standard AM-radio broadcast band); 54-88 MHz and 174-216 MHz (the VHF-TV bands); 88-108 MHz (the standard

FM-radio broadcast band); about 150 and 450 MHz (land-mobile bands); and 470-890 MHz (the UHF-TV bands). The signals in each band were received with separate antennas specifically designed for each band. Measurements in the AM-radio broadcast band were not included in the analyses because that band was below the then prevailing 10-MHz lower frequency limit of the 1974 ANSI standard.

The median exposures ranged from 0.002 $\mu W/cm^2$ (for San Francisco and Chicago) to 0.020 $\mu W/cm^2$ (for Portland), while the population-weighted median for all 15 cities was 0.0048 $\mu W/cm^2$. Also, the percentages of the population exposed to less than 1 $\mu W/cm^2$ in each city ranged from 97.2% (for Washington, D.C.) to 99.99% (for Houston), with a mean for all cities of 99.44%. The major contributions to those exposure values were from FM-radio and TV stations.

In addition, the EPA measured RFR levels at sites near to single or multiple RF emitters, for example, at the bases of transmitter towers and at the upper stories (including the roof) of tall buildings or hospital complexes in the vicinity of transmitter towers. At the base of an FM tower on Mount Wilson, California, the fields were found to range from about 1 to 7 mW/cm^2 [35]. Measurements in tall buildings close FM and TV transmitters yielded values well below 0.01 mW/cm^2 (10 $\mu W/cm^2$), but a few values were close to or slightly exceeded 0.2 mW/cm^2 (e.g., 0.23 mW/cm^2 on the roof of the Sears Building in Chicago).

12.8 SURVEY FOR RF INTERFERENCE

Electromagnetic interference (EMI) is a rapidly growing discipline in all areas of electrical engineering. EMI is part of the bigger subject of electromagnetic compatibility (EMC). EMC explores the capability of electronic devices to function properly in an EM environment [36]. The frequent use of sensitive electronics in all areas of daily life, or the high circuit density in communication systems, makes equipment highly susceptible to interference with EM sources.

Radio frequency interference (RFI) refers to interference from RF fields that are coupled from a source to an electric or electronic device through the air. RFI results in an electronic signal being propagated into and interfering with the proper operation of electrical or electronic equipment. Interference may be experienced on communication equipment such as radios, televisions, and telephones. It may also be experienced on other electronic equipment such as personal computers, stereos, electronic organs, doorbells, and medical electronic equipment. Medical equipment, which has been found susceptible to interference, includes wheelchairs, cardiac pacemakers, ventilators, defibrillators, infusion pumps, blood warmers, and infant incubators. Also, a specific type of interference involving FM broadcast stations is called *blanketing*. It occurs when electrical devices are very close to the transmitter and when the FM signal is very strong.

Many wireless facilities have been constructed at well-located sites; frequently high-power FM and TV broadcast antennas, BTSs, and other wireless stations. In addition, portable wireless systems, such as cellular phones and vehicle-mounted transceivers, are another major source of RFI. These facilities have created a kind of electromagnetic environment (EME). RFI occurs whenever the EME exceeds the equipment immunity of the home or business electronic device. In such situations, there is a real threat that the high-level RF will cause interference problems throughout a wide range of transmitting and receiving equipment.

12.8.1 RFI of Medical Devices

Medical devices such as infant apnea monitors, powered wheelchairs, implanted cardiac pacemakers, and ventilators are often more sensitive to RFI because they incorporate low power integrated electronics. It has been found that RFI could cause critical-care medical devices to malfunction with serious consequences. Reports of medical device failure from RFI have increased [37-40]. The consequences of interference have ranged from inconvenience to serious injuries and death. Other incidents may occur but are not reported because most users of medical devices are unaware that RF fields are present when problems are recognized. Circuitry of newer instruments is much more sensitive to RF energy than their electrical and electromechanical predecessors. There has also been a significant rise in the use of electronically controlled medical devices outside the clinical environment. These devices are often used in homes, attached to patients, or implanted in their bodies.

Besides the frequency and distance between RF sources and susceptible medical devices, two major RFI factors affect medical equipment [41]:

1. Coupling between a source of interference and medical equipment.
2. Modulation imposed on fields from each source.

Coupling

Coupling means interaction between an RF source (interference source) and an affected electronic device. Effects of coupling usually occur when the susceptible device is in the near field of the source. Capacitive coupling occurs in a region near the source where the electric field is dominant, such as the tip of mobile antenna. In contrast, inductive (magnetic) coupling between the base of a cellular phone antenna and implanted cardiac pacemakers has been demonstrated by Carillo et al. [42] to prevail over capacitive coupling for this situation. While coupling is a critical factor for RFI under near-field conditions, in the far-field region it is the carrier frequency that is crucial to the introduction of RF into a device. Generally, the frequencies with the greatest ability to induce RFI are those whose wavelengths are comparable to the maximum dimension of a medical device's physical dimension.

Modulation

The modulation technique also affects the degree of interference. Amplitude modulation (including pulsed RF) is usually the most significant for RFI. A RF carrier with AM may induce RF voltages in the circuitry of medical equipment. The amplitude-modulated RF carrier may be detected at the semiconductor junctions in the device. Significant interference occurs if the modulating frequencies are within the physiological passband (range of frequencies associated with the events of a physiological process) of the device. The presence of objects near medical equipment may create motion-induced multipath reflections. These reflections might combine with the original signal, for example CW, to produce AM on the RF fields near the medical device. If the AM is within the frequency of the physiological band of the signal that the equipment is designed to detect, interference may occur.

RF Susceptibility

Susceptibility is a condition where equipment shows an undesired function due to RF exposure. During the 1980s, the FDA had become aware that approximately 60 infants died in the United States while being monitored for breathing cessation by one model of an apnea monitor. Subsequent tests have shown that this particular monitor is extremely susceptible to low-level RF fields [43]. Other apnea monitors have been shown to be similarly susceptible to malfunction. This has resulted in voluntary recall of more than 16,000 apnea monitors.

Another device that has demonstrated RFI susceptibility is the electrically powered wheelchair. Unintended motion has been initiated by RFI from transceivers in nearby emergency vehicles [44], causing persons to be ejected from their wheelchairs or propelled into traffic. New draft performance standards for wheelchairs are being developed by the Rehabilitation and

Assistive Technology Society of North America (RESNA) to address these serious problems; many manufacturers are developing products that conform to these standards.

Problems also involve implanted cardiac pacemakers and defibrillators. Teams of engineers and cardiologists in several countries have independently studied these equipment, either inpatient or tissue-simulating models, demonstrating that nearby digital cellular phones sometimes induce unwanted effects [45, 46]. The dominant effect observed has been the loss of pacemaker adaptive control. Interference with pacemakers has not been observed when the phones are held at the ear. In this regard, a panel of researchers has concluded that phone/pacemaker interference should not be considered a major public health concern and has offered specific recommendations for pacemaker users [47, 48].

Cellular phones have also been shown to cause unintended firings of implantable cardiac defibrillator [49]. Handheld digital cellular phones that use pulse-modulated TDMA have been found to disrupt the proper operation of in-the-ear hearing aids. TDMA phones include GSM and North American Digital Cellular (NADC) pulse modulation formats, which utilize schemes that produce 100% amplitude modulated pulses of the RF carrier at frequencies within the audible hearing range. Subjective perception of interference varies from barely perceptible to annoying and loud, starting when the phones are within one meter of the hearing aid and becoming louder when the phones are several centimeters away [50]. This type of interference also occurs in behind-the-ear hearing aids, making it difficult for wearers of this device to be able to use this type of phone.

12.8.2 Recommendations

Extensive measurements should be made to determine the field strengths produced by common RF sources in actual or simulated clinical environments. Standardized RFI test methods have been developed to enable engineers in clinical environments to estimate the susceptibility of medical devices to specific RF transmitters in a setting comparable to that of actual use [51]. Such methods should be used to identify potentially problematic situations in hospitals where transmitters are repeatedly used in close proximity to critical medical devices.

Wireless systems may be optimized for compatibility with medical electronics. Modulation frequencies of RF transmitters should be outside the physiological passband of medical devices. Digital techniques that use TDMA, and the associated AM pulses, should be carefully designed to avoid RFI.

The radiated power of many modern mobile and portable cellular phones is under the control of a BTS. When close to a BTS, such devices may operate at power levels far lower than the maximum power of 0.6 W (for handheld phones) or 3.0 W (for portable-bag phones). Thus, when a BTS is located near a health care facility or when a low power BTS (microcell) is used within the facility, cellular phones will normally operate at low power. However, the BTS itself must be properly situated to avoid causing RFI. If deemed necessary, RF sources can be restricted from the more sensitive areas of a hospital, such as intensive care units.

IEEE Committee on Man and Radiation (COMAR) recommends that manufacturers and users of both medical devices and RF transmitters work together to ensure that medical devices can operate in a safe and effective way in the presence of RF fields. Medical equipment manufacturers should design and test their products to ensure conformance with current RFI standards so that their devices are not excessively sensitive to RFI. This requires that the products are shielded in electrically conductive, or conductor coated enclosures that include feed through filters and other techniques to increase EMC. Even when medical devices conform to existing standards, manufacturers should warn both medical professionals and patients of situations where RFI failure may occur. The caution includes information that describes how to recognize the symptoms of RFI, how to deal with RFI, and how to report incidents.

REFERENCES

[1] Federal Focus National Symposium on Wireless Transmission Base Stations Facilities, A WTR LLC Tutorial, 1996.

[2] Bonte, M., and R. W. Y. Habash, Standards for Safety Levels with Respect to Human Exposure at Radio Frequency Radiation, Technical Report on Surveying Few Base Stations of Sonera, RF Survey Report, Mikkeli, Finland, 1999.

[3] Thansandote, A., G. B. Gajda, and D. W. Lecuyer, Radiofrequency Radiation in Five Vancouver Schools: Exposure Standards Not Exceeded, *Canadian Medical Association Journal* 160, pp. 1311-1312,1999.

[4] Mann, S. M., T. G. Cooper, S. G. Allen, R. P. Blackwell, and A. J. Lowe, Exposure to Radio Waves Near Mobile Phone Base Stations, National Radiation Protection Board, UK, 2000.

[5] McKenzie, D. R., Y. Yin, and S. Morrell, Childhood Incidence of Acute Lymhoblastic Leukaemia and Exposure to Broadcast Radiation in Sydney-A Second Look, *Australia and New Zealand Journal of Public Health* 22, pp. 360-367, 1998.

[6] Hocking, B., I. Gordon, H. Grain, and G. Hatfield, Cancer Incidence and Mortality and Proximity to TV Towers, *Medical Journal of Australia* 65, pp.

601-605, 1996.

[7] Baird, R. C., R. L. Lewis, D. P. Kremer, and S. B. Kilgore, Field Strength Measurements of Speed Measuring Radar Units, NBSIR 81-2225, National Bureau of Standards, Washington, DC, 1981.

[8] Traffic Radar Power Densities: Summary of Findings, Institute of Police Technology and Management (IPTM), University of North Florida, Jacksonville, FL, 1991.

[9] Fisher, P. D., Microwave Exposure Levels Encountered by Police Traffic Radar Operators, MSU-ENGR-91-007, Michigan State University, Michigan, IL, 1991.

[10] Fisher, P. D., Microwave Exposure Levels Encountered by Police Traffic Radar Operators, *IEEE Transactions on Electromagnetic Compatibility* 35, pp. 36-45, 1993.

[11] Lotz, W. G., R. A. Rinsky, and R. D. Edwards, Occupational Exposure of Police Officers to Microwave Radiation from Traffic Radar Devices, PB95-261350, National Institute for Occupational Safety and Health, 1995.

[12] IEEE Recommended Practice for the Measurement of Potentially Hazardous Electromagnetic Fields-RF and Microwave, IEEE Standard C95.3, Institute of Electrical and Electronic Engineers, New York, NY, 1991.

[13] Balzano, Q., J. A. Bergeron, J. Cohen, J. M. Osepchuk, R. C. Petersen, and L. M. Roszyk, Measurement of Equivalent Power Density and RF Energy Deposition in the Immediate Vicinity of a 24-GHz Traffic Radar Antenna, *IEEE Transactions on Electromagnetic Compatibility* 37, pp. 183-191, 1995.

[14] Fink, J. M., J. P. Wagner, J. J. Congleton, and J. C. Rock, Microwave Emissions from Police Radar, *American Industrial Hygiene Association Journal* 60, pp. 770-76, 1999.

[15] Stuchly, M. A., M. H. Repacholi, D. Lecuyer, and R. Mann, Radiation Survey of Dielectric (RF) Heaters in Canada, *Journal of Microwave Power* 15, pp. 113-121, 1980.

[16] Bini, M., A. Checcucci, A. Ignesti, L. Millanta, R. Olmi, N. Rubino, and R. Vanni, Exposure of Workers to Intense RF Electric Fields that Peak from Plastic Sealers, *Journal of Microwave Power* 21, pp. 33-40, 1986.

[17] Human Exposure to Microwaves and Other Radio Frequency Electromagnetic Fields-Entity Position Statement, IEEE-USA COMAR, Washington, DC, 1991.

[18] Williams, M. A., and K. H. Mild, Guidelines for the Measurement of RF Welders, Report No. 1991:8, National Institute of Occupational Health, Department of Medicine, Umea, Sweden, 1991.

[19] Olsen, R. G., T. A. Griner, and B. J. Van Matre, Measurement of RF Current and Localized SAR Near a Shipboard RF Heat Sealer, In *Electricity and Magnetism in Biology and Medicine* (ed. Blank, M.), San Francisco Press, San Francisco, CA, pp. 927-929, 1993.

[20] Gandhi, O. P., D. Wu, J. Y. Chen, and D. L. Conover, Induced Current and SAR Distributions for a Worker Model Exposed to an RF Dielectric Heater Under Simulated Workplace Conditions, *Health Physics* 72, pp. 236-242, 1997.

[21] Human Exposure to Electric and Magnetic Fields from RF Sealers and Dielectric Heaters-A COMAR Technical Information Statement, *IEEE Engineering in Medicine and Biology* 18, pp. 88-90, 1999.

[22] Radiofrequency (RF) Sealers and Heaters: Potential Health Hazards and Their Prevention, National Institute for Occupational Safety and Health, 1979.

[23] Ruggera, P. S., and D. H. Schaubert, Concepts and Approaches for Minimizing Excessive Exposure to Electromagnetic Radiation for RF Sealers, Rockville, MD: Food and Drug Administration, DHHS Publication No. (FDA) 82-8192, 1982.

[24] Murray, W. E., D. L. Conover, R. M. Edwards, D. M. Werren, C. Cox, and J. M. Smith, The Effectiveness of a Shield in Reducing Operator Exposure to Radiofrequency Radiation from a Dielectric Heater, *Applied Occupational and Environmental Hygiene* 7, pp. 586-592, 1992.

[25] Stuchly, M. A., M. H. Repacholi, and D. Lecuyer, The Impact of Regulations on Microwave Ovens in Canada, *Health Physics* 37, pp. 137-144, 1978.

[26] Miller, T. M., Results of Microwave Oven Radiation Leakage Surveys at Fermilab, *American Industrial Hygiene Association Journal* 48, pp. 77-80, 1987.

[27] Moseley, H., and M. Davison, Radiation Leakage Levels from Microwave Ovens, *Annals of Occupational Hygiene* 33, pp. 653-654, 1989.

[28] Matthes, R., Radiation Emission from Microwave Ovens, *Journal of Radiological Protection* 12, pp. 167-172, 1992.

[29] Thansandote, A., D. W. Lecuyer, A. Blais, and G. B. Gajda, Compliance of Before-Sale Microwave Ovens to the Canadian Radiation Emitting Devices Regulations, *32nd Microwave Power Symposium Proceedings*, July 14-16, Ottawa, Ontario, Canada, 1997.

[30] Heynic, L. N., and P. Polson, Human Exposure to Radiofrequency Radiation: A Review Pertinent to Air Force Operations, U.S. Air Force Armstrong Laboratory (AL/OER), Brooks Air Force Base, TX, 1996.

[31] Janes, D. E., R. A. Tell, T. W. Athey, and N. N. Hankin, Radiofrequency Radiation Levels in Urban Areas, *Radio Science* 12, pp. 49-56, 1977.

[32] Tell, R. A., and E. D. Mantiply, Population Exposure to VHF and UHF Broadcast Radiation in the United States, *Proceedings of the IEEE* 68 (1), pp. 6-12, 1980.

[33] Hankin, N. N., The Radiofrequency Radiation Environment: Environmental Exposure Levels and RF radiation Emitting Sources, U.S. EPA Technical Report EPA 520/1-85-014, 1985.

[34] Federal Radiation Protection Guidance; Proposed Alternatives for Controlling Public Exposure to Radiofrequency Radiation; Notice of Proposed Recommendations, pp. 27318-27339, EPA, Federal Register (Part II) 51 (146), 1986.

[35] Tell, R. A., and P. J. O'Brien, An Investigation of Broadcast Radiation Intensities at Mt. Wilson, California, Note ORP/EAD 77-2, U.S. Environmental Protection Agency, 1977.

[36] Evaluation of Interference Between Hand-Held Wireless Phones And Implanted Cardiac Pacemakers: Recommendations For Corrective Intervention, WTR LLC Progress Report, 1996.

[37] Silberberg, J. L., Performance Degradation of Electronic Medical Devices Due to Electromagnetic Interference, *Compliance Engineering* 10, pp. 25-39, 1993.

[38] Silberberg, J. L., Medical Device Electromagnetic Interference Issues, Problem

Reports, Standards, and Recommendations, *Proceedings of the Health Canada Medical Devices Bureau Round-Table Discussion on Electromagnetic Compatibility in Health Care*, Ottawa, Canada, pp. 11-20, 1994.

[39] Joyner, K., V. Anderson, and M. Wood, Interference and Energy Deposition Rates from Digital Mobile Phones, *Abstracts Annual Meeting of the Bioelectromagnetics Society* 16, pp. 67-68, 1994.

[40] Tan, K. S., and I. Hinberg, Malfunction in Medical Devices Due to RFI from Wireless Telecommunication Devices, *Proceedings of the Annual Meeting and Exposition of the Association for the Advancement of Medical Instrumentation* 13, p. 96, 1995.

[41] Bassen, H. I., RF Interference (RFI) of Medical Devices by Mobile Communications Transmitters, In *Mobile Communications Safety* (eds. Kuster, N., Q. Balzano, and J. C. Lin), pp. 65-91, Chapman & Hall, London, UK, 1997.

[42] Carrillo, R., B. Saunkeah, M. Pickels, E. Traad, C. Wyatt, and D. Williams, Preliminary Observations on Cellular Telephones and Pacemakers, *PACE* 18, p. 863, 1995.

[43] Ruggera, P., and E. O'Bryan, Studies of Apnea Monitor Radiofrequency Electromagnetic Interference, *Proceedings of the Annual International Conference IEEE Engineering in Medicine and Biology Society* 13, pp. 1641-1643, 1991.

[44] Witters, D., and P. Ruggera, Electromagnetic Compatibility (EMC) of Powered Wheelchairs and Scooters, *Proceedings of the Annual International Conference IEEE Engineering in Medicine and Biology Society* 16, pp. 894-895, 1994.

[45] Barbaro, V., P. Bartolini, C. Militello, G. Altamura, F. Ammirati, and M. Santini, Do European GSM Mobile Phones Pose a Potential Risk to Pacemaker Patients: *In Vitro* Observations, *PACE* 18, pp. 1218-1224, 1995.

[46] Barbaro, V., P. Bartolini, A. Donato, and C. Militello, Electromagnetic Interference of Analog Cellular Telephones with Pacemakers, *PACE* 19, p. 1410, 1996.

[47] Hayes, D., R. Carrillo, G. Findlay, and M. Embrey, State of the Science: Pacemaker and Defibrillator Interference from Wireless Communication Devices, *PACE* 19, p. 1419, 1996.

[48] Irnich, W., L. Batz, R. Miller, and R. Tobisch, Electromagnetic Interference of Pacemakers by Mobile Phones, *PACE* 19, p. 1431, 1996.

[49] Bassen, H., H. Moore, and P. Ruggera, Cellular Phone Interference Testing of Implantable Cardiac Defibrillators *In Vitro*, *Circulation* 92 (8 Suppl I), p. 3547, 1995.

[50] Joyner, K., M. Wood, E. Burwood, D. Allison, and R. Strange, Interference to Hearing Aids by the New Digital Mobile Telephone System, Global System for Mobile (GSM) Communications Standard, National Acoustic Laboratories, Australian Hearing Services, Sydney, Australia, 1993.

[51] Recommended Practice for an On-Site, Ad-Hoc Test Method for Estimating Radiated Electromagnetic Immunity of Medical Devices to Specific Radio Frequency Transmitters, ANSI Standard C63.18, 1997.

13

Internal Field Dosimetry

13.1 INTRODUCTION

Internal field dosimetry was originally developed for ionizing radiation [1]. It was based on a relationship between dose (energy absorbed per unit mass) and biological effect. Since the energy absorbed is directly related to the internal EM fields (EM fields inside the object, not EM fields incident upon the object), dosimetry is interpreted to mean the determination of EM fields inside the biological body.

Internal fields rather than incident fields and currents are responsible for interactions with living systems independently of whether these interactions are thermal or nonthermal. The internal and incident EM fields can be quite different, depending on the size and shape of the object, its electrical properties, its orientation with respect to the incident fields, and its operating frequency. Since any biological effect is related directly to the internal fields, any cause-and-effect relationship must be formulated in terms of these fields only, not the incident fields.

Dosimetry in this manner considers the measurement or determination by calculation of the internal fields, induced current density, specific absorption (SA), or specific absorption rate (SAR) distributions in objects like models (phantoms), animals, humans, or even parts of human body exposed to RFR. It is very difficult to entirely characterize the propagation of EM fields in human body, keeping in mind the complexity and nonhomogeneous character of biological tissues.

Internal dosimetry can be divided into two categories [2]: *macroscopic* and *microscopic* dosimetry. In macroscopic dosimetry, the EM fields are determined as an average over some volume of space, such as in mathematical cells that are small in size. For example, the **E** field in a given mathematical cell of one mm is

345

assumed to have the same value everywhere within 1 mm^3 volume of the cell. The same is applied for **B** fields. While, in microscopic dosimetry, the fields are determined at a microscopic (cellular) level. Or the other way, the mathematical cells over which the EM fields are determined are microscopic in size.

A large body of work has been done on macroscopic dosimetry; however, work on microscopic dosimetry has been carried out only recently. The right approach to adopt is to evaluate fields in the macroscopic level, and then move deep to find fields in the microscopic level. Microscopic dosimetry is useful for studies at the cellular level, which may throw light on EM interaction mechanisms. This kind of dosimetry is not easy to achieve due to the huge number of data and factors involved at the dynamic cellular level of the living system.

13.2 SPECIFIC ABSORPTION RATE

The intensity of RFR in the environment is measured in units such as mW/cm^2. However, the intensity provides little information on the biological consequence unless the amount of energy absorbed by the irradiated object is known. This is generally given as the specific absorption rate (SAR) [3]. SAR generally quantifies absorption of EM energy from an incident EM field by a biological body.

13.2.1 Types of SAR

In general, there are two types of SAR [4]. First is the whole-body average SAR, which is defined as the total energy, transferred to the body per unit time, divided by the total mass. The whole-body SAR represents the spatial mean value for the body in any specified configuration and orientation. It is effective for objects that have complex shapes and large spatial variations of constituents because it is a quantity that can be measured experimentally without the need for data on the internal SAR distribution.

Under certain conditions, SAR of various parts of the human body, such as head, torso and limbs, also require attention. This type of SAR is the localized (partial-body) SAR, which refers to a small part of the body. Primarily, the localized SAR is applied to exposure from small radio equipment such as cellular phones.

Both whole-body SAR and localized SAR characterize a measure of RF absorption as heat. It is also used as a measure of the internal field intensities in studies classified as athermal or nonthermal, in which the heat generated by the RFR is insignificant.

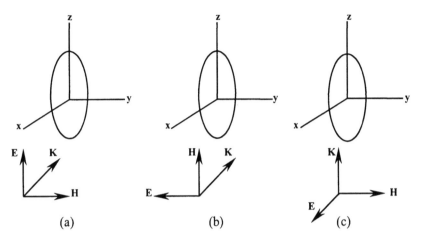

Figure 13-1 (a) E polarization. (b) H polarization. (c) K polarization. (Adapted from Figure 5.1 [2]).

13.2.2 Parameters Related to SAR

The value of SAR in any biological material depends on several exposure parameters: characteristics of the incident fields such as frequency, modulation, amplitude, and direction of its components; spatial distribution of complex dielectric and thermal properties of the system including those of the site and its location within the object; and the configuration of the entity and its orientation relative to the incident fields.

The technical problem, which must be addressed while considering these parameters, is difficult, because biological systems are quite inhomogeneous, lossy, and vary from person to person.

Polarization

The polarization of an EM wave is the direction of lines of force in the electric field. The whole-body average SAR varies as a function of incident field orientation with respect to the object [3]. For objects of rotation (those with circular symmetry about the long axis), three polarizations are considered: E, H, and K, as illustrated in Figure 13-1. E polarization corresponds to the electric field parallel to the main axis of the body; H polarization corresponds to the magnetic fields parallel to the main axis of the body, and K polarization to the wave propagation vector parallel to the long axis of the body. For the human body, which is not a subject of rotation (ellipsoid), three additional polarizations are considered. SAR would also be calculated for circularly polarized RFR. Such

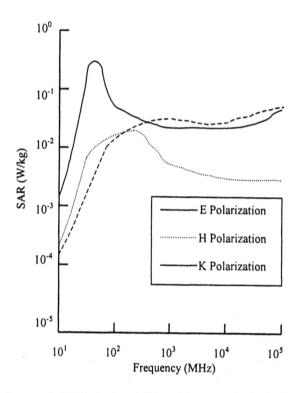

Figure 13-2   Average whole-body SAR as a function of frequency for model of average man in free space exposed to a plane wave with a power density of 10 W/m² for three types of polarization [5].

radiation can be resolved into two mutually perpendicular components, each has half the total power density. Therefore, a body exposed to circularly polarized RFR would have lower resonant SAR values than it would have if exposed to linearly polarized RFR.

Frequency

For all the three types of polarization, SAR varies approximately as the square of frequency at low frequencies [2]. For E polarization, absorption of power and accordingly SAR peaks occur at about 70-80 MHz. This frequency corresponds to ungrounded man and should be higher for smaller animals. The variation of the whole-body average SAR with the frequency and polarization is shown in Figure 13-2. For a man in contact with RF ground, the resonant frequency becomes about 30-40 MHz. At resonant frequency, the power absorbed is a few times greater than that obtained by multiplying the surface area of the body cross section by the incident power density [5]. Thus, the human body has absorption characteristics quite identical to those of a lossy dipole antenna in free space.

At frequencies above resonance, SAR varies approximately as the inverse of the frequency. Generally, the whole-body SAR at frequencies below resonance in the E polarization is approximately proportional to f^2, however, at frequencies above resonance, the whole-body SAR is approximately proportional to $1/f$ for about one decade of frequency and exhibits smaller relative secondary resonance at higher frequencies.

Size and Shape

The average SAR depends also on the size and shape of the body. Figure 13-3 shows the SAR for three species for E polarization for an incident power density of 10 W/m². It is observed that the average SAR for monkey and mouse is many times higher than that of human when both are exposed to the same frequency. If biological effect is observed in mouse at a given power density, a greater power density is needed to cause the same effect in human. In addition, the spatial distribution of SAR varies from point to point inside the human body because of the different anatomical features. Nevertheless, the spatial distribution inside the monkey and rats are different from that of human.

SAR in a body can also be affected by the presence of other bodies. The presence of a ground plane or other reflecting surfaces shifts the resonant frequencies downward and can produce higher values of whole-body SAR at lower resonant frequencies. For example, placing a human body on a perfectly conducting plane will cause the resonant frequency to approximately cut to half compared to that of body in free space. This is due to the effect of *imaging*, where the body looks twice as tall. For a human standing on not perfectly conducting ground, the resonant frequency would be lower than for free space, but not half, as it would be for perfect conductor. Placing insulator between the human body and the ground, for example, shoes, further affects the resonant frequency [2].

Electrical Properties of Tissues

SAR calculations or measurements depend largely on the electrical properties of the irradiated body. As discussed in Section 7.2, the electrical properties of tissues are specified in terms of permittivity and conductivity. These parameters depend on frequency, temperature, and local tissue distribution inside the biological body. In humans, the local tissue distribution for different individuals varies largely and might even change with time. Also, the electrical properties depend on other characteristics such as level of physical and metabolic activity, anatomy, health, and age.

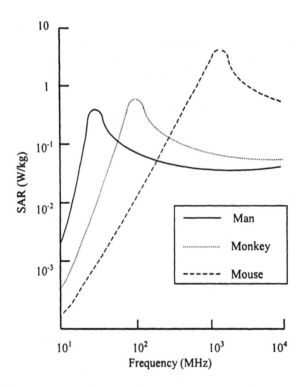

Figure 13-3 SAR in spheroidal models of a man, monkey, and mouse exposed to a plane wave of 10 W/m² for E polarization [5].

13.2.3 Estimation of SAR

SAR is not easily measurable in practice, but can be determined empirically or theoretically despite the limitations of these methods. Basically, SAR is measure of the rate at which energy is absorbed by the body. It may also be defined as the time derivative of specific absorption (SA), which corresponds to the incremental energy (dW) absorbed by an incremental mass (dm) within a volume element (dV) of a given density (ρ). It is defined as [6]

$$SA = \frac{dW}{dm} = \frac{dW}{\rho dV} \tag{13.1}$$

SA is expressed in units of joules per kilogram (J/kg).

However, SAR is measured in watts per kilogram (W/kg) or milliwatts per gram (mW/g). It is defined as

$$\text{SAR} = \frac{d}{dt}\frac{dW}{dm} = \frac{d}{dt}\frac{dW}{\rho dV} \qquad (13.2)$$

Also, SAR could be defined as the power absorbed by a unit mass of biological system. SAR can be represented in terms of electric field strength E in V/m, conductivity σ in mhos/m, and density of tissue ρ in kg/m^3 (this is usually given in units of g/cm^3, for example, ρ for water is about 1 g/cm^3). It is given by

$$\text{SAR} = \frac{\sigma E^2}{\rho} \qquad (13.3)$$

An integral of SAR over a volume of tissue containing a given mass presents the absorbed power. This is expressed in mW/g (for certain tissue density) averaged over 1 g or 10 g, depending on the adopted safety standard.

The initial rate of temperature increase at the body (neglecting heat losses) is directly proportional to the SAR

$$\frac{dT}{dt} = \frac{\text{SAR}}{C} \qquad (13.4)$$

where T is the temperature in °C, t is the time in seconds, and C is the specific heat capacity (energy needed to raise the temperature of one gram of substance by one degree Celsius).

Several biological effects of RFR, which have substantial implications on human health, can be related to induced heating. Heating from RFR best relates to SAR rather than to power density to account for differences in coupling. Temperature rise and specific absorption are related as shown

$$T = \frac{SA}{\hbar \times 4180} \qquad (13.5)$$

where T is the temperature rise (°C), and $\hbar$ is the relative heat capacity (= 0.85).

13.3 THEORETICAL DOSIMETRY

The internal field in any biological material irradiated by RFR is calculated by solving Maxwell's equations. Practically, this is a difficult task and can be done for only a few special cases. Because of the mathematical difficulties encountered in the process of calculation a combination of techniques is used to find the SAR.

Each technique gives information over a limited range of parameters in such a way that suits the chosen model. Various models such as blocks, spheroidal, and cylindrical with suitable electromagnetic and thermal characteristics have been used in many studies [7-11] to represent different parts of the human body such as the head and limbs.

In general, computational methods for analyzing EM problems fall into three categories [12]: analytical techniques, numerical techniques, and expert systems. Analytical techniques apply assumptions to simplify the geometry of the problem in order to apply a closed-form solution. Numerical techniques attempt to solve basic field equations directly, due to boundary conditions posed by the geometry. However, expert systems estimate, but do not calculate, the values of fields for the parameters of interest based on a rules database.

In bioelectromagnetics, one or more computational methods are employed for the computation of internal fields, and therefore the SAR, in the human body. First, involves the use of analytical techniques for calculations of absorbed energy in simplified biological geometries such as plane slabs, spherical, cylindrical, and prolate spheroidal or elliptical models. Second, involves the use of numerical techniques for analyzing the coupling of RF fields with various biological structures.

13.3.1 Analytical Techniques

The mathematical techniques currently used to characterize and determine absorption rates inside biological systems are often quite demanding. The whole-body and partial-body SARs were initially found by considering homogenous objects of different shapes exposed to plane waves. Various analytical techniques have been implemented to calculate the fraction of the incident field that gets deposited at the human body. This, in turn, requires one to model the human body, or part of the body, which is a complicated biomass structure. Any one of the following models may be used:

1. Planar multilayer model. The human body is regarded as a stratified medium composed of isotropic homogenous lossy dielectric layers of planar geometry.
2. Spherical, cylindrical, and prolate spheroidal or elliptical models. The human body or any of parts are regarded as sphere, cylinder, ellipsoid of an isotropic, or homogeneous lossy dielectric medium.
3. Block model. The human body or any part of it is modeled as an assembly of a number of independent cells of lossy dielectric media.

The choice of suitable model depends on the frequency of operation, the purpose of study, the portion of the body to be investigated, and the ease of analytical formulation. For cellular phone dosimetry, for instance, the operating frequency is very small compared to the dimensions of the human body, especially if the torso, flat shoulder, chest, back, or thigh is considered. Hence, the simplest model could be the planar multilayer model.

Various theoretical methods were applied in literature to calculate the power absorption by biological models. Among the methods [4]:

1. Transmission-line model for one-dimensional isotropic infinite plane tissue layers.
2. Plane wave spectrum analysis for semi-infinite homogeneous slab.
3. Mie theory for three-dimensional spherical and multilayered spherical models.
4. Extended boundary condition method (EBCM) up to approximately resonance (80 MHz) and iterative extended boundary condition method (IEBCM) an extension of the EBCM, up to 400 MHz.
5. Long-wavelength approximation method for two-dimensional infinite circular cylinder (up to frequencies of about 30 MHz), and three-dimensional prolate spheroid models.

Several early analytical studies have been carried out employing the plane wave transmission-line model approach to evaluate the EM fields and determine the energy deposited in a lossy, semi-infinite, and homogenous target (man and animals) at high frequency RFR [12, 13]. Other models have also been employed, such as spheres [14], prolate spheroidal [15-17], ellipsoids [18, 19], and multilayer elliptic cylinder [20, 21]. For very high frequencies, a geometrical optics method has been developed to estimate the power absorption in cylindrical models [22], and in prolate spheroidal [23] of man. Values of field, absorbed energy in human body and effect of layering on energy deposition have been also obtained [24-27].

Analytical studies on homogeneous models were the main resources of information regarding RF energy deposition inside the human body or any part of it. These studies provided the required dosimetric data needed in setting RF exposure limits and the relevant protection guidelines.

13.3.2 Numerical Techniques

In the field of electromagnetics, we come across many complex problems, the solutions of which are extremely difficult and usually not possible by analytical methods. In such cases the solutions lie at the use of numerical techniques. Different numerical techniques have been investigated over the past several years.

Numerical methods are often divided into basic ones such as finding the root of an equation, integrating a function or solving a linear system of equations to intensive ones. Intensive numerical methods are regularly needed for the solution of practical problems and they often require the systematic application of a range of elementary methods, often millions of times over. Such techniques generally fall into two major categories: domain techniques and boundary techniques. Domain techniques discretize the whole computational domain and solve differential equations within the volume; boundary techniques discretize only the boundary of the computational domain and solve integral equations.

Although the theory behind these methods have has available for many decades, the real introduction of early numerical techniques goes back to the 1960s, just after the arrival of the mainframe computers. A number of numerical techniques were developed during this period to solve various electromagnetic problems. These range from the traditional solutions that involve determination of electric field distribution to more modern hybrid methods that employ a variety of techniques, each of which is applicable over different regions of the problem. Some of these may produce the right solutions but require large computational resources.

During the 1990s, many numerical methods were developed and organized toward certain applications. In this discussion, only methods applied to electromagnetics in general and bioelectromagnetics in particular are discussed. A few commercial codes, which run simulations of bioelectromagnetic phenomena in order to ensure high performance and safety, are also included.

Method of Moments

Richmond [28] and Harrington [29] first introduced the *method of moments* (MOM) (or moment method) in the 1960s. Initially, the MOM was presented as a general procedure to solve partial differential equations through a linear system of equations. However, MOM today relates to an approach that solves complex integral equations by reducing them to a system of simple linear equations. It employs a technique called the *method of weighted residuals*. It continues to be probably one of the popular modeling techniques used in electromagnetics.

MOM is very commonly used to analyze problems with conducting subjects such as antenna structures and a number of different applications. First it finds currents or charges on the surface and then integrates these quantities over the entire surface to find fields. MOM is a frequency domain technique. It will only analyze a single frequency at a time, although popular software codes allow the solution to iterate over a number of frequencies.

MOM requires that the entire structure under modeling be broken down into wires and/or metal plates. Each wire is subdivided to a number of wire segments, which must be small compared to the wavelength. Each metal plate is subdivided into a number of surface patches, which must be small compared to the wavelength. Once the model is defined, a source is imposed (a plane wave approaching, or a voltage source on one of the wire segments). The current on every wire segment and surface patch due to the source and all the other currents (or the other wire segments and surface patches) is then determined. When these currents are known, the electric field at any point in space is calculated from the sum of all contributions from all wire segments and surface patches.

MOM is a very versatile and intuitive modeling technique. Users may easily understand how to use it, and know what to expect from a given model. They can picture the RF currents on a structure and realize how they would lead to electric and magnetic fields. But the main drawback of this method is the large computational resources required.

A widely used numerical EM modeling method based on MOM is the NEC. Many versions of NEC have been released. It was developed at Lawrence Livermore National Laboratory few years ago and has been compiled and run on various computer systems. The version NEC4WIN is particularly effective to simulate, analyze, and optimize antennas. This version is based on the MININEC3 algorithms developed by the Naval Ocean Systems Center during the 1980s [30]. Meanwhile, these codes are not applicable for lossy dielectric materials and therefore not suitable for RF dosimetry.

Finite Difference Time Domain

The *finite-difference time-domain* (FDTD) concept was first introduced by Yee [31] in 1966. With the improved capacity of computers, Taflove and Brodwin [32] implemented it for the first time in 1975 for solving scattered fields from a dielectric cylinder. The FDTD method belongs to the general class of differential time domain numerical modeling methods. It involves the discretization of the differential form of Maxwell's equations in time and space using second-order accurate central differences. The resulting *difference equations* are then solved in a time marching sequence by alternately calculating the electric and magnetic fields on an interlaced Cartesian grid. The FDTD method has been applied to many problems involving scattering or radiation in open domain.

FDTD is one of the most popular modeling techniques currently being used for EM interactions and SAR analysis. There are many reasons for this popularity: it is easy to understand and implement in software, and since it is a time-domain technique it can cover a wide frequency range with a single simulation run. It possesses the advantages of simple implementation for relatively complex problems and high accuracy. However, it may unexpectedly cause serious errors due to inappropriate modeling of radiation source and inadequate setting of calculation conditions. In 1976, Taflove and Brodwin [33] published first application of the FDTD method to calculate the induced fields and temperature in the human eye model exposed to RFR.

A few more books have been published in the FDTD method [34-36]. Professor O. P. Gandhi at the University of Utah presented a chapter entitled, "FDTD in Bioelectromagnetics: Safety Assessment and Medical Applications," in the book edited by Taflove [36].

Sullivan et al. [37, 38], Gandhi et al. [39], and Spiegel et al. [40] applied the FDTD technique for modeling biological systems exposed to RFR.

Kuwano and Kokubun [41] employed the FDTD method to calculate SAR distribution in a cylindrical human body model placed near a wall due to RFR. Also, Kuwano and Kokubun [42] calculated the power absorption of a cylindrical man model placed near a flat reflector exposed to RFR.

Watanabe and Taki [43] and Watanabe et al. [44] applied the FDTD to calculate the frequency characteristics of whole-body averaged SARs in a homogeneous human model exposed to the near field of an electric dipole or a magnetic dipole.

Several commercial EM modeling codes employing the FDTD are also available. Among those, which can be applied to bioelectromagnetics are:

1. XFDTD [45].
2. MAFIA-4 (based on the finite integration method (FIM), which leads to the same numerical scheme as FDTD) or CST Microwave Studio (using a perfect boundary approximation, which is also based on the FEM) [46].
3. EMIT [47].

Finite Element Method

The *finite element method* (FEM) is usually applied to complex nonlinear problems for electrical, mechanical, and civil engineering. The application of FEM to electromagnetics came in the 1990s [48, 49]. FEM requires complete volume of the configuration to be meshed as opposed to surface integral techniques, which only require surfaces to be meshed. Each mesh element can have different material properties from those of neighboring elements. The corners of the elements are called *nodes*. The aim of the FET analysis is to determine the field quantities at the nodes. The drawback of this method is that for complicated bodies it will be very difficult and sometimes impossible to carry out the integration procedure over the entire body.

There are many general textbooks on numerical methods for applied electromagnetics in which the FEM is discussed, however other books [50] could be a rich resource on FEM.

Several commercial EM modeling codes employing the FEM are available. Among those that can be applied to bioelectromagnetics are Maxwell Eminence and HFSS simulator [51, 52]. They employ the FEM and the *boundary element method* (BEM). Other codes are HP HFSS [53] and EMAS.

Generalized Multipole Technique

The *generalized multipole technique* (GMT) is a new method for analyzing EM problems. Like the MOM, GMT is based on the method of weighted residuals, where a system of linear equations is made and solved to find coefficients of the expansion functions that produce the answer. Unlike the MOM, GMT does not have singularities within the boundary.

Generally, GMT is a method for the solution of partial differential equations like *Laplace equations* or the scalar and vector *Helmholtz equations* in piecewise linear, isotropic and homogeneous media. The solution is approximated by a set of base functions that are analytical solutions of the respective differential equations. Multipoles are the most effective expansion functions.

GMT can be applied to various dielectric and conducting configurations. A comprehensive textbook about the GMT technique is authored by Hafner [54]. Commercial codes are also available such as the MMP (Multiple MultiPole) code, which is a semi-analytical field calculation technique, first been proposed in 1980 by Christian Hafner [55, 56]. The MMP has been applied for many dosimetric studies [57-60]. Also, MaX-1: containing GFD and MMP is a new graphic platform for PCs under Windows 95/NT designed by Hafner [61].

13.4 EXPERIMENTAL DOSIMETRY

Although many theoretical methods have been developed for dosimetry, it is useful to confirm the theoretical data experimentally. Experimental methods provide a viable means for estimating SAR under environments that exceed the capabilities of the existing theoretical techniques.

Measuring SAR is simple in theory, but very difficult in practice. The main difficulty arises from the intrusive nature of the ideal methodology. Practically, SAR is measured directly as a temperature increase in a localized area of tissue. Probes may need to be inserted into a live human's head or any part of the body under radiation to map SAR directly. This is impractical; therefore, physical or mathematical models of exposed heads or other parts of the body seem the only viable option for estimating SAR. Theoretical models, however, have their own problems, and building a model for head or any part of the human body involves a lot of approximations in tissue, blood, and other contents.

13.4.1 Phantom Models

Because of the difficulty in measuring actual SAR in the human body, SAR is estimated by measurements using *phantom* models. Phantoms are tissue-equivalent synthetic materials simulating biological bodies. They may be simple or complex depending on the tissue composition as well as the shape [62, 63].

All human tissues have electrical characteristics that are different from air but not so different between each other [64]. For example, at the frequencies used in today's cellular technologies (up to 2.4 GHz), the dielectric constant is in the range of 40 plus and conductivity is around 1 S/m. Regarding phantom material, both high relative permittivity ε and high dielectric loss tangent (tan δ) are required to simulate human tissues.

There are two types of formulations for preparing simulated high water-content tissues such as skin, muscle, various brain tissues, blood, and cerebrospinal fluid [65-67]. First, a moist jelly-like material consisting of saline water, polyethylene powder, and a gelling agent called TX-151. The other type is a liquid consisting of water, sugar, salt, and a compound called HEC, which adjusts the viscosity of the liquid. The jelly-like material is usually used for SAR evaluations with high power applications using temperature measurement methods. The liquid material is transparent, which offers advantages in setting up measurements by allowing only one type of tissue. The liquid tissue material is contained in a shell of the simulated part, about 1-3 mm thick, usually molded from fiberglass or other plastic material with very low RF absorption. Generally, it is difficult to prepare tissue material with the exact properties, so it is desirable to prepare the material with rather higher conductivity and lower permittivity to avoid SAR shortcoming.

In addition, a dry phantom material composed of ceramic powder, graphite powder, and bonding resin also has been developed to simulate tissues for SAR measurement [63]. Multilayered tissues can be simulated by one homogeneous liquid whose electrical properties match those of the tissue that is of most interest [64]. The IEEE SCC 34 SC-2, the group in charge of developing the SAR testing procedures, has agreed this.

Many factors affect the SAR distribution. The shape, for example, should be an engineered representation of the human body. The phantom should allow repeatable measurements of RF energy absorbed by the simulated tissues. Other factors include the shape and radiation characteristics of the source, especially those of antenna, and the relative position of the phantom and the source. In addition, it is necessary to imitate the actual exposure situation as closely as possible in order to ensure the accuracy of the measurements.

There are a variety of phantoms used in SAR measurement [64]: flat, spherical, human-like and a combination of conical shape-universal head phantoms. Flat phantoms are used to represent few parts of the human body. They are also used for experimental setup verification and probe calibration. Spherical phantoms are mainly used for head simulation. Human-like phantoms are used for simulating the human body. They are very complicated due to the variety of models of different sizes and shapes. The combination of canonical shapes-universal head phantom can be used as a head or a body simulator. It contains curved and flat parts. The curved areas represent the upper head (above the ear) and the chin, while the flat parts represent the cheek side of the head.

13.4.2 Measurement Methods

To ensure the accuracy of SAR measurement as precisely as possible, it is necessary to clarify each factor of errors or uncertainty, such as the standard output error of the equipment, errors due to the use of homogeneous phantoms, and errors caused by the vessel of the liquid phantoms. Some unavoidable measurement errors must be left finally, considering them as permissive errors. The IEEE SCC34/SC2 and CENELEC [67] have recently developed standard SAR measurement methods. Through these standardization processes the accuracy of SAR measurement will be enhanced.

Electric Field Measurement Method

SAR distribution in the phantom is derived from the measurement of electric field strength inside the body with implantable isotropic electric field probes (small antennas). SAR is then calculated from Equation (13.3). An electric field probe often consists of electrically short dipole with a diode sensor across its terminals and highly resistive lines to carry the detected signal for measurement. Sensors of the probe are designed to function as true square-law detectors where the output voltage is proportional to the square of the electric field [68-70].

Because of the deviation from the ideal probe and the variation of probe construction, it is useful to characterize the probes to know their limits in terms of *isotropy, spatial resolution, linearity,* and *offset error* [70]. The isotropy of the probe means a constant response of the probe regardless the direction of the electric field vector. Probe uncertainty depends on the direction of the E-field vector relative to the axis of the probe. Isotropy is better in the plane perpendicular to the probe axis and poor in the plane passing through the probe axis. The isotropy can be assessed within the corresponding media in a spherical bowl by rotating the probe around its axis, rotating the field polarization from normal to parallel to the incident plane, and varying the incidence angle from 0 to $90°$, therefore, obtaining hemispherical receiving pattern.

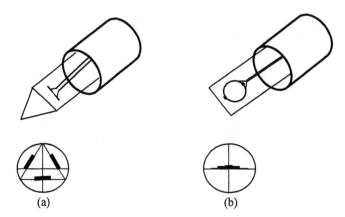

Figure 13-4   (a) Miniature E-field probe. (b) Miniature H-field probe [71].

The spatial resolution of the probe measures its capability to discriminate two RF sources in close proximity. Due to the finite dimensions of the probe, the measured field is not related to field strength at one point but depends on the field in a certain volume around the probe sensors.

Probe linearity is due to the diode detector used to rectify the dipole sensor voltage output. For CW and modulated fields, any nonlinearity must be compensated accurately according to the temporal characteristics.

Offset error is the DC voltage shift even when there is no RF field. This error can be measured and compensated for in the system.

Instruments needed to assemble an electric field measurement system for the measurement of SAR include electric field probes, A/D converters or voltmeters, computer-controlled systems, and phantoms. Such instruments are commercially available. Typical probes are on the order of 3-5 mm in diameter and about 20-30 cm long.

The electric field probes must be calibrated together with the system instrumentation. The calibration should be conducted in the type of tissue media formulated for the test frequency and at that frequency. Some probes are calibrated in two phases, first in air and then in the tissue media. However, a one-phase calibration is possible using a waveguide filled with appropriate biological material and the output voltages of the probe are compared against the calculated field values.

Figure 13-4(a) shows configuration of a miniature E-field probe. The probe is enclosed in a protective sleeve to avoid contact with the simulated media. The probe does not perturb the field being measured. It is isotropic; therefore, the sum of the outputs of the three dipoles gives the same value regardless the position of the probe relative to the electric field.

Magnetic Field Measurement Method

Another way to estimate SAR distribution in the phantom is through the measurement of magnetic field strength. Instrument for measuring magnetic fields consists of two basic components, a loop and a detector. The loop is sensitive only to magnetic field components perpendicular to the plane of the loop. A time- varying magnetic field produces a voltage in the loop that is proportional to the area of the loop and the operating frequency. Therefore, at low frequencies the loop must be large enough in order to be sensitive to weak fields [4]. Figure 13-4(b) shows the configuration of a miniature H-field probe.

Temperature Measurement Method

The SAR distribution in the phantom is also derived from the measurement of the temperature increase due to the absorbed RF energy by using a miniature temperature probe and then calculating SAR from Equation (13.4). This method is suitable for high RF exposure so that heat transfer within and out of the body does not influence the temperature significantly.

13.4.3   SAR Measurement System

As discussed earlier, SAR is measured using isotropic small insertion probes (for electric and magnetic fields) in a volume grid of test points. However, the common measurement practice involves electric field measurement with electric field probes. A multiple-axis probe positioning system and additional instrumentation regarding data processing and calibration are needed for this purpose. Probe placement is conducted either manually or by a robot. A probe supported by a nonmetallic robotic arm moves from one point to another in a homogeneous liquid simulating tissue. The liquid is contained in a *manikin* (a RF transparent shell for the phantom) simulating a human head or another part of the human body. The head model, for example, is usually placed on its side (left or right ear) that allows a handset to be placed underneath the head to facilitate field measurement. A SAR measurement system is illustrated in Figure 13-5 [71- 73].

A few factors influence the results of SAR measurements: isotropic probe response, probe calibration in tissue-equivalent models, tissue properties, phantom shape, sample position, and scan and data acquisition system. In addition, the whole SAR measurement system is usually approved before each SAR measurement using fixed procedures by comparing against some defined results. A known cellular phone, for instance, could be used as a reference to carry out SAR test to determine if previous measurements can be achieved with a

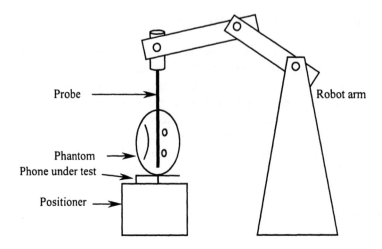

Figure 13-5 A schematic of a SAR measurement system.

certain margin of error. It is also possible to use a reference dipole to irradiate the phantom, or a spherical or rectangular phantom to make similar measurements. Such procedures are necessary for confirming system accuracy and to determine if the system is performing as expected before taking a measurement.

13.5 MOBILE AND PORTABLE WIRELESS DEVICES

Mobile and portable wireless transmitting devices include those operating in the cellular and personal communication networks, satellite communication services, and maritime communications. The above devices, especially handheld cellular phones, are of concern by the public. It is agreed that such devices should be subject to routine RF environmental evaluation prior to use.

13.5.1 Power Ratings

RF exposure is significant from cellular handsets because of the presence of the phone-transmitting antenna close to the head. A very common question that often arises is whether there are potential health risks to users of handheld phones due to their exposure to RFR used for cellular transmissions. The answer to this question lies with the amount of power transmitted by such phones. In general, the transmitted power from a handheld unit determines the operating range of the equipment, which is limited by the available battery power. Further, the output power of the phone is a function of frequency, with more power being permitted at lower frequencies.

Although more power is desirable for longer range, it may cause spurious emissions, which can affect the network as well as the user. Usually, handheld cellular phones operate at low-power levels (several milliwatts to several watts). However, all of this power never enters the user's head. GSM for example, uses a time division multiplexing (TDM) technique with eight time slots. This means that the transmitter is only ever switched on for an eighth of the time. Therefore, the maximum average power output is 0.25 W for a 900 MHz GSM phone. Also the BTS to which it is talking controls the transmitted power of the phone. This allows for a scenario where it is handling eight conversations, one per time slot, with some users very close to the BTS and others far away. The idea is to equalize the strength of the received signals. So 0.25 W is likely to be emitted from a handset that is around 20 km away from the BTS. In addition, the power used while receiving is a small fraction of the transmitted power.

There are also questions as to the potential for the time-division power pulsing of GSM system (signals flash 217 times per second, and this flashing is punctuated at the much slower rate of 8.34 per second) to be the source of the claimed health problems. This is indeed the main cause of electrical interference with computers, car radios, and other electronic equipment. Eight GSM phone users can share a pair of 200 kHz wide-band channels, because each user is given access only to a single time-slot of 576 μs duration in a 4.6 ms frame that is repeated 217 times a second. This 217-Hz cycle of power pulses is in the range of the normal bioelectrical functions both in, and between, cells, so it may induce low-frequency power surges causing health problems rather than the 900-MHz RF frequencies, which probably do not cause health problems. This also applies only to handsets, not to the BTSs: The BTS transmits a steady stream of RFR.

The transmitted power from cellular phones depends on the cellular system and manufacturer. Kuster [74] measured 16 different European digital phones. He could observe wide variation in the SAR values. The phone with lowest SAR, when averaged over 10 g tissue, had a SAR of 0.28 W/kg, while the highest had 1.33 W/kg, all normalized to an antenna input power of 0.25 W. The above measurements were done under normal user conditions. According to the author, the value may go from 0.2 to 3.5 W/kg if the phone is slightly tilted. Therefore, the way the phone is placed widely affects SAR values.

Manning [72, 73] compared SARs from 3 cellular phones with and without personal hands-free kits. The phones were first tested in the four standard positions recommended by CENELEC [67]. Tests were conducted at the left ear. The phone was spaced away from the head using a circular ring spacer of 3.6-mm thickness and 20 mm diameter. This ensures that the phone is placed at a constant of 6 mm from the phantom liquid inside the shell. A significant reduction was observed in the maximum SAR in the head through the use of the personal hands-free as compared with the phone used without personal hands-free (60%-96%).

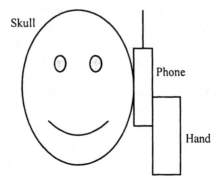

Figure 13-6   A simplified configuration of a human head and a cellular phone.

Even though cellular phones transmit much less power than BTSs, the user's body absorbs more power from the handset antenna. Unlike the mobile phone (car or bag) where the antenna can be separated from the transceiver, the handset exposes the user's head and hand, which are located in the reactive near-field region of the antenna to the highest localized RFR from the antenna. Figure 13-6 shows a simplified configuration of a human head and a cellular phone.

13.5.2   Factors of Concern

RF energy from a cellular phone is transmitted through body tissues, scattered, and attenuated as it passes through, and maximum energy absorption is expected in tissues with high-water content near the surface of head and hand.

In fact, there are three main sources of concern. The first is related to the SAR in the head. From the limited body of literature on dosimetry for cellular phones, it is known that such equipment can generate considerable SAR in the head. But it is difficult to predict or measure the SAR at the user's head because the head is a nonhomogeneous object. In some cases up to 50% of the device output power is deposited in the user's head.

Second, the head is subject to increased energy absorption (hot spots). The location of hot spots depends on the size of the head, the EM characteristics of its layers, and the wavelength of the incident field. Usually, hot spots occur inside lossy spheres that model brain tissue with radii between 0.1- 8 cm for frequencies between 300 MHz and 12 GHz [75]. Similar results were obtained for a multilayered spherical model [76]. It is believed also that keeping a cellular phone clipped to the waist leads to hot spots of radiation, which might be pumped into organs located in that part of the body; for example, the liver and the kidneys. Many users are now attaching cellular phones to their belts as they switch to hands-free kits falsely believing they are safer!

A third issue is related to new technologies, which improve the efficiency and channel utilization through digital modulations. This results in amplitude (pulse) modulation at extremely low-frequency (ELF) signal. Because certain bioeffects have been observed at RF amplitude modulated at ELF and at exposures to ELF alone, there is uncertainty regarding the possibility of RF health risks.

The main concern regarding the potential exposure of the user's head to RFR is brain tumors. Structures such as the vestibulum, cochlea, acoustic nerve, and other cranial nerves are also exposed under these circumstances. It is useful to examine the absorption characteristics of the brain itself. The brain is a tissue rich in water, but with a significant amount of fatty tissue. The brain has a metabolic rate about 16 times higher than that of muscle tissue and consequently generates much more heat than muscle tissue. This is largely compensated by a 20-fold higher rate of blood flow and a somewhat higher thermal conductivity. Therefore, the rate of heat dissipation in brain tissue is higher than that of muscle.

For cellular phones, no commonly agreed calculation or measurement method has been established so far. Since the antenna is in close vicinity to the body, the derived limits for RF exposure are not applicable. Instead, SAR by the body must be determined. Therefore, measurement and computational methods to estimate SAR have been proposed in the scientific literature. The SAR values obtained have to be compared with the basic limits given in the RF protection guidelines.

13.6 DOSIMETRIC STUDIES OF CELLULAR PHONES

There have been several research papers published in peer reviewed scientific journals that show SARs above the exposure limits associated with exposure to cellular phones. These are referred to as positive studies. On the contrary, there have been other studies that have failed to show SARs beyond the limits and are referred to as negative studies.

13.6.1 SAR Investigations

Gandhi [77] used both computational and experimental techniques to estimate SARs in human head for ten cellular phones from four different manufacturers. The computation results were verified using a head-shaped model made of tissue-equivalent materials. Gandhi's results were summarized as follows: peak SAR over any 1 g of tissue 0.09 - 0.29 W/kg; peak SAR over any 1 g of brain tissue 0.04 - 0.17 W/kg; and whole body SAR 0.5 - 1.1 mW/kg.

These figures differ sharply with those obtained by other researchers. For example, by using FDTD calculations on 5×105 cells in 2 mm^3 voxels in an MRI acquired image of a human head, Dimbylow [78] showed SAR values 3.1 W/kg averaged over 10 gm tissue inside the head. SAR averaged over 1 gm of tissue was 4.7 W/kg for a quarter-wave monopole antenna at 900 MHz. When operating at 1.8 GHz the maximum SAR values along the side of the head were 4.6 and 7.7 W/kg for 10 and 1 gm of tissue, respectively. According to the estimated SARs, maximum power that would be required to be emitted to meet the ANSI/IEEE guidelines for public environments (1.6 W/kg) would be 0.34 W at 900 MHz.

Lovisolo et al. [79] reported SAR values of 1.9 W/kg averaged over 10 gm of liquid brain-equivalent material in a cylindrical phantom head exposed to a 0.6-W cellular phone operating at 900 MHz. Their measurements show peak SAR levels of 3.5 and 2.5 W/kg at depths in the head of 5 and 10 mm, respectively. Bone of 5-mm thickness reduced SAR by less than 15%.

Balzano et al. [80] measured SAR induced in human-equivalent phantoms by two types of Motorola cellular phones. They found SAR as high as 1.4 W/kg for "Flip" phones (phones with a very thin radio case and a collapsible antenna; when the antenna is extended, the radiation emitted is slightly further away from the head and this results in lower SAR).

Gandhi et al. [81] described some recent developments in both numerical and experimental methods for determination of SARs and radiation patterns of handheld phones, with emphasis on comparison of results using the two methods. For numerical calculations, it was possible to use the Pro-Engineer CAD Files of cellular phones for a realistic description of the device. Also, they used the expanding grid formulation of the FDTD method for finer-resolution representation of the coupled region, including the antenna, and an increasingly coarser representation of the more-distant, less-coupled region. Automated SAR and radiation pattern measurement systems were used to validate both the calculated 1-g SARs and radiation patterns for several telephones, including some research test samples, using a variety of antennas. Even though widely different peak 1-g SARs were obtained, ranging from 0.13 to 5.41 W/kg, agreement between the calculated and the measured data for these telephones, five each at 835 and 1900 MHz, was excellent and generally within ±20% (±1 dB). An important observation was that for a maximum radiated power of 600 mW at 800/900 MHz, which may be used for phones using AMPS technology, the peak 1-g SAR could be higher than 1.6 W/kg. This may be reduced carefully designing the antenna and placing it further away from the head.

13.6.2 Warmth Sensation

A warmth sensation could occur while using a cellular phone for many reasons: because of radiation from the phone, heat from the battery, blocking of heat radiation from the head, and other aspects of phone's use.

Anderson and Joyner [82] measured electric fields induced within a phantom head from exposure to three different AMPS handheld phones using an implantable probe. Measurements were taken in the eye nearest the phone and along a lateral scan through the brain from its center to the side nearest the phone. During the measurement, the phones were positioned alongside the phantom head as in typical use and were configured to transmit at maximum power (600-mW nominal). SARs induced in the eye ranged from 0.007 to 0.21 W/kg. Metal-framed spectacles enhanced SARs in the eye by 9-29%. In the brain, the maximum levels were recorded at the measurement point closest to the phone and ranged from 0.12 to 0.83 W/kg. Thermal analysis of the eye indicated only 0.022°C maximum steady-state temperature rise in the eye from a uniform SAR loading of 0.21 W/kg. Thermal analysis in the brain also indicated a small temperature rise of 0.034°C for a local SAR loading of 0.83 W/kg.

Törnevik et al. [83] measured temperature increases around the ear on human volunteers holding cellular phones. The maximum temperature readings ranged between 37 and 41°C for analog phones and between 36 and 39°C for GSM phones.

Van Leeuwen et al. [84] evaluated the 3D-temperature rise induced by a mobile phone inside a realistic head model. This was done numerically using an FDTD model to predict the absorbed electromagnetic power distribution, and a thermal model describing bioheat transfer both by conduction and by blood flow. The researchers calculated a maximum rise in brain temperature of 0.11°C for antenna with an average emitted power of 0.25 W. Maximum temperature rise was at the skin. A maximum averaged SAR characterized the power distributions over an arbitrarily shaped 10-g volume of approximately 1.6 W/kg. Although these power distributions are not in compliance with all proposed safety standards, temperature rises are far too small to have lasting effects.

Wainwright [85] developed a finite element thermal model of the head to calculate temperature rises generated in the brain by radiation from cellular phones and similar EM devices. A 1-mm resolution MRI dataset was segmented semiautomatically, assigning each volume element to one of ten tissue types. A finite element mesh was then generated using a fully automatic tetrahedral mesh generator developed at the NRPB. There were two sources of heat in the model: first, the natural metabolic heat production; and second, the power absorbed from the EM field. The SAR was derived from an FDTD model of the head, coupled to a model mobile phone, namely a quarter-wavelength antenna mounted on a metal box. The steady-state temperature distribution was calculated using the standard *Pennes bioheat equation*. It was observed that in the normal cerebral cortex the high blood perfusion rate serves to provide an efficient cooling mechanism. In the case of equipment generally available to the public, the maximum temperature rise found in the brain was about 0.1°C.

13.6.3   Exposure Systems

A carrousel irradiator for mice, which delivers a headfirst and near-field RF exposure that closely simulates cellular phone use, was developed by Swicord et al. [86] in Motorola. Mouse cadavers were placed on the carrousel irradiator and exposed with their nose 5 mm from the feed point of a 1.6 GHz antenna. Local measurements of SAR in brain regions corresponding to the frontal cortex, medial caudate putamen, and mid hippocampal areas were 2.9, 2.4, and 2.2 W/kg per watt of irradiated power, respectively. The average SAR was estimated to be 3.4 W/kg per watt along the sagittal plain of the brain, 2.0 W/kg per watt along the sagittal plane of the body, and between 6.8 and 8.1 W/kg per watt at peak locations along the sagittal plane of the body surface.

Chou et al. [87] developed an animal exposure system for bioeffect studies of RFR from handheld telephones, with energy deposition in animal brains comparable to those in humans. The FDTD method was initially used to compute SAR in an ellipsoidal rat model exposed with various size loop antennas at different distances from the model. A 3×1-cm rectangular loop produced acceptable SAR patterns. Sprague Dawley rats were exposed with a 3×1-cm loop antenna tuned to 837 or 1957 MHz for thermographically determined SAR distributions. Point SARs in brains of restrained rats were also determined thermometrically using fiberoptic probes. Calculated and measured SAR patterns and results from the various exposure configurations were in general agreement. The FDTD computed average brain SAR and ratio of head to whole body absorption were 23.8 W/kg/W and 62% at 837 MHz, and 22.6 W/kg/W and 89% at 1957 MHz. The average brain to whole-body SAR ratio was 20 to 1 for both frequencies. At 837 MHz, the maximum measured SAR in the restrained rat brains was 51 W/kg per watt in the cerebellum and 40 W/kg per watt at the top of the cerebrum. According to the authors, two-tenths of a watt input power to the loop antenna will produce 10 W/kg maximum SAR, and an estimated 4.8 W/kg average brain SAR in a 300 g medium size rat.

13.7   RECENT AUTHORITATIVE CONCLUSIONS

Over the years, a large body of work regarding the possible harmful effects of radiation from mobile phones has been conducted, but the puzzle still remains; many experts interpret the available evidence from the above studies and come to conclusions that may not tell the whole story.

13.7.1   Vienna EMF-Resolution

In 1998, Vienna EMF-Resolution [88] was passed by representatives from the United States, New Zealand, Germany, Canada, Sweden, Poland, and Belgium who have attended the Mobile Phones and Health Symposium at the University of Vienna, Austria. According to the resolution: "The participants agreed that biological effects from low-intensity exposures are scientifically established. However, the current state of scientific consensus is inadequate to derive reliable exposure standards. The existing evidence demands an increase in the research efforts on possible health risk and on an adequate exposure and dose assessment."

Regarding cellular phones and ways to improve situation of the users, the resolution states: "Technical data should be made available to the users to allow comparison with respect to EM exposure. In order to promote prudent usage, sufficient information on the health debate should be provided. This procedure will offer opportunities for the users to manage reduction in RFR exposure. Also, this process could stimulate further developments of low-intensity emission devices."

13.7.2   The Food and Drug Administration

In October 1999, the U.S. Food and Drug Administration (FDA) released a consumer update on mobile phones. This update was an answer to questions that have been raised about cellular phones. The FDA stated that little was known about the possible health effects of repeated or long-term exposure to low-level RFR of the type emitted by cellular phones. Nevertheless, the FDA has urged the mobile phone industry to take a number of steps to assure public safety. The agency has fixed the following recommendations for the industry [89]:

1. The need to support research into possible biological effects of RFR of the type emitted by mobile phones.
2. Mobile phones need to be designed in a way that minimizes any RF exposure to the user that is not necessary for device function.
3. Cooperation is required to provide users with the best possible information on what is known about bioeffects of mobile phone use.

13.7.3   The Independent Expert Group on Mobile Phones

The British government had asked the Chairman of the National Radiological Protection Board (NRPB) to establish an independent group of experts to evaluate possible adverse health effects of mobile phones. The Independent Expert Group on Mobile Phones (IEGMP) was set up under the chairmanship of Sir William Stewart and represented a wide spectrum of expertise with leading figures from physics, radio engineering, biology, medicine, and epidemiology, in addition to lay members.

In May 2000, the Britain's Independent Expert Group presented its report (http://www.iegmp.org.uk/IEGMPtxt.htm). According to the IEGMP: "We conclude therefore that it is not possible at present to say that exposure to RF radiation, even at levels below national guidelines, is totally without potential adverse health effects, and that the gaps in knowledge are sufficient to justify a precautionary approach."

Also, the report presented a number of recommendations:

1.   Telecommunication network operators must notify the local authority of the proposed installation of BTSs (macrocells, microcells, and picocells).
2.   Operators should avoid situating BTSs near schools.
3.   Phone companies should provide information (for example, SAR) for consumers to allow them to make informed choices about personal exposures resulting from their use.
4.   Companies should be discouraged from promoting the use of cellular phones by children.

13.7.4   The American Cancer Society

In May 2000, the American Cancer Society bulletin says: "No solid evidence yet exists regarding cell phones and cancer." The bulletin also stated that a scientific panel that was commissioned by the British government to evaluate research to date on health risks of cell phones warns that children may be at greater risk of injury from cell phone radiation because their central nervous system (CNS), including the brain, is still developing.

13.7.5   The World Health Organization

According to the Fact Sheet No. 193 released by the World Health Organization (WHO) in June 2000: "Most studies have examined the results of short-term, whole-body exposure to RF fields at levels far higher than those normally associated with wireless communications. With the advent of such devices as walkie-talkies and mobile phones, it has become apparent that few studies address the consequences of localized exposures to RF fields to the head."

Regarding cancer, WHO states: "Current scientific evidence indicates that exposure to RF fields, such as those emitted by mobile phones and their base stations, is unlikely to induce or promote cancers. Several studies of animals exposed to RF fields similar to those emitted by mobile phones found no evidence that RF fields causes or promotes brain cancer. While one 1997 study found that RF fields increased the rate at which genetically engineered mice developed lymphoma, the health implications of this result is unclear."

13.8 CONCLUDING REMARKS

Today, most people have either portable phone in the home, cell phone for away-from-home use or both. New data transmission protocols with higher data rates over the existing GSM system (e.g., GPRS) will also lead to higher mean output power. These devices are connecting people in convenient ways as their cost continues to drop as the market increases in size and technologies become more capable and increasingly cheaper to operate.

The idea of health effects from cellular phones or other devices is fast becoming the focus of much research. As health concerns surrounding wireless networks in general and cellular phones in particular grow, the public is demanding that government, industry, and the scientific communities should address this matter seriously. Over the years, governments and industries, mostly in cooperation with research communities, are sending out indefinite and often conflicting messages, raising a number of difficult questions. On the other hand, the cellular phone industry has been giving assimilated messages regarding safety. The industry continues to downplay the risk and hold off on more research. The public always seeks proof, and habitually interprets scientific evidence oppositely from scientists. The strict proof required is changing the basics of the life sciences. This will occur when the impact of low-level RF energy is understood. Waiting for the proof does not reassure the public. Apprehension and bad feelings command the discourse, and these feelings are generally pointed at the industry.

The "precautionary principle" could be the right answer for an age in which technology is advancing and the impact of that technology may not be known for years. However, because of uncertainty in the medical and scientific communities concerning nonionizing radiation, it is recommended that law enforcement agencies implement a policy of "prudent avoidance," including purchasing equipment with the lowest published maximum power densities.

While uncertainty continues, it is fair to exercise some prudence in the use of cellular phones. It is, of course, the user's choice as to whether they have a cellular phone in the first place and how much they choose to use it. If individuals are very concerned about the potential health risk that might result from the use of a RF-emitting device to the side of their head, they may simply choose to avoid or minimize their usage pattern. An alternative solution, which may be more practical, is to keep a greater distance between the antenna and the user's head. This may be easily accomplished by the use of kits that connect an earpiece to the phone by means of a cable.

However, any technique or procedure that modifies the design, construction, or operation of the radiating system in order to prevent undesired radiation could be considered to be a radiation source control.

In addition, certain procedures might be useful for users to follow:

1. Reducing the use of cellular phones is regarded as the best step. As a perceptional matter, avoid speaking for long periods on the phone.
2. Use by children should be eliminated because of their developing nervous system.
3. Avoid using the phone in areas where the signal is weak. For example, indoor use, which involves weak signals from the base station, increases exposure significantly because the signal strength requires creating a stronger connection from inside a car or building.
4. Keep the antenna away from the head and point it away from the body.
5. Place the phone in the *intended use position* as was suggested by a working group of CENELEC under the EU mandate M/032 [1]. The intended use position is established by fully pulling out the antenna from the mobile phone. The center of the earpiece should be placed directly at the entrance of the auditory canal. The intended use position is defined by an angle of 80° between the reference line of the phone (the line lies within the reference plane defined by the auditory canal openings of both ears and the center of the closed mouth) and the line connecting both auditory canal openings.
6. Unless a cellular phone is switched off it is in constant use, and may adversely affect the user's body if carried in clothing or attached to a belt. Accordingly, keep the phone away from the body when in standby mode. For example, avoid carrying the phone in the belt around the waist. It is worthless to expose the deposits of bone marrow in the hips and the testicles to RFR.

REFERENCES

[1] Kuster, N., and Q. Balzano, Experimental and Numerical Dosimetry, In *Mobile Communications Safety* (eds. Kuster, N., Q. Balzano, and J. C. Lin), pp. 13-58, Chapman & Hall, London, UK, 1997.
[2] Durney, C. H., and D. A. Christensen, *Basic Introduction to Bioelectromagnetics*, CRC Press, Boca Raton, FL, 1999.
[3] Erdreich, L. S., O. P. Gandhi, H. Lai, and M. C. Ziskin, Assessment of Public Health Concerns Associated with Pave Paws Radar Installations, The Massachusetts

Department of Public Health, MA, 1999.

[4] Durney, C. H., H. Massoudi, and M. F. Iskander, *Radiofrequency Radiation Dosimetry Handbook*, Electrical Engineering Department, The University of Utah, Salt Lake City, Utah, 1986.

[5] Elder, J. A., P. A. Czerski, M. A. Stuchly, K. H. Mild, and A. Sheppard, Radiofrequency Radiation, In *Nonionizing Radiation Protection* (eds. Suess, M. J., and D. A. Benwell-Morison), WHO Regional Publications, European Series 25, pp. 117-173, 1989.

[6] IEEE Standard for Safety Levels with Respect to Human Exposure to Radio Frequency Electromagnetic Fields: 3 kHz to 300 GHz, IEEE Standard C95.1-1999, IEEE, New York, NY, 1999.

[7] Joines, W.T., and R. J. Spiegel, Resonance Absorption of Microwaves by Human Skull, *IEEE Transactions on Biomedical Engineering* 21, pp. 46-48, 1974.

[8] Lin, J. C., Microwave Properties of Fresh Mammalian Brain Tissues at Body Temperature, *IEEE Transactions on Biomedical Engineering* 22, pp. 74-76, 1975.

[9] Wu, C. L., and J. C. Lin, Absorption and Scattering of electromagnetic waves by Prolate Spheroidal Models of Biological Structures, *IEEE Antenna and Propagation Society International Symposium Digest*, pp. 142-145, 1977.

[10] Hagmann, M. J., and O. P. Gandhi, Numerical Calculations of Electromagnetic Energy Deposition in Models of Man with Grounding and Reflector Effects, *Radio Science* 14 (6S), pp. 23-29, 1979.

[11] Karimullah, K., K. -M. Chen, and D. P. Nyquist, Electromagnetic Coupling Between a Thin-Wire Antenna and a Neighboring Biological Body: Theory and Experiment, *IEEE Transactions on Microwave Theory Technology* 28, pp. 1218-1225, 1980.

[12] Hubing, T. H., Survey of Numerical Electromagnetic Modeling Techniques, Electromagnetic Compatibility Laboratory, Report No. TR91-1-001.3, 1991.

[13] Habash, R. W. Y., Non-Invasive Microwave Hyperthermia, PhD Thesis, Indian Institute of Science, Bangalore, India, 1994.

[14] Lin, J. C., A. W. Guy, and C. C. Johnson, Power Absorption in a Spherical Model of Man Exposed to 1-20 MHz Electromagnetic Field, *IEEE Transactions on Microwave Theory and Techniques* 21, pp. 791-797, 1973.

[15] Johnson, C. C., C. H. Durney, and H. Massoudi, Long Wavelength Electromagnetic Power Absorption in Prolate Spheroid Models of Man and Animals, *IEEE Transactions on Microwave Theory Techniques* 23, pp. 739-747, 1975.

[16] Barber, P. W., Electromagnetic Absorption in Prolate Spheroidal Models of Man and Animals at Resonance, *IEEE Transactions On Biomedical Engineering* 24, pp. 513-521, 1977.

[17] Durney, C. H., Electromagnetic Dosimetry for Models of Humans and Animals: A Review of Theoretical and Numerical Techniques, *Proceedings of the IEEE* 68(1), pp. 33-40, 1980.

[18] Massoudi, H., C. H. Durney, and C. C. Johnson, Long Wavelength Analysis of Plane Wave Irradiation of an Ellipsoidal Model of Man, *IEEE Transactions on Microwave Theory and Techniques* 25, pp. 41-46, 1977.

[19] Barber, P. W., Resonance Electromagnetic Absorption by Non-Spherical Dielectric Objects, *IEEE Transactions on Microwave Theory and Techniques* 25, pp. 373-381, 1977.

[20] Caorsi, S., M. Pastorino, and M. Raffetto, Analytic SAR Computation in a Multilayer Elliptic Cylinder for Bioelectromagnetic Applications, *Bioelectromagnetics* 20, pp. 365-371, 1999.

[21] Caorsi, S., M. Pastorino, and M. Raffetto, Analytic SAR Computation in a Multilayer Elliptic Cylinder: The Near-Field Line-Current Radiation Case, *Bioelectromagnetics* 21, pp. 473-479, 2000.

[22] Massoudi, H., C. H. Durney, and C. C. Johnson, The Geometric Optic Solution and the Exact Solution for Internal Fields in a Cylindrical Model of Man Irradiated by Electromagnetic Plane Wave, *International Symposium on Biological Effects of Electromagnetic Waves*, p. 49, Airlie, VA, 1977.

[23] Rowlandson, G. I., and P. W. Barber, RF Energy Absorption in Biological Models: Calculations Based on Geometerical Optics, *International Symposium on Biological Effects of Electromagnetic Waves*, p. 50, Airlie, VA, 1977.

[24] Livesay, D. E., and K. M. Chen, Electromagnetic Fields Induced Inside Arbitrary Shaped Biological Bodies, *IEEE Transactions on Microwave Theory and Techniques* 22, pp. 1273-1280, 1974.

[25] Chen, K. M., and B. S. Guru, Internal EM Field and Absorbed Power Density in Human Torso Induced by 1-500 MHz EM Waves, *IEEE Transactions on Microwave Theory and Techniques* 25, pp. 746-756, 1977.

[26] Barber, P. W., O. P. Gandhi, M. J. Hagmann, and I. Chatterjee, Electromagnetic Absorption in Multilayered Model of Man, *IEEE Transactions on Biomedical Engineering* 26, pp. 400-405, 1979.

[27] King, R. W. P., Electromagnetic Field Generated in Model of Human Head by Simplified Telephone Transceivers, *Radio Science* 30, pp. 267-281, 1995.

[28] Richmond, J. H., Digital Computer Solutions of the Rigorous Equations for Scattering Problems, *Proceedings of the IEEE* 53, pp. 796-804, 1965.

[29] Harrington, R. F., Matrix Methods for Field Problems, *Proceedings of the IEEE* 55, pp. 136-149, 1967.

[30] Logan, J. C., and J. W. Rockway, The New MININEC (Version 3): A MiniNumerical Electromagnetic Code, Naval Ocean Systems Center, NOSC TD 938, San Diego, CA, 1986.

[31] Yee, K. S., Numerical Solution of Initial Boundary Value Problems Involving Maxwell's Equations in Isotropic Media, *IEEE Transactions on Antennas and Propagation* 14, pp. 302-307, 1966.

[32] Taflove, A., and M. E. Brodwin, Numerical Solution of Steady State Electromagnetic Problems Using the Time Dependent Maxwell's Equations, *IEEE Transactions on Microwave Theory and Techniques* 23, pp. 623-660, 1975.

[33] Taflove, A., and M. E. Brodwin, Computation of the Electromagnetic Fields and Induced Temperatures Within a Model of the Microwave Irradiated Human Eye, *IEEE Transactions on Microwave Theory and Techniques* 23, pp. 888-896, 1975.

[34] Kunz, K. S., and J. L. Raymond, *The Finite Difference Time Domain Method for Electromagnetics*, CRC Press, Boca Raton, FL, 1993.

[35] Taflove, A., *Computational Electrodynamics: The Finite-Difference Time-Domain Method*, Artech House, Norwood, MA, 1995.

[36] Taflove, A., *Advances in Computational Electrodynamics: The Finite-Difference Time-Domain Method*, Artech House, Norwood, MA, 1998.

[37] Sullivan, D. M., D. T. Borup, and O. P. Gandhi, Use of the Finite Difference Time Domain Method in Calculating Absorption in Human Tissues, *IEEE Transactions on Bioemedical Engineering* 34, pp. 148-157, 1987.

[38] Sullivan, D. M., O. P. Gandhi, and A. Taflove, Use of the Finite Difference Time Domain Method in Calculating EM Absorption in Man Models, *IEEE Transactions on Microwave Theory and Techniques* 35, pp.179-185, 1988.

[39] Gandhi, O. P., Y. –G. Gu, J. –Y. Chen, and H. I. Bassen, Specific Absorption Rates and Induced Current Distributions in an Anatomically Based Human Model for Plane-Wave Exposures, *Health Physics* 63, pp. 281-290, 1992.

[40] Spiegel, R. J., M. B. A. Fatmi, S. S. Stuchly, and M. A. Stuchly, Comparison of Finite-Difference Time-Domain SAR Calculations with Measurements in a Heterogeneous Model of Man, *IEEE Transactions on Biomedical Engineering* 36, pp. 849-855, 1989.

[41] Kuwano, S., and K. Kokubun, Calculation of SAR in a Human Body Model with a Reflecting Wall for Microwave Irradiation, *International Symposium on Electromagnetic Compatibility*, Sendai, Japan, pp. 238-240 1994.

[42] Kuwano, S., and K. Kokubun, Microwave Power Absorption in a Cylindrical Model of Man in the Presence of a Flat Reflector, *IEICE Transactions on Commununications* E78-B, 11, pp. 1548-1550, 1995.

[43] Watanabe, S., and M. Taki, Distributions of Specific Absorption Rate of Human Model Exposed to Near-Field of a Small Radiation Source, *International Symposium on Electromagnetic Compatibility*, Sendai, Japan, pp. 421-424, 1994.

[44] Watanabe, S., M. Taki, and Y. Kamimura, Frequency Characteristics of Energy Deposition in Human Model Exposed to Near Field of an Electric or a Magnetic Dipole, *IEICE Transactions on Communications* E77-B 6, pp. 725-731, 1994.

[45] XFDTD Remcom Inc., State College, PA, USA.

[46] CST GmbH, Computer Simulation Technology, CST, Darmstadt, Germany.

[47] EMI Toolbox Modeling Software, EMIT, SETH Corporation, Johnstown, PA, USA.

[48] Jin, J. -M., *The Finite Element Method in Electromagnetics*, John Wiley and Sons, Piscataway, NJ, 1993.

[49] Silvester, P. P., and G. Pelosi, *Finite Elements for Wave Electromagnetics*, IEEE Press, New York, NY, 1994.

[50] Silverster, P. P., and R. F. Ferrari, *Finite Elements for Electrical Engineers*, Cambridge University Press, New York, NY, 1996.

[51] Maxwell Eminence, Ansoft Corporation, Pittsburgh, PA, USA.

[52] Ansoft HFSS, Ansoft Corporation, Pittsburgh, PA, USA.

[53] HP HFSS Designer Version 5.2, Hewlett Packard, 1998.

[54] Hafner, C., *The Generalized Multipole Technique for Computational Electromagnetics*, Artech House, Norwood, MA, 1990.

[55] Hafner, C., *2-D MMP: Two Dimensional Multiple Multipole Analysis Software and User's Manual*, Artech House, Norwood, MA, 1990.

[56] Hafner, C., and Bomholt L., Demo Version of the 3D MMP Codes for Personal Computers, *ACES Short Course Notes*, Monterey, CA, 1992.

[57] Kuster, N., and Q. Balzano, Energy Absorption Mechanism by Biological Bodies in the Near Field of Dipole Antennas Above 300 MHz, *IEEE Transactions on Vehicular Technology* 41, pp. 17-23, 1992.

[58] Tay, R. Y., and N. Kuster, Performance of the Generalized Multipole Technique (GMT/MMP) for Antenna Design and Optimization, *Applied Computational Electromagnetics Journal* 9, pp. 79-89, 1994.

[59] Haueisen, J., C. Hafner, H. Nowak, and H. Brauer, Neuromagnetic Field Computation Using the Multiple Multipole Method, *International Journal of Numerical Modelling: Special Issue on Computational Magnetics* 9, 145-158, 1996.

[60] Martin, A., R. Villar, and M. Martinez-Búrdalo, Using the Generalized Multipole Technique to Study the Interaction Between Electromagnetic Fields and Dielectric Objects, *International Union of Radio Science*, Lille, France, 28 August-5 September 1996.

[61] Hafner, C., *MaX-1: A Visual Electromagnetics Platform*, John Wiley & Sons, Chichester, UK, 1998.

[62] Kuster, N., and Q. Balzano, Experimental and Numerical Dosimetry, In *Mobile Communication Safety* (eds. Kuster, N., and Q. Balzano), pp. 13-64, Chapman & Hall, London, UK, 1997.

[63] Tamura, H., Y. Ishikawa, and T. Kobayashi, A Dry Pahntom Material Composed of Ceramic and Graphite Powder, *IEEE Transactions on Electromagnetic Compatibility* 39, 1997.

[64] Phantom Definition-Contribution to IEEE SCC34 SC2 WG1 to Faciliate Preparation of Section 2 and 4, APREL, Spectrum Sciences Institute, RF Dosimetry Research Board, Ontario, Canada, 1998.

[65] Guy, A. W., Analyses of Electromagnetic Fields Induced in Biological Tissues by Thermographic Studies on Equivalent Phantom Models, *IEEE Transactions on Microwave Theory and Techniques* 19, pp. 205-214, 1971.

[66] SAR Measurements Requirements SSI/DRB-TP-D01-030, APREL, Spectrum Sciences Institute, RF Dosimetry Research Board, Ontario, Canada, 1998.

[67] Considerations for the Evaluation of Human Exposure to Electromagnetic Fields (EMFs) from Mobile Telecommunication Equipment (MTE) in the Frequency Range 30 MHz-6 MHz, CENELEC European Specifications ES 59005, 1998.

[68] Smith, G. S., Limitation on the Size of Miniature Electric-Field Probes, *IEEE Transactions on Microwave Theory and Techniques* 32, pp. 594-600, 1984.

[69] Chou, C. K., RF Dosimetry for Mobile Telephone Handsets, Motorola Florida Research Laboratories, Fort Lauderdale, FL, 1998.

[70] Chan, K., R. F. Jr. Cleveland, and D. L. Means, Evaluating Compliance with FCC Guidelines for Human Exposure to Radiofrequency Electromagnetic Fields, Supplement C (Edition 97-01) to OET Bulletin 65, Edition 97-01, Federal Communications Commission Office of Engineering and Technology, 1997.

[71] Wojcik, J. J., and P. G. Cardinal, New Advanced Methodology for Near Field Measurements for SAR and Antenna Development, *IEEE Symposium on EMC*, Seattle, Washington, 2-6 August 1999.

[72] Manning, M., SAR Tests of Two Mobile Phones with Personal Hands-Free Kits, SARTest Report 75/00 (Report prepared by SARTest Ltd for Vodafone), 2000.

[73] Manning, M., SAR Tests of Two Mobile Phones with Personal Hands-Free Kits, SARTest Report 77/00 (Report prepared by SARTest Ltd for One2One), 2000.

[74] Kuster, N., Swiss Tests Show Wide Variation in Radiation Exposure from Cell Phones, *Microwave News*, pp. 10-11, 1997.

[75] Kritikos, H. N., and H. P. Schwan, The Distribution of Heating Potential Inside Lossy Spheres, *IEEE Transactions on Biomedical Engineering* 22, pp. 457-463, 1975.

[76] Kritikos, H. N., and H. P. Schwan, Formation of Hot Spots in Multilayer Spheres, *IEEE Transactions on Biomedical Engineering* 23, pp. 168-172, 1976.

[77] Gandhi, P. O., ANSI Radiofrequency Safety Guide: Its Rationale, Some Problems and Suggested Improvements, In *Biological Effects and Medical Applications of Electromagnetic Energy* (ed. Gandhi, O. P.), pp. 29-46, Prentice Hall, Engelwood, NJ, 1990.

[78] Dimbylow, P. J., FDTD calculations at the SAR for a Dipole Closely Coupled to the Head at 900 MHz and 1.9 GHz, *Physics in Medicine and Biology* 38, pp. 361-368, 1993.

[79] Lovisolo, G. A., L. Raganella, S. Nocentini, F. Bardati, A. Gerardino, and P. Tognolatti, Hand-Held Cellular Telephones: SAR Deposition in Phantoms, *The Bioelectromagnetics Society Meeting* (Abstract), p. 65, 1994.

[80] Balzano, Q., O. Garay, and T. J. Manning, Electromagnetic Energy Exposure of Simulated Users of Portable Cellular Telephones, *IEEE Transactions on Vehicular Technology* 44, pp. 390-403, 1995.

[81] Gandhi, Om. P., L. Gianluca, A. Tinniswood, and Q. -S. Yu, Comparison of Numerical and Experimental Methods for Determination of SAR and Radiation Patterns of Handheld Wireless Telephones, *Bioelectromagnetics* 20, pp. 93-101, 1999.

[82] Anderson, V., and K. H. Joyner, Specific Absorption Rate Levels Measured in a Phantom Head Exposed to Radio Frequency Transmissions from Analog Hand-Held Mobile Phones, *Bioelectromagnetics* 16, pp. 60-69, 1995.

[83] Törnevik, C., V. Santomaa, and Q. Balzano, Evaluation of the Temperature Increase at Ear of Cell Phone Users, *The Bioelectromagnetics Society Meeting*, St. Pete's Beach, Florida, 1998.

[84] Van Leeuwen, G. M., J. J. Lagendijk, B. J. Van Leersum, A. P. Zwamborn, S. N. Hornsleth, and A. N. Kotte, Calculation of Change in Brain Temperatures Due to Exposure to a Mobile Phone, *Physics in Medicine and Biology* 44, pp. 2367-2379, 1999.

[85] Wainwright, P., Thermal Effects of Radiation from Cellular Telephones, *Physics in Medicine and Biology* 45, pp. 2363-2372, 2000.

[86] Swicord, M, J. Morrissey, D. Zakharia, M. Ballen, and Q. Bazano, Dosimetry in Mice Exposed to 1.6 GHz Microwaves in a Carrousel Irradiator, *Bioelectromagnetics* 20, pp. 42-47, 1999.

[87] Chou, C. K., K. W. Chan, J. A. McDougall, and A. W. Guy, Development of a Rat Head Exposure System for Simulating Human Exposure to RF Fields from Handheld Wireless Telephones, *Bioelectromagnetics* 20, pp. 75-92, 1999.

[88] Workshop on Possible Biological and Health Effects of RF Electromagnetic Fields, Vienna EMF Resolution, University of Vienna, Austria, October 25-28, 1998.

[89] FDA Center for Devices and Radiological Health, Consumer Update on Mobile Phones, October 1999.

Acronyms and Abbreviations

1G	first generation
2G	second generation
3G	third generation
4G	fourth generation
5G	fifth generation
AC	alternating current
AC	authentication center
ACA	Australian Communications Authority
ACGIH	American Conference of Governmental Industrial Hygienists
AD	Alzheimer's Disease
ALARA	as low as reasonably achievable
ALL	acute lymphoblastic leukemia
ALS	amyotrophic lateral sclerosis
AFOSH	Air Force Occupational Safety and Health
AM	amplitude modulation
AML	acute myeloid leukemia
AMPS	Advanced Mobile Phone Service
ANSI	American National Standards Institute
ARL	Australian Radiation Laboratory
ARRL	American Radio Relay League
ASA	American Standard Association
BBB	blood-brain barrier
BEI	biological exposure indice
BEM	boundary element method
BMR	basal metabolic rate
BSC	base station controller
BTS	base transceiver station
CAD	computer-aided design
CCG	Children's Cancer Group
CDC	Centers for Disease Control and Prevention
CENELEC	Comite Europeen de Normalisation Electrotechnique
CDMA	code division multiple access
CDRH	Center for Devices and Radiological Health

CFIDS	chronic fatigue and immune dysfunction syndrome
CFS	chronic fatigue syndrome
CGS	centimeter-gram-second
CLL	chronic lymphocytic leukemia
CNS	central nervous system
COMAR	Committee on Man and Radiation (IEEE)
COST	European cooperation in the field of science and technical research
CRT	cathode ray tube
CST	Computer Simulation Technology
CT	cordless telephone
CTIA	Cellular Telecommunications Industry Association
CW	continuous wave
dB	decibel
D-AMPS	Digital AMPS
DCS	Digital Communications Services
DECT	Digital European Cordless Telephone
DEN	diethylnitrosamine
DNA	deoxyribonucleic acid
DOD	Department of Defence
DOE	Department of Energy
EBCM	extended boundary condition method
ECG	electrocardiogram
EEG	electroencephaography
EIA	Electronic Industries Association
ELF	extremely low frequency
EM	electromagnetic
EMF	electromagnetic fields
EMF-RAPID	Electric and Magnetic Fields Research and Public Information Dissemination
EMC	electromagnetic compatibility
EMI	electromagnetic interference
EMIT	electromagnetic interference toolbox
ENU	neurocarcinogen ethylnitrosourea
EPA	Environmental Protection Agency
EPA-OPPE	EPA's Office of Policy, Planning, and Evaluation
EPA-ORP	EPA's Office of Radiation Program
ERP	effective radiated power
ES	electrical sensitivity
ETACS	Extended Total Access Telecommunication System
ETDMA	Enhanced TDMA
ETSI	European Telecommunications Standards Institute
EU	European Union

eV	electron volts
FCC	Federal Communications Commission
FDTD	finite difference time domain
FDA	Food and Drug Adminstration
FDA-CDRH	FDA's Center for Devices and Radiological Health
FDMA	frequency division multiple access
FEM	finite element method
FIM	finite integration method
FM	frequency modulation
FRG	Federal Republic of Germany
GM	geometric mean
GFD	generalized finite difference
GIC	geomagnetically induced currents
GMT	generalized multipole technique
GPRS	General Packet Radio Service
GSD	geometric standard deviation
GSM	Global System for Mobile Communication
HAPS	High Altitude Atmospheric Platform Station
HF	high frequency
HFSS	high frequency structure simulator
HLR	home location register
Hz	hertz, originally cycles per second
IEBCM	iterative extended boundary condition method
IEEE	Institute of Electrical and Electronics Engineers
IEGMP	Independent Expert Group on Mobile Phones
ICINRP	International Commission on Non-Ionizing Radiation Protection
INIRC	International Nonionizing Radiation Committee
IPTM	Institute of Police Technology and Management
IR	infrared
IRI	inter-response intervals
IRIDIUM	Low Earth Orbit Satellite Cellular System
IRPA	International Radiation Protection Association
ISM	industrial scientific medical
ITS	intelligent transport systems
ITU	International Telecommunication Union
JDC	Japanese Digital Cellular
JTACS	Japanese Total Access Telecommunication System
LCD	liquid crystal display

LF   low frequency

MEE   maximum exposure energy
MF   medium frequency
MKSA   meter-kilogram-second-ampere
MMP   Multiple MultiPole
MOM   method of moment
MPE   maximum permissible exposure
MPT   Ministry of Posts and Telecommunications (Japan)
MRI   magnetic resonance imager
MS   mobile station
MSC   mobile switching centre
MTE   mobile telecommunication equipment
MTSO   mobile telecommunication switching office

NADC   North American Digital Cellular
NAS   National Academy of Sciences
NATO   North Atlantic Treaty Organization
NBS   National Bureau of Standards
NCGIH   National Conference of Governmental Industrial Hygienists
NCRP   National Council on Radiation Protection and Measurements
NGO   nongovernment organization
NH & MRC   National Health and Medical Research Council
NIEHS   National Institute of Environmental Health Sciences
NIOSH   National Institute for Occupational Safety and Health
NIST   National Institute of Standards and Technology
NMT   Nordic Mobile Telephone
NRC   National Research Council
NRPB   National Radiological Protection Board
NTIA   National Telecommunications and Information Administration

ODC   ornithinedcarboxylase
Oe   oersted
OER   observed/expected ratio
OR   odds ratio
OSHA   Occupational Safety and Health Adminstration

PACS   Personal Access Communications Services
PC   personal computer
PCS   Personal Communications Radio Service
PDC   Personal Digital Cellular
PHS   Personal Handyphone System
POCSAG   Post Office Code Standardization Advisory Group
PPE   personal protective equipment
PS   portable station

PSTN	public switched telephone network
RADAR	radio detecting and ranging
RESNA	Rehabilitation and Assistive Technology Society of North America
RF	radio frequency
RFI	radio frequency interference
RFR	radio frequency radiation
RLS	radio location station
RMS	root mean square
RNA	ribonucleic acid
ROW	rights-of-way
SA	specific absorption
SAR	specific absorption rate
SD	standard deviation
SF	shielding factor
SIM	subscriber identification module
SIR	standardized incidence ratio
SMR	standardized mortality ratio
SP	slow brain potentials
TACS	Total Access Telecommunication System
TDM	time division multiplexing
TDMA	time division multiple access
TLV	threshold limit value
TNF	tumor necrosis factor
TV	television
TWA	time-weighted average
UHF	ultra high frequency
U.K.	United Kingdom
UMTS	Universal Mobile Telecommunication System
UNEP	United Nations Environment Program
U.S.	United States
USABRDL	U.S. Army Biomedical Research and Development Laboratory
USAF	United States Air Force
USASI	United States of America Standard Institute
USSR	Union of the Soviet Socialist Republics
UV	ultraviolet
VDT	video display terminal
VGA	video graphics array
VHF	very high frequency
VLF	very low frequency

VLR	visitor location register
VOR	VHF omnidirectional range

WBP	whole body peak
W-CDMA	Wide-band CDMA
WHO	World Health Organization

Index

9 780824 706777

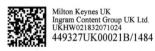
Milton Keynes UK
Ingram Content Group UK Ltd.
UKHW021832071024
449327UK00021B/1484